Food Makes the Difference

A Parent's Guide
to Raising a Healthy Child

PATRICIA KANE, Ph.D.

Simon and Schuster
New York

FOR APRIL
who reached out to me
in a most precious way
and guided me
through the creation
of this book

Published by Simon and Schuster
A Division of Simon & Schuster, Inc.
Simon & Schuster Building
Rockefeller Center
1230 Avenue of the Americas
New York, New York 10020
SIMON AND SCHUSTER and colophon are registered trademarks of
Simon & Schuster, Inc.
Designed by Jacques Chazaud
Manufactured in the United States of America
1   3   5   7   9   10   8   6   4   2
Library of Congress Cataloging in Publication Data
Kane, Patricia.
Food makes the difference.
Bibliography: p.
Includes index.
1. Food allergy in children—Diet therapy.
2. Diet therapy for children.   3. Children—Nutrition.
4. Cookery for the sick.   I. Title.
RJ386.5.K36   1985   618.92′00654   85-18374
ISBN: 0-671-54323-7

CONTENTS

PART I

Searching

Without an appreciation of the importance of the internal environment—how nutrition works and how adverse elements can creep in and interfere with metabolism—the solution to many individual health problems is hopeless.

DR. ROGER WILLIAMS

ONE

Beyond Our Touch

For many of us the road through parenthood is longer and rockier than we ever imagined, yet there is by far no greater pain than standing by helplessly watching an ill or troubled child struggle through life. This pain seems to touch all of us at one time or another, if not our own children, then the children of our friends and relatives. Our hopes for these children are unfulfilled, our dreams dashed away . . .

You really are not alone with a child suffering a physical, mental, and/or emotional problem. It is a burden many of us carry: fearing that we are the only one who suffers such agonizing pain over a troubled child for whom doctors just don't seem to have any real answers. And so it was for Aaron and his parents as they struggled to find a solution to his frustrating behaviors.

Aaron was an exceptionally active baby even before he was born, tossing and kicking within his mother's womb so that she often wondered if he was training for the Olympics. As a small child, Aaron did seem well-prepared for the world, as his physical development was months ahead of schedule. He didn't walk, he ran. He spoke not single words, but sentences. He wanted not baby food, but table food. He refused to take time to do anything; it was as if he were in a headlong rush. Aaron's health seemed fairly good—nothing worse than a little colic in infancy, diarrhea and a running nose on and off as a toddler, and the flu on occasion. He did tend to overreact with anger, tears, tantrums, and silliness, but his parents felt he would outgrow these outbursts.

As Aaron grew older, his parents realized that his behavior was not smoothing out as they had hoped. His attention span was quite short, he was clumsy, and he developed sleeping problems. His parents blamed themselves for letting Aaron "get away with murder." He seemed to understand right from wrong, but was unable to control his negative behaviors. Aaron's mother often remarked that she felt unable to reach him through words—it was as if his eyes were glazed and he looked right through her. Aaron's kindergarten teacher and pediatrician verified his parents' worst fear: he was hyperactive.

Aaron's mother decided to try a special diet (Feingold) instead of the medication suggested by the doctor because he did crave sweets and always complained of being thirsty. But as a year passed, Aaron's problems seemed to intensify. He often had periods of giddiness and would laugh hysterically over things that just weren't that funny. He was forgetful, wiggled a great deal, and always seemed to have headaches, stomachaches, leg aches. Finally Aaron's parents tried the drug Ritalin in hopes of calming him down, but the medication seemed only to intensify his problems.

Aaron was unable to control himself at school as well as at home, and his schoolwork continued to slip. Homework was a nightmare, with his parents sitting for hours beside him while he fidgeted, twisted, or whined. Aaron's handwriting was indecipherable, and reading was an uphill battle for him; his teacher suspected a learning disability. When this proved to be true, Aaron's concerned parents placed him in a private school that used special teaching techniques. After two years, Aaron is still pretty much the same—just older, and now angry and frustrated with himself. The psychologist he sees says to "give him time." There just doesn't seem to be anywhere for Aaron and his parents to turn; special diet, teaching techniques, medications, and talk therapy have failed, and Aaron's parents wonder if they are failures as parents. Maybe they didn't love him enough? Maybe they weren't strict enough? Maybe, maybe . . . but what is to be done about Aaron? . . .

Jordan seemed to enter the world ill prepared—a pale, colicky infant who cried a great deal. Jordan's mother switched him from one formula to another trying to find one he could tolerate. Jordan's sister had been an allergic baby too, but Jordan's problems were far worse. He had suffered from cradle cap, vomiting, thrush, severe diaper rash, and diarrhea before he was three months old. At five months of age he had a bad cold and ear infection that became a vicious cycle for the next eighteen months; he would finish a round of antibiotics and decongestant and then a few weeks later develop another cold/ear infection, which signaled yet another round of antibiotics.

Many foods upset Jordan, and he was an extremely picky eater. But it was hard to isolate which foods actually bothered him because he would eat a food one day and seem to tolerate it, only to eat it the next and have it bother him. At two Jordan was a listless, whiny child whose illnesses with colds, flu, and coughs seemed to blur together. The doctor labeled Jordan an allergic, delicate child and said he would grow out of it.

As Jordan grew older, he continued to be ill much of the time and was always exhausted. He suffered from eczema, wheezing, stomachaches, abdominal bloating, and a habit of constantly clearing his throat. Conventional allergy testing and treatment did not yield much improvement, nor did the removal of his tonsils and adenoids. Jordan was a bright child, but missed so much school as a result of illness that he found it hard to keep up with his schoolwork. His pale, withdrawn little face brought tears to his mother's eyes, but Jordan's parents felt their only recourse was to learn to live with Jordan's chronic illness as his doctors suggested.

Melissa's parents were at first apprehensive over having a child again at such a late time in their lives. After raising two boys and cleaning the attic of the crib, bottles, and toys, they had thought their family complete. But here was Melissa cuddled in their arms, a ray of unexpected sunshine. Melissa grew to be a bright, happy child with dimples and sparkling blue eyes. An extremely well-mannered and responsible child, Melissa, at three, understood and respected the rules of the house—especially those concerning the family swimming pool.

On one fateful summer afternoon, a tragedy occured that was to change the life of Melissa and her family forever. Melissa and her mother were sitting by the pool when the telephone rang. As her mother talked on the phone inside the house, Melissa decided to bathe her doll in the pool. The doll floated away from her, and in reaching for it she fell into the water. When Melissa's mother returned a few minutes later, she realized with horror that the child was drowning. She attempted to resuscitate the child and then called an ambulance. Melissa was severely brain-damaged, and the pediatrician informed her parents gently that the child should be placed in an institution and forgotten. Her parents, riddled with grief and guilt at the hopeless situation, have vowed to find something, anything that will help their daughter . . . if only they knew what . . .

Garret was a happy-go-lucky kid, but he had a secret he didn't want anyone ever to find out. He wet his bed. Garret's parents were sure he would outgrow the problem any day now and tried not to make a big deal of it, but at the age of ten they were becoming quite concerned. His health seemed to be okay—he had a few cavities at each dental checkup, colds now and then, a bad flu one year. And, oh, leg cramps and stomachaches that bothered him sometimes; but these things were normal, weren't they? Garret and his parents tried everything they could think of to help him stop wetting the bed, but he continued to have the problem on into puberty. One of his friends discovered his secret, and now the kids at school teased him. The bed-wetting problem really began to upset Garret's life, and he felt himself a failure . . .

Alex was a somber baby who was fiercely independent. As a toddler he began acting out in a destructive manner by kicking, spitting, and screaming if he did not get his way. His explosive temper became legendary in the neighborhood. At school his grades were erratic and his behavior was tense, anxious, and irritable, but within the confines of the schoolyard he did manage to control most of his angry outbursts.

At home, Alex constantly caused havoc within his family by ignoring the rules, tormenting his brother, and insisting he never got his share of anything. Alex' parents were deeply concerned by his sullen, restless, defiant behavior and spoke to the family doctor about it several times. At first, the doctor implied that Alex was just spoiled and should be pulled into line. Alex' parents felt helpless in making the doctor understand that they could not control Alex—he refused to change his "Is that all there is?" attitude or conform to normal behavior no matter what tactics they tried.

Alex was given a thorough examination by a specialist whom his family doctor finally recommended. The eleven-year-old appeared in good health, but the doctor did discover that Alex had unusual eating habits. He loved milk and would drink a gallon a day if it was available. Cheese and ice cream were also favorite foods—so much so that Alex would often awaken in the middle of the night to gobble cheese, milk, or ice cream. Alex would gorge on food for days at a time and then refuse to eat much of anything for a week or more. The specialist recommended that the family seek the help of a pyschiatrist, but Alex' father was totally opposed to this idea. A few months later, however, Alex set a nearby field on fire and his father agreed that the child needed help. The psychiatrist suggested long-term talk therapy, based on the feeling that Alex's parents "didn't really love him" and that this was the reason for his behavior. Or was it? Alex's parents did love him, no matter what his problems or what the psychiatrist believed! . . .

Emily lived in a world of her own. No one seemed able to penetrate the glass wall she had built around herself. How and when had it all begun? Emily's mother had felt from the very beginning that something was wrong with her child. At first it was a nagging uneasiness, but as the months slipped by Emily's mother knew that her baby's development was not normal. The pediatrician joked about worried mothers and insisted that babies develop differently. But when Emily at the age of two still did not speak, made odd gestures, was terrified of being dirty, had suffered two mild convulsions, and made no attempt to socialize with others, the pediatrician finally agreed that the child should be evaluated.

The specialist concluded that Emily was "probably autistic, with schizophrenic tendencies." He suggested that her parents "wait and see." Wait and see what? For the child to receive an exact label? Emily was slipping farther away from her family every day. Her parents did not want to wait and see. Emily needed help now . . . .

Hopeless problems, hopeless children? No, there are answers for these special children who live in a mentally dormant, floating state just beyond our reach. Some children are labeled hyperactive, underachieving, learning-disabled, incorrigible, allergic, schizophrenic, sickly, autistic, delicate, brain-injured, deviant. But often no such label is slapped upon the child. Instead the parents harbor a creeping uneasiness that something is wrong with their child—until a crisis occurs. However, even if the child does receive a descriptive label, the problem remains unchanged. This is because parents and child are experiencing a phenomenon about which most doctors understand very little—the biochemical relationship between body and mind.

Enshrouding the Cause

There is no gauge to determine what your child could have been or could become. No magic drug exists that can solve your child's problems, for your child is expressing symptoms of an inadequately nourished body and mind. The solution of your children's problems is difficult only because many doctors in this country still refuse to believe that food has a profound effect on an individual's level of health, and especially the mind. Can you really believe that a hyperactive child's problems can be solved by administration of Ritalin, a child with recurrent illnesses should be treated with one round of antibiotics after another, a disturbed child "managed" with antidepressants and/or locked away and forgotten? This approach does not touch the root cause of the problem! Do you really believe what "experts" often tell parents—that their children's difficulties are caused by parental rejection or spoiling? Our reluctance to accept these kinds of evasive answers is supported by our own gut-level feeling that something is wrong with our children and more than anything in the world we wish to help them.

In the past, you may have accepted the conventional doctor's diagnosis and treatment as infallible, but now you are ready to search for other options. You may be going from one doctor to another and reading everything you can find that pertains to your child's unpleasant behavior or problems, all to no avail. Those who try diet as a means of control often become turned off when they try only one aspect—such as eliminating artificial colorings and flavorings—and can see no significant change. The problem is rarely so simple as removing a few of many potential troublemakers from the diet. It is multifaceted, and requires a thorough understanding of what is going on within each child's body. Finding the right pieces to fulfill your child's unique biochemical and nutritional needs is essential, but does not have to be a complicated task. Your child holds the answers.

Shades of Gray

The responses occurring in children are too alarming to ignore any longer. It isn't that we purposely avoid facing the moodiness, chronic illnesses, hyperactivity, abnormal fears, learning difficulties, night cries, irritability, and other sensitivities children demonstrate. No. We simply have no "cure"; hence they must be tolerated.

Parents often discover that the conventional doctor has little time to offer in resolving their child's problem. Instead, the problem is promptly dropped back on the parents in the form of painful guilt. Therefore, we as parents must become knowledgeable enough to make a positive change in our children's health.

Turning Point

Having worked closely with many parents and children in a clinical setting, I have seen patients with minor difficulties as well as many frustrating, upsetting, debilitating, and seemingly hopeless disorders that responded exceptionally well to a nutritional/ecological regime. It is to this approach—finding the cause of disturbances in the body and finding answers to these biochemical puzzles—that I have dedicated my life. I believe in it. I live it. I have experienced it to the fullest degree as I watched my own child pronounced "hopeless" after a severe brain injury and then saw nutrient therapy return him to normal. Through clinical practice, I have seen wonderful things happen. To be sure, there have been problems which did not improve to the degree I would have liked, but I have never observed anyone who did not benefit from nutritional intervention to some degree.

You will not find a single magic pill to smother your child's symptoms. Instead one finds that the nutritional/ecological approach is one of learning, questioning, and becoming stronger through the discovery of how one can take care of oneself with the guidance of an informed physician. Therefore, this book was written for those who wish to know why children are experiencing such an array of negative physical and mental changes; and what can and *is* being done about it.

Average Is Not Normal

It is increasingly difficult to identify "normal" health these days, since we tend to confuse normal with average. Most of us consider ourselves to be healthy if we experience just a moderate level of fatigue and have only a few bouts with colds and flu, heartburn, cold sores, and constipation. And we may consider our children healthy even though they wet the bed occasionally, have frequent growing pains, complain now and again of headaches, have seasonal hay fever, and develop perhaps two cavities a year. These danger signals (for that's what they are) are considered normal simply because everyone has them, and as long as everyone experiences the same thing, it is acceptable.

Many children, as well as adults, exist on the borderline between their true potential and detectable dysfunction. There is no measure of how much is being suppressed as a result of inadequately nourished bodies and minds. As more and more children are affected by diets that fail to supply essential nutrients, truly good health is lost in the shuffle. Far too many children live in a physically and mentally dormant state.

Connecting your child's problems with nutrient deficiencies, imbalances, and/or sensitivities requires an understanding of what you are up against. What are our children doing and feeling? Let's take a good look at the forms some of these problems take.

The Incredible Hulk Response

Outbursts of unprovoked and uncontrolled anger are often the prelude to such intense actions as biting, kicking, screaming, spitting, crying, hitting, or bizarre behavior. Mood swings with no apparent cause may be explained as grand-mal tantrums. Dealing with the more severe forms of this response is usually automatic for most of us (a firm hand applied to the apparent seat of the problem), but often we find the child's strength and pain threshold are astonishingly high during this time. The child is completely out of control and can no longer respond to anything but the turmoil within.

The Tummy Blues Response

Complaints of tummyaches are common in sensitive children, as are vomiting, abdominal bloating, gas, constipation, indigestion, and nausea. Most frequently, a response such as this is food-related and due to the body's inability or limitation in handling particular foods.

The Bottomless Pit Response

When the body does not receive the nutrients necessary to function properly, you remain hungry even though you are stuffed with empty (non-nutrient) foods. And so it is with sensitive children who seemingly are unable to fill themselves with enough food. These children eat and *eat* and EAT, trying to obtain nutrients their bodies desperately need to attain normality. Their stomachs are unable to handle the huge amounts of empty food necessary to meet the bodily requirements—and the child's needs are left unfulfilled. Some children possess an abnormally large need for particular nutrients, which further aggravates the problem. Clinical ecologists also have observed that allergenic food (specific to the individual) may be craved and consumed in huge quantities—in itself an allergic response.

The Isolation Response

There are two ways in which children may respond when they isolate themselves from others. They may appear detached, quiet, shy, withdrawn, or they may be hostile, sullen, disruptive. What the two have in common is that the child is unhappy, without friends, and tends to shut himself off from the world. In most severe cases, we see autistic children—alone in a world all their own.

The Bogeyman Response

Children usually go through phases of being frightened of a self-invented bogeyman. In our house it was "monsters" which grab, hurt, and eat little boys. We heard quite a bit about monsters, but finally they drifted off. Sometimes such fears go beyond the normal and envelop the child, such as fears of leaving the house, of being alone in a room, or possibly being poisoned. If there is no occurrence of emotional trauma as a cause for such anxiety, then a thorough search is necessary for nutritional deficiency, imbalance, and/or sensitivity.

The Eruption Response

Some children respond with a skin eruption—blisters, eczema, hives, itchiness, roughness, pallor, scaling, rashes, welts, red patches on the cheeks, or blemishes. We tend to be more familiar with skin eruptions as a response because, unlike the case with a headache or a "strange" feeling, we can see them. We can associate the reaction with an allergen if it occurs quickly after exposure to the offending substance. Doctors cannot very well ignore such visual evidence. The problem may be resolved with the elimination of strawberries, for instance. But what if it isn't? What if the cause cannot be found by standard tests? Instead of smothering or ignoring the response, we must apply new ways of finding the answer.

The Night Cry Response

The problems children experience at night may involve tossing and turning, nightmares, sleepwalking, night sweats, bed-wetting, crying. Some children are simply unable to fall asleep; they remain awake without making any noise until well past midnight. Dealing with night disturbances is possible only if we can understand what is actually wrong—and act upon it.

The Low Defense Response

The "cold that doesn't go away" has become far too prevalent in children. Frequent or prolonged illness is an indication that the body's defenses are low; thus the child's health is not what it should be. The only abnormality may be swollen lymph tissues. At times, this response may appear in the form of not being sick, yet not being well either. The doctor cannot find anything wrong, yet the child feels, looks, and *is* sick.

The Pick-Bite-Wipe Response

Habits can be particularly irritating, and the urge to shout, *"STOP IT!"* is frequently too overpowering to ignore. Shouting, threats, spanking, and other varied punishments don't help much, since if we do achieve the cessation of a particular habit, a new one pops up. Much to our dismay, this new habit is often far worse than its predecessor. Habits may establish themselves as hair twisting, nose or bottom picking, snorting, rocking, facial grimaces, continual clearing of the throat, wiping of the face, chewing, handshaking, or other nerve-racking actions. What is actually happening is that the child is trying to block out stimuli that are too intense. The cause may be emotional or biochemical in origin, or both.

The Trip Response

Clumsiness and lack of coordination often are looked upon with disdain because they are conspicuous and therefore embarrassing. The child who trips, drops, and spills, has difficulty doing normal tasks (such as shoe tying, buttoning, writing, playing ball) and usually is downright accident-prone may lack proper coordination as a result of sustained damage to the nervous system or faulty development, as well as nutritional deficiency, sensitivity, and/or imbalance.

The Grouchy Bear Response

Pulling a grouchy bear out of bed in the morning is no easy task. This inability to fully awaken may continue through breakfast and early morning with irritability, moodiness, and exhaustion. It is not uncommon for these responses to remain with the child throughout the day, often accompanied by outbursts of anger or depression. A child with these problems usually consumes a diet that is severely inadequate; the brain and body consequently suffer.

The Eyes, Ears, Nose, Throat Response

The sensitive child frequently suffers with:

Eye problems—puffy, itchy, blurry, watery, dull, tired, glazed, black circles or wrinkles under, double vision, painful, twitching, swollen, light sensitivity, night-blindness, blurring, crusty lids, frequent blinking, bloodshot, spots before eyes, lazy eye muscles.

Ear problems—fluid behind the eardrum, infections, earaches, ringing, dizziness, clicking, ear popping, on-and-off hearing, itching, imbalance, flushed earlobes, cracks and scaliness behind.

Nose problems—sneezing, mouth breathing, rubbing, wiggling, snorting, stuffiness, watery, itchiness, hay fever, nosebleeds.

Throat problems—throat clearing, coughing, gulping sounds, dryness, itchiness, swelling, feeling of a lump in the throat, hoarseness.

Suppressing these obvious symptoms with drugs merely masks the existing problem, and inadequately at that. Why not explore and treat the root cause so that these responses may be eliminated without side effects?

The Wild Wiggles Response

Hyperactive children who are fidgety, wiggly, touchy, excitable, feisty, uncontrolled, aggressive, impulsive, and uncoordinated are all too familiar. To sum it all up, they bounce off the walls. They may also possess short attention spans, low frustration tolerance, sleeping difficulties, speech problems, and inability to get along with others. Removal of artificial coloring and flavoring is not a complete approach to helping these children, although it does inadvertently improve the diet by removing some of the empty foods, since most of them contain chemicals. Refined sugar (a notorious empty food) often remains in the diet, and this, as well as allergens and an inadequate diet, may block the child's recovery. Removal of allergens, control of nutrients, mobilizing of heavy metals (such as lead) out of the body, and a diet that fulfills the child's needs must be adhered to in order to reach the source of the problem and eliminate it.

The Hunger Strike Response

Often sensitive children simply don't eat because when they do they feel bad. This is especially so if they are sensitive to many foods. They engage in an unconscious fast to stop the allergic reactions. This response also involves the child who is starving an hour or two before dinner, yet when dinner finally comes has no appetite. The cause for this is that the blood sugar has dropped, bringing on headache, nausea, and irritability. Equally frustrating for us, as parents, is when the child announces, soon after the dishes are done and the food put away, that he or she is hungry. Of course the child doesn't want the neglected dinner, but requests cookies or some other sweet goodie. At this point, although it is difficult to admit, do you give in so that the child will eat *something* and let you alone to relax after dinner? You are not the only one.

The Cringe Response

Extreme sensitivity to noise, light, odor, touch, and temperature may occur in some children. Responses may include putting the hands over ears or eyes, squinting, shivering, or sweating, complaints of being hot or cold when others are comfortable, bizarre behavior, or a feeling of impending doom. Perfumes, gas, glue, paint, and other chemicals that have penetrating odors can cause severe reactions. Strange as it may seem, the odor of foods to which a child is sensitive can cause the same responses as eating that particular food.

The Tearful Response

The child who is easily hurt and moved to tears is difficult to live with, and the resultant crying, whining, moaning, and pouting are trying indeed. Some would explain this as the child's way of manipulating parents, or more simply label the child a spoiled brat. Nevertheless, such children are telling us something is amiss; thus the problem requires that we search for what is actually wrong instead of trying to resolve the problem by insisting they shut up.

The Blah Droopies Response

Usually the listless, depressed, drowsy, sluggish, exhausted, lethargic child is thought to be anemic. Although that may be part of the problem, it is only one piece of a very large puzzle.

I recall visiting a woman who had several children, one of whom exhibited this response. As we sat talking, she suddenly got up to check on this child, who was taking a bath. She was back in a minute signaling for me to follow her. There in the bathtub lay the child, fast asleep. I might not have been so disturbed had it been in the evening and if the child had been very young, but it was the middle of the afternoon and this child was eight years old. The mother, not disturbed at all, assured me the child fell asleep like that all the time and was the quiet one in the family. Since the child's doctor could not find a reason for the child to be exhausted all the time, the mother considered the response to be normal.

Exhaustion in children is not normal and should be given serious attention. A child's cry for help may be silent, but we must take action to determine the cause of his symptoms.

The Ache-Twitch-Cramp Response

Headaches, tics, backaches, tremors, leg aches, twitches or cramps may trouble your children to varying degrees. Trying to explain away leg aches as growing pains or tics as nervousness or headaches as too much running around seems easier for many doctors than really finding out what is wrong. Mineral deficiencies and imbalances are often involved in this problem.

The Crave Response

The craving for sugar and other highly refined foods is characteristic of many children and eventually brings on a refined-carbohydrate overload and nutritional deficiencies as empty foods are repeatedly thrust upon the body. It is important to understand that this craving becomes a physical as well as emotional *need* and the removal of refined foods from the diet may bring on withdrawal symptoms.

The Addictive Response

Deficiencies, imbalances, and sensitivities all intertwine to bring about an addictive response. Addiction as we know it is usually related to alcohol and drugs, but for many children, addiction to sugar and foods to which they are allergic are also overpowering problems.

The "Open Wide" Response

Some of the more frequent responses are canker sores, taste distortion, coated tongue, puffy and bleeding gums, bad breath, itchy roof of the mouth, cracks at the corners of the mouth, dry cracked lips, grooves on the tongue. These problems are usually closely associated with a lack of friendly bacteria in the intestine as well as a deficiency of B vitamins (along with other nutrients) and sensitivities to certain foods.

The Molecules in Motion Response

Dizziness, light-headedness, inner trembling, heart palpitations, spaciness, fuzziness, and an accompanying visual phenomenon that puts molecules in motion before the child's eyes are due to a drop in blood sugar. This response may be one factor or a combination of many, but often it is the body's response when the child has failed to eat a food that has become addictive (allergenic).

One child told me he frequently felt this type of response when he awoke in the morning. He stopped it with a large glass of milk, his addiction, although he was totally unaware that it was. At one time, I would have believed milk to be an appropriate food to stop a drop in blood sugar, but this child consumed milk by the quart instead of by the glassful and proved to be highly sensitive to it. When he failed to drink milk, he saw "molecules in motion." (More about this allergy/addiction in Chapter Three.) To avoid perpetuating an allergic reaction, one must be aware of the addiction and withdrawal phenomenon in the allergic state.

The Garbled Response

When the brain is inadequately supplied with nutrients because of deficiencies, imbalances, and/or sensitivities, it will respond in some way. Sometimes this response takes the form of stuttering, slurring, or garbled speech or explosive, constant, repetitive speech. Have you ever noticed that when you are very tired or hungry you are unable to get out clearly what you want to say? The feeling is similar in sensitive children, but to a far greater degree. In the most extreme case the loss of speech is total.

The Obsessive-Compulsive Response

For some children, obsessive-compulsive behavior is evident in rituals such as excessive hand washing, repeatedly walking up and down stairs, or drawer opening and closing. These actions, thoughts, or urges yield a sort of solace and are repeated over and over uncontrollably. The fear of "something bad happening if I don't do this again and again" is the child's usual explanation, although these actions and feelings are kept carefully hidden whenever possible.

The Disconnected Response

A child with perceptual disorders of time, sound, space, and reality is unable to tell us about it because the child believes everyone has the same dysperceptions, or becomes too frightened to talk about it when made aware others *don't* feel the same things. Children who often appear to be overly confused, indecisive, disoriented or who experience an impaired ability to remember things desperately need help, but are incapable of expressing what is happening. Sensitivities to certain foods, inhalants, or chemicals may bring on a feeling of the mind's being separate from the body, as if they no longer interact. The child struggles to regain control, but until the response recedes, the child is locked into the confusion and unable to respond in a normal pattern.

The Smothered Response

Most of us are familiar with asthma and the resultant wheezing and gasping for breath. But even without asthma, the feeling of not being able to breathe can occur in some children when they are exposed to substances to which they are highly sensitive. Pulmonary-function tests, however, may show no abnormalities of lung capacity. The feeling is similar to that of being smothered and is a frightening one that fresh air does not always immediately alleviate.

The Intestinal Response

Being unable to properly break down particular foods and therefore allergic to them, sensitive children may experience intestinal problems. But when children experience diarrhea, constipation, or an itchy bottom, many parents don't become particularly alarmed. Empty refined foods tend to be severely lacking in fiber; thus fecal matter tends to stick to the wall of the large intestine. This buildup is very detrimental, since waste that should be released from the body instead accumulates to form inconsistencies and distensions that interrupt proper excretion.

The "Mentally Dormant" Response

Children labeled schizophrenic, autistic, learning-disabled, or (the broad term) "retarded in development" are not necessarily unreachable. Mentally dormant, the term applied by Dr. Carl Pfeiffer, refers to a state that is reversible when the right key is found to release the child's capabilities by stimulation, removal of allergic substances, the addition of missing nutrients, or all of these forces combined.

The "Is That All There Is?" Response

Children who are never satisfied no matter what you offer them can be difficult for any parent to endure. Their pessimistic attitude permeates the entire household, and no special treat or event appears to hold their interest for long. The child may complain "Is that all you got me?" "That's no fun," "Big deal," "What are we doing after this?" or utter similar phrases so frequently that the child's parents are at their wit's end. Spoiled? Maybe. . . . But perhaps there are other reasons beyond spoiling. The child may actually be expressing symptoms of depression, apathy, or irritability resulting from nutrient inadequacy.

The Puffy Response

Bloating, swelling, or puffiness may occur in any part of the body as a result of an allergic response. Bloating of the abdomen is frequently observed, as is puffiness of the face and hands. Just as the abdomen swells, so does the brain, producing severe headaches, as the brain lies in the rigid confines of the skull and pressure is built up in this very delicate part of the body. This swelling response of the brain may stimulate some nerve pathways while inhibiting others, thus affecting thinking, emotions, and behavior in any way imaginable and to any degree.

A Closer Look

Of all these responses, I have personally experienced more than half. The most painful part of being a sensitive person is the feeling that you alone live with these responses, since no one else ever speaks of having similar feelings. As a young girl, I was puzzled and sometimes frightened by my need to repeatedly open and close drawers, by the sensation of being smothered, by nausea, unexplained moodiness, inner trembling, food binges, exhaustion, skin eruptions, bloating, dizziness, visual disturbances, and a feeling of panic when in an enclosed space where strong odors of perfume, smoke, gas, or paint were present.

After many years of unexpressed turmoil, my search to understand what caused these overpowering responses produced the enlightening discovery that other people experienced the same feelings and responses—I was *not* alone. The search for knowledge brought understanding, with understanding came acceptance, and with acceptance a commitment to do something to relieve these intense responses.

Working Together

Observing intense behavioral changes in my son after he was exposed to certain foods, I began to explore deeper into the intricacies of the biochemical body/mind relationship. A decade of study and working as a clinical nutritionist with many sensitive patients helped me recognize the multifaceted problems that are involved in resolving health problems. The mind as well as the body responds when we fail to supply what is necessary for optimal function. To obtain information is one thing, but to apply it, as in modifying the diet to wholesome foods, is quite another, *especially* with children. Just as we understand and accept the origin of their problems, so must they, but in simple terms. Working together, the search for answers to their problems will go much more smoothly if they are involved and aware of what we are looking for and why. The search moves on.

TWO

From Foods to Moods

There are some things about your children you cannot see or feel or even get them to talk about. This leads to a kind of helplessness that often gives in to "It will go away," "The child is just not normal," "There's nothing a good spanking won't cure," or "I can't [or won't] deal with it."

The most misunderstood responses children experience are those involving the brain, because children have great difficulty relating what they are feeling. How do you tell someone you feel your brain is no longer connected with your body or that you are overcome with the feeling of impending doom? With the child's belief that no one else has these feelings (since no one ever talks about them), fear of discovery is omnipresent. Or nothing may be mentioned about bizarre responses because the child believes everyone experiences them, hence accepts them as normal. If the child does attempt to describe these or other mental changes, it may be as "feeling bad," throwing us completely off course because we associate feeling bad with such things as the flu or a fight with a playmate, not a nutritional imbalance or deficiency and/or food sensitivity that involves the brain.

The Hungry Brain

The brain is an exquisite, sensitive organ that controls mood, thought, perception, emotion, and behavior. Composed primarily of lipid (over one-half the total dry weight) and proteins, the brain is dependent upon the body for supplying energy and other nutritional factors by the blood flowing through it. Functioning of the brain is the result of electrical impulses that move in sequence from neuron (nerve cell) to neuron which are stimulated by neurotransmitters (between-nerve-cell communicators). Approximately thirty different substances are known or believed to be neurotransmitters, each possessing the ability to excite or inhibit the functioning of the brain. The manufacture of these neurotransmitters is controlled by the production of energy through the breakdown of blood sugar in brain tissue, helped by essential nutrients. Thus wide fluctuations in the blood-sugar level can alter brain function.

The brain has a protective barrier called the blood/brain barrier that selectively transports nutrients and other substances that are appropriate for brain function. The production of neurotransmitters is directly linked to this uptake from the blood, and if these nutrients are inadequate, imbalances of these neurochemicals may occur, resulting in disturbed mood, thought, perception, emotion, or behavior. This phenomenon may occur with excessive or inhibited release of neurotransmitters and is directly related to brain-cell nutrition. In 1982, Iverson[1] reported in *Lancet* that eight neurotransmitter substances regulating behavior have been closely associated wtih certain patterns of food intake, while Wurtman[2] described the behavioral effects of nutrients in *Lancet* in 1983. Dhopeshwarker wrote a highly informative book[3] on the effect of nutrition on the brain which was published in 1983. More and more research is under way to gain insight into the function of the brain and the effects of nutrients upon it.

Psychological disturbances are one of the first indications of nutritional deficiency.[4] Disturbances in brain function induced by a deficiency or imbalance of essential nutrients depend upon the degree of the problem, how long it has existed, the body's ability to deal with the inadequacy, and the portion of the brain most severely affected. The tissues of the brain and nervous system are believed to be the most sensitive in the body in relation to chemical reactions, and this is why prominent researchers such as Linus Pauling, Abram Hoffer, and Roger Williams contend that when nutrient insufficiency occurs, mental changes often become apparent before the physical symptoms.

Brain Allergy

Factors other than an inadequate supply of nutrients may also affect the brain. Sensitivities to foods, inhalants, and/or chemicals may induce changes in brain chemistry in susceptible individuals. Although most of us relate an allergy to sneezing, a rash, swelling of the throat, hay fever, or asthma, allergy does in fact encompass a far wider realm. An allergic reaction may occur in any system of the body, including the brain.

The brain may suffer either immunological reactions (allergy) or non-immunologic reactions (intolerances). Food allergy or intolerance may affect different areas of the brain, precipitating reactions within the brain on a wide individual spectrum. Cerebral, or brain, allergy is so specific that it is possible to directly relate individual responses to particular sensitizing agents. As amazing as it may seem, common foods like wheat may be identified as inducing a hyperactive reaction, egg to unprovoked hostility, milk to confused thinking, or orange to exhaustion.

The connection between brain allergy and partial digestion of food has been described by Hemmings.[5] Children with food allergies or intolerances invariably do not completely break down the foods they eat. The incomplete-protein-breakdown products (called IPBs) may enter the bloodstream unchanged from the intestinal tract to lodge in target areas (tissues) such as the brain, inducing allergic effects. These reactions may appear in the brain as disturbances of mood, thought, perception, emotion, or behavior. Sensitivities are often registered in the brain first because it receives more blood than any other organ—25 percent. Even with the protection of the blood/ brain barrier these allergic offenders, or incomplete-protein-breakdown products, have been demonstrated to enter the brain.

Sensitive children may have moderate to severe impairment of brain function due to a brain allergy. Therefore, it is imperative that we identify any food sensitivities a child may have so that these allergic stress factors on the brain can be removed.

The Hungry Body = The Hungry Brain

What children eat or don't eat is crucial to the health of their bodies and their minds. Emotional stress cannot be ruled out as a contributing factor because it has an effect on well-being. But emotional stress is by no means the sole explanation for the way our children act.

Many children suffer from an inability to handle carbohydrates properly because of the overwhelming amount and kinds of carbohydrates chosen. This is further complicated by the usual American diet, which is sadly lacking in essential nutrients. The ingestion of refined sugar increases the need for many nutrients, but to cite one study by Lonsdale and Shamberger,[6] a group of youths expressing symptoms of insomnia, chornic fatigue, headache, aggression, irritability, and hostility were found to be suffering from thiamine deficiency due to the consumption of large amounts of refined carbohydrate. (This deficiency was isolated through studies of an enzyme, erythrocyte transketolase.) Thiamine is needed to metabolize, or break down, sugars—the higher the intake of refined sugar, the higher the need for thiamine. To reverse the effects of high sugar/low thiamine deficiency, the researchers administered large doses (150–300mg.) of thiamine for three weeks. Thiamine levels (and enzyme activity) were monitored in the blood, and as these levels rose, the behavior difficulties disappeared.

In whole foods, vitamins and minerals are normally present to handle the important balance of carbohydrates to nutrient levels, but empty carbohydrates (refined flour and grains, refined sugar) do not provide this balance and actually end up drawing on the body's reserves to be metabolized. The continued ingestion of refined sugar and flour drains these reserves, leaving the body ill equipped to handle a surge of empty carbohydrates. A deficiency of B-complex vitamins and/or the mineral zinc may actually cause an individual to crave more and more sugary foods.[7] Sugar is addictive: the more you eat, the more you want; thus the cycle is locked into place. Blood-sugar problems and often allergies are intertwined in this cycle in a mild, moderate, or even severe degree, and they too must be reckoned with.

Inadequate intake of nutrients, allergic or food-intolerance difficulties, digestive disturbances, and/or flooding the body with refined carbohydrates may bring about hypoglycemia (low blood sugar) or hypoglycemic reactions, which interfere with the level of glucose (energy) available to the brain. Heavy consumption of refined sugar, caffeine, and foods to which an individual is sensitive produces a lift by raising the blood-sugar level. The relief that is achieved, however, is only temporary, as it is followed by a steep decline in blood sugar, often to below the original level. Thus another stimulant is used; the vicious circle which continues may be expressed as an addiction (the person has to have it) to refined sugar, allergy-provoking foods, and/or caffeine.

Our children's nutritional needs are intricate, and the addition or removal of one nutrient or food may play a part in well-being, but it is not the approach we are searching for. All nutritional needs must be observed and difficulties overcome with a total approach, one that involves the body in all aspects, including the brain. One factor may affect a child more severely than others, but the problems cannot be resolved until we establish what foods the child is sensitive to, what nutrients are called for, what digestive support is needed, and the proper balance of foods for optimal health. Since it is estimated that a child's brain has double the energy needs of the adult brain, it becomes even more essential for children to receive all the nutrients they require for good health.

The Beginning of Understanding

The next six chapters will closely examine some of the more common syndromes that manifest themselves in children as the result of nutritional inadequacies and biochemical abnormalities.

What is in store for our sensitive, overreactive children? Only we as parents can ensure that our children's problems will be dealt with head on instead of being smothered with drugs or smoothed over with excuses.

THREE

Cookie Monster Blues

The surge of refined carbohydrates into children's diets is appalling. Food processors and manufacturers strip away nutrients by refining. The remaining products—white sugar and flour—have little more to offer than empty calories. For many children, refined carbohydrates are the predominant foodstuff ingested each day, and their entry is often beyond parental control as children encounter Grandma's sugar cookies, Santa's candy cane, the Great Pumpkin's goodies, the Easter Bunny's chocolate rabbit, the grocer's lollipop, the ice cream man's coated bar, the birthday child's cake, the baker's doughnuts, the neighbor's artificially flavored, colored, sugared "juice."

On and on it goes. "Just this once," the special occasion for sweets, has a tendency to grow and grow.

Meals are more within our control. Much of the time, though, we opt for convenient food that children will accept without a fuss. This, in turn, translates to a diet high in refined sugar, as more than 70 percent of processed foods contain added sugar. Yet as parents, we are often in a quandary as to what children will or will not eat. This problem may begin at a very early age when we offer it's-good-for-you food such as liver and spinach that ends up on the floor or spewed into our faces.

There are not many things more frustrating than trying to get a child to eat who doesn't like what is being served. Something becomes better than nothing. Just what a child chooses to eat is the problem.[1] Researchers from Cornell University observed that for every two hours of television that young children watched they consumed another sugary food. A study of 5-to-12-year-olds indicated that the younger children are, the higher the percentage of refined sugars they consume.[2] The major sources of refined-sugar intake for these children—95 percent—were found to be 1) soft drinks and sweetened beverages, 2) candy, 3) cookies, cakes, pies, 4) ice cream, 5) sugared cereals, and 6) salty and caramel snacks. An examination of dietary data by the Department of Agriculture and the Department of Health, Education, and Welfare[3] has pushed the figure for sugar and sweetener consumption up over 130 pounds of sugar per American per year!

That's more than one-third of a cup of sugar per day! And most of that sugar (70 percent) is hidden in the cloak of processed foods. So even if a family tosses out the sugar bowl, its members still may consume copious amounts of hidden sugar in processed foods.

The choices children make are strongly influenced by a kaleidoscope of colors, flavors, and prizes. Television with its "Sugar is fun" commercials makes other food seem boring and dull. And parents also are influenced by what television tells them. Is white toast, a sugary fruit-flavored drink, milk, and sugared cereal a good breakfast? Is lunch a good time for the great (refined) taste of white-bread hamburgers, deep-fried potatoes, and sugary soft drink? Is a good snack one that has a big (sugary) delight in every bite? It is shocking how many people offer this "food" to children and think that it is balanced.

Living on the Nutritional Edge

The changeover in this century from unrefined whole-carbohydrate foods (whole grains, fruit, vegetables) to refined carbohydrates (white sugar, white flour, white rice) has placed the health of our children in jeopardy. Now there is a gross imbalance between the amount of *carbohydrate* consumed and the amount of *nutrients* consumed. In 1980, Americans consumed 43 percent less complex carbohydrate and 45 percent more refined carbohydrate than in 1910.[4] Two-thirds of the calories in the average diet come from low-nutrient refined carbohydrate and fat. That means that the remaining one-third of the diet must supply most of the nutrients required to maintain good health. Times are changing but not in the right nutritional direction.

Even the staff of life is no more. Whole wheat has been changed into a denatured flour stripped of its eighteen or more nutrients and "enriched" with a select four (niacin, thiamine, pyridoxine, iron). Even bread labeled whole-wheat often contains a large percentage of white flour (termed "flour" on the ingredient list). Our children are being denied the full spectrum of nutrients and fiber essential for their health.

We are so preoccupied with the shelf life of fat that we have forgotten to ask what kind of fat is in our food supply. Thus the fat that is now available to our children is largely hydrogenated fat found in infant formulas, processed foods, margarine. This man-made fat, foreign to the human body, extends the shelf life of processed foods, but offers no nutritional value other than calories. Lacking essential fatty acids vital to the health of the entire body and especially the brain, hydrogenated fat may be the most serious nutritional error of our time.

In addition to the stress imposed by altered basic staples, our children's bodies must contend with more than sixty-five thousand food additives. To be sure, many are harmless; but some are questionable; some are potentially dangerous; some are dangerous to certain individuals, even though not to others. Yet by thrusting diets composed of refined and synthetic "foods" at our children, we are taking unknown risks with their well-being.

And what about the actual intake of nutrients? Examining data from the U.S. Department of Agriculture, Pao and Mickle[5] found that out of 6,545 children between one and eleven years of age, most were eating diets far below the government's Recommended Dietary Allowances. The most serious deficiencies were in Vitamin A, Vitamin C, pyridoxine, zinc and iron. These findings, the authors concluded, suggest "that the typical eating patterns of American children are not at recommended levels." The Recommended Dietary Allowances (RDAs) are the levels of "adequate nutrients judged by the Food and Nutrition Board to meet the nutritional needs of "practically all healthy persons." Of the 44 known nutrients required by the human body, only about a third are suggested in the Recommended Dietary Allowances. And what about each child's unique nutritional needs? Growth spurts, illness, climate, stress, and many other factors affect a child's nutritional needs. Many researchers and physicians now recognize that biochemical individuality makes nutritional needs individual. The Recommended Dietary Allowances are helpful as guidelines (for gathering information in a nutritional survey), but they are not geared to individual needs. Our view of the health of children in America has been sharply distorted. If our children are not even receiving diets that supply close to the Recommended Dietary Allowances (and *these* suggestions are low), one can clearly see the seriousness of our children's health situation.

Dr. Jeffrey Bland, Director of Research at the Linus Pauling Institute, describes this situation as the "overconsumption-undernutrition" syndrome. Our children are eating too much (empty calories) of too little (nutrients). The time has come to change our diets.

Snap-Crackle-Plop!

The "American breakfast" so heavily promoted on television fills children with food that fails to supply enough essential nutrients to build health. The toast/flavored-drink/sugared-cereal breakfast presents a tremendous amount of filler food offering little more than empty calories;

The toast. More often than not, the bread chosen to make toast is of the white or caramel-colored Styrofoam variety, smeared with a buttery-looking substance and usually topped off with sugar, jelly, or jam.

Carbohydrate yield: 2 slices of white toast plus 4 teaspoons jelly equals 34 grams of refined carbohydrate.

The drink. "Fruit" drinks are widely used because they are advertised as containing Vitamin C. Some even contain a whopping amount of real fruit juice—10 percent! Vitamin C is the only nutrient these artificial drinks do supply. The remainder is artificial color (visual appeal), artificial flavor (taste appeal), and sugar (addictive appeal). Artificial juice is cheaper than real juice but does not compare in nutritional content.

Carbohydrate yield: 8 ounces of artificial juice equals an average of 30 grams refined carbohydrate.

The milk. Milk is the only nutritious part of the American breakfast. Protein, vitamins, and minerals are contained in milk. Be aware, though, that many children are allergic to milk, and this may cause problems in sensitive individuals.

Carbohydrate yield: 8 ounces equals 30 grams of natural carbohydrate.

Protein yield: 8 ounces contains 9 grams of complete protein (the only complete protein found in this breakfast).

The sugared cereal. The most disturbing part of the breakfast that is supposed to start our children's day off right is the sugared cereal that can supply as much refined sugar as candy. This is a conglomeration of refined grain, refined sugar, artificial colors, artificial flavors, and preservatives. Five or six nutrients may be added, whereas three times that many were removed in processing. Take into account as well that refined-sugar intake increases the need for nutrients, especially for thiamine.

Carbohydrate yield: 1 ounce equals 26 grams of refined carbohydrate.

The carbohydrate content of this meal, most of it refined, is between 85 and 108 grams, while the protein content is at best 12 grams, not all of it complete protein. At the present time no exact carbohydrate requirement has been determined for children or adults. The Food and Nutrition Board of the National Academy of Sciences suggests at least 50 to 100 grams of carbohydrate per day. Notice that the common breakfast consumed by American children contains 85 to 108 grams of carbohydrate at breakfast alone. The amount of carbohydrate required, however, is dependent upon many factors such as age, physical activity, growth, size, climate, and individual metabolic needs. Our greatest concern lies in the amount of refined carbohydrate (white sugar, white flour) children are eating and its imbalance in relation to the nutrient content of the foods they are eating. The effects of refined sugar on behavior have jumped to the medical forefront as researchers such as Fishbein[6] and Schoenthaler[7] have demonstrated a connection between refined-sugar intake and maladaptive behaviors.

Common variations of the advertised "American breakfast" also often prove to be inadequate nutritionally. A survey in my own community revealed some other common breakfast choices:

A bowl of sugared cereal
Breakfast rolls (sugar, white flour)
Doughnuts and cocoa
Pop-Tarts and fruit-flavored drink
Pancakes or waffles (frozen) with maple-flavored sugar syrup
Sugar-cinnamon toast and tea with sugar

Instant Breakfast or Ovaltine
Oatmeal with sugar and milk
Granola (brown-sugar-sweetened) and milk
No breakfast at all

For many children it is not unusual to be sent to school without having eaten breakfast. The government recognizes this problem and subsidizes breakfast programs in schools to provide breakfast for students. But the foods offered are often refined carbohydrates such as white bread, sugared cereal, or sweet rolls accompanied by some milk. At school or at home, the breakfasts many children receive don't supply what their bodies need.

One of the major reasons children eat such poor breakfasts is that what you want them to eat and what you have time to fix doesn't always coincide with what they are willing to eat. No one knows better than I what it is like to rush around in the morning before work to prepare a nutritious meal and have the child say, "I'm not hungry." Once he's taken the bite you beg him to take, the first comment is followed by an inevitable second: "Yuk!" Why bother? Who has the time to make a breakfast that no one will eat or the money to throw away good food? You find yourself falling into the trap of getting your children to eat something—anything—that is quick, that tastes good (which translates to sweet), and preferably that they can make themselves so you can get a little extra sleep.

The Cycle Continues

Breakfast often starts the day out wrong, but lunch and dinner don't always help much either. The home lunches of my childhood remain vivid in my memory—the "old reliables" which continue to be the mainstay of many children's lunches (in other words, it's cheap and they'll eat it):

Monday—Canned ravioli and cheese puffs
Tuesday—Peanut butter and jelly on white bread, Jell-O
Wednesday—Bologna on white bread with mustard and potato chips.
Thursday—Canned spaghetti with one tiny meatball and a piece of white bread with butter.
Friday—Hot dogs on a white bun with ketchup and corn chips.
Saturday—Canned chicken-noodle or tomato soup with saltines.

Desserts usually followed in the form of small cakes with whipped chemical filling, pink snowballs, chocolate cupcakes, sugar-layered chocolate cookies, and the like. Beverages were soft drinks, milk, powdered mixes with artificial flavors, and the like.

The lunches children eat at home today are basically the same, but the deluge of refined foods is on a far wider scale. The bread may be dyed with caramel coloring to make it look more natural, although white bread is still going strong with advertisers touting, "Good nutrition doesn't have to mean whole-wheat." Think again! There is much more available in the way of chips, main dishes (pasta in different shapes and small chemicalized casseroles that need only water added), brightly colored and sugared beverages, and quite a selection of desserts containing sugar as the main ingredient. Many of these cereals, cookies, drinks, and mini-cakes list sugar as the first ingredient, meaning these products contain more sugar than flour! At one time we had sugar-layered chocolate cookies; now we have "double stuff" (double-sugar) cookies.

The school cafeteria provides a lunch comparable to that at home. The accent is on:

Hamburgers, tacos, breaded meat loaf, pizza, hot dogs, spaghetti, breaded fish.
White rice, white bread, instant mashed potatoes.
Overcooked, oversalted vegetables that no one ever eats.
Salads made almost exclusively of iceberg lettuce, cole slaw, or canned sweetened fruit cocktail
Pasteurized, homogenized milk—plain and chocolate.
Empty foods such as gelatin (85 percent sugar), cookies, cake, cobbler, ice cream, chips, puddings.
Once in a while an apple or a banana!

This starchy, overcooked lunch presents another problem: You never really know what part of the lunch your child actually ate. If meat loaf, cole slaw, and milk were consumed, the meal was passable. But if instead gelatin, white bread, and instant potatoes were eaten, topped off with ice cream, the meal was a nutritional disaster. And don't forget the matter of lopsided meals due to traveling food. Bartering, buying, and trading are big business at the lunch table.

Dinner is frequently a hectic time, especially for those of us who work. Our ongoing battle with saving time leads to more and more dependence on convenience foods. This reliance is difficult to shake, since the alternatives don't look too promising. For many, it is inconceivable to give up such "delicacies" as:

Frozen, nondairy whipped topping instead of freshly whipped cream.
Canned, frozen, or "missing" vegetables instead of raw vegetables.
Dry, boxed mixes to add to ground beef instead of using whole-grain pasta and natural seasonings.
Ready-to-make cookie and cake mixes to which you need only add water instead of making them from wholesome ingredients.
Canned, overcooked soup instead of soup you cook at home from fresh vegetables, lean meats, and poultry.
Processed instant potatoes instead of cooking your own.
Canned, syrupy fruits instead of fresh fruit.
A frozen dinner in a tray or plastic bag that you heat and eat instead of a wholesome meal you prepare yourself.

The meals you prepare for dinner reflect more than just your concern for time. Meals are an expression of your ability, creativity, and enjoyment in cooking; of the energy and effort you are capable of putting forth; of what you are able to afford for food. What you prepare is influenced by foods your parents served—and of course, what your family is willing to eat.

The emphasis always seems to be on what families are not willing to eat —a matter that limits food choices severely. It's really quite basic—either they will eat the food you serve or they will not. Your priority becomes finding something they will accept without a fuss so that you don't end up begging, yelling, and bribing with ultimately only one mouthful to show for it. This can become so exasperating you may take the "Give yourself a break" approach by jumping into the car and heading for fast food.

Fill in this mealtime pattern with nutrient-free between-meal snacks, both liquid and solid, and you have a refined-carbohydrate overload that is threatening children's well-being. The pattern is moving against us.

Breaking out of the fast-food trap is not an impossible task, but it does require that you learn how to free yourself, as well as your children, from its grasp.

Games Children Play: or, Strategy in Full Swing?

The tactics children use to avoid eating foods such as vegetables and liver are gems carried from one generation to the next. But whether your child feeds his "It's good for you" food to the dog, gags and feigns strangulation, or pouts, mutters, and complains, it all comes down to the fact that the foods children refuse to eat are usually the most nutritious ones and are replaced with filler foods—foods that fill the stomach but offer little nutritionally.

Filler foods have an addictive quality and lead to a "The more you eat the more you want" cycle. Children fall into this pattern easily, since food that is fun and appeals to them is almost always heavily sugared, and sugar consumption creates a craving for more sugar.

To deal with this addictive situation, children learn to use the "I'm hungry/I'm not hungry" technique: They are not hungry at mealtime, but become suddenly ravenous at inopportune moments when nutritious food is unavailable. They know that between meals it's easier for you to give them a cookie or some other filler food than to fix another meal. This manipulative approach is usually not a conscious one, but it fulfills a self-perpetuating craving. The body is in control; the mind merely follows along.

The "I'm hungry/I'm not hungry" technique occurs with allergenic as well as refined foods. Since the most distinctive characteristic of cerebral allergy is craving the very food the victim is allergic to, it is not surprising that allergy is involved in this area. Refined and allergenic foods evoke the same response: each sets up a cycle of craving for the very food that is not needed by the body. This occurs because the body is constantly trying to reach a state called homeostasis—an internal stability.

When the body is bombarded with something it cannot handle, such as refined sugar or an allergenic food, it responds by adapting to the substance —in effect, becoming dependent on it. An analogy can be made to alcoholism and drug abuse in adults. The situations are not identical, of course, but the point is that refined sugar and allergenic foods can also evoke a protective, homeostatic response. This dependent or addictive cycle can be broken only by avoidance of those foods or substances to which the body reacts unfavorably. Withdrawal from sugar and allergenic food usually occurs in about two days after their removal from the diet, but one often can observe withdrawal symptoms much sooner if the child demands very frequent snacks of his troublemaking food. For example, a child who demands and ingests sugary foods all throughout the day would tend to have a greater addictive problem than a child who eats sugary food only once a day. Once the addictive cycle is broken you can see the reaction the child *really* has to the food he cannot handle because the protective addictive shield of homeostasis is down.

"I'm hungry/I'm not hungry" is in full swing when children frequently must eat refined foods to give them a lift. Since most children don't have free access to the refrigerator, they must rely on food Mother offers. If this does not measure up to their expectations, the child goes on a hunger strike at mealtimes, hoping for a settlement between meals of the more desirable.

Sometimes it seems children are almost instinctive about when you are most likely to give them the refined foods they crave. For example:

> One hour after dinner, with the dishes washed and everything put away. You are just sitting down to relax after an exhausting day when they complain of hunger. You ask why they hardly touched their dinner, and they say, "But Mom, I wasn't hungry then!"
> When you're rushing through the market trying to finish grocery shopping quickly. They know you're an easy mark when you're in a hurry—and there are so many goodies around.
> When you are on the telephone. An excellent time to ask for sugar cookies or candy because you don't want to be interrupted—and boy, do they know it!

The child's search for goodies begins with breakfast. This isn't much of a problem, since many foods offered at breakfast are largely carbohydrate anyway—"Keep 'em home for breakfast" with doughnuts, sweet rolls, sugared cereal, white toast and jelly, sugar syrup on pancakes—and the desired lift is achieved. Soon this lift wears off, so the child eats a candy bar or chews sugared gum at school or, at home, whines and begs for cookies. Lunchtime might provide an acceptable meal, but usually it is largely carbohydrate too, such as spaghetti or white bread and bologna. If the child has eaten some protein for lunch, it will hold for a little longer than breakfast. Snacktime after school or nap may again fail to supply little more than calories. The time before dinner, and dinner itself, often becomes the setting for intense responses, since this is the one time parents tend to be adamant about goodies' spoiling appetites. Insistence that your children wait for dinner when they are "starving" an hour beforehand may cause a great deal of turmoil. The dip in their blood-sugar levels can bring on headaches, nausea, irritability, and/or depression[8] which kills the appetite for what is often the only nutritious meal of the day. The symptoms ease up about an hour after dinner, and the child is asking for something to eat—but only something sweet will do. And so the search for something sweet continues.

Excuses, Excuses (but Good Ones!)

Our world is rapidly changing along with our food choices. Parents find that convenience food is necessary for the lives we lead. We all may basically agree that the food we offer our children needs to be selected with care, and strive to do so, but often lack of time and knowledge seem to put that goal beyond our reach.

Time is a critical factor, particularly in families where both parents work. Children (small ones especially) demand a great deal of attention, and this often provides little time for choosing foods. As one mother put it:

"I used to read labels and carefully prepare meals, but now with the two toddlers I just run into the store and *grab*—and I'm darn lucky to be able to do that!"

Unfortunately, the food you do grab is often full of substances that do not belong in your child's body (or your own) and accomplishes little more than a fill-up on empty calories. The child's need for essential nutrients remains unfulfilled.

To extend your knowledge of nutrition in order to feed your children properly is often difficult because of the many conflicting theories extant. Furthermore, it isn't easy to escape refined foods in America; so just getting your children off such foods long enough to see any results is a major accomplishment. Success in fulfilling your children's nutritional needs usually requires an entire revamping of the idea of good nutrition, but this knowledge can be helpful only if we know how to go about it—and that is what this book is all about.

What ever happened to the basic foods of yesteryear? Homemade soups, whole-grain breads, fresh fruits and vegetables? Once upon a time, breakfast was the meal the whole family shared, laden with scrambled eggs, buckwheat pancakes with real maple syrup, milk, oatmeal, homemade sausage, fresh fruit. Lunch may have been a big bowl of homemade vegetable soup, a hunk of cheese, a whole-grain muffin, and an apple. Dinner was perhaps roast chicken, yams, green beans, and homemade custard for dessert. Obviously, many of us do not have the time nor inclination to prepare large or complex meals on a daily basis; but it is still possible to provide healthful, convenient, kid- (and husband-) acceptable meals!

Up, Down, Round, and Round

The draining effect produced by bombarding the body with more re-fined carbohydrate, altered fats, chemical additives, and allergenic food-stuffs than it can handle is a severe stress on all bodily processes. Nutrients are used up and wasted needlessly; the need for particular nutrients can skyrocket while the body fights desperately to balance itself. Pinpointing the source of dysfunction is difficult, since the body's response to food is a complex interaction; what affects one part will affect the entire body. In addition, each of our bodies responds uniquely to stress. Whereas the major source of difficulty in one person might appear to be in the adrenal glands, in another it may originate in the pituitary glands, the pancreas, the thyroid, or other areas.

The stability of the blood-sugar level is so vital that the body possesses an intricate system for balancing it; any deviation in the blood-sugar level can be counteracted by many different mechanisms. The protective process begins with the endocrine system, ductless glands that send hormones, or messages, directly into the bloodstream to regulate the metabolic and other functions of the body. The endocrine system includes the adrenals, the pancreas, the thyroid, the pituitary, the gonads, and the thymus. If abused, however, this system may not perform properly, which plays havoc with the blood-sugar level and thereby the proper functioning of the body and the mind.

For instance, the pituitary gland may initiate the release of hormones to the adrenals, signaling them to correct an imbalance in the blood sugar. But if the adrenals are exhausted from overstimulation due to a high-refined-sugar carbohydrate diet they cannot respond properly because they lack essential nutrients necessary to follow through with the pituitary's commands.

There is evidence that the endocrine glands also may be influenced by allergic responses to foods, chemicals, and inhalants.[9] These irritants can inhibit the function of the glands, but excitation may also occur. To relieve the inhibited-function symptoms, adrenal and thyroid hormones are some-times administered. But the application of these hormones does not solve the problem of why the imbalance occurred. Furthermore, it has been ob-served that the function of the endocrine glands may return to normal with the removal or rotation of the allergens. Thus these hormones are often used unnecessarily.[10]

What you are or are not ingesting is the critical factor in maintaining your body's unique biochemical balance. To understand what may be un-balanced, it is helpful to explain what goes on in different glands of the body. Separating body functions in this way is hypothetical, but can help us in a clearer understanding of what goes on within.

The Panicked Pancreas

The pancreas is a long, narrow gland that supplies digestive juices to the small intestine, where most absorption of nutrients takes place. It also plays a major part in blood-sugar regulation. It secretes the hormone glucagon, which raises the blood-sugar level, and the hormone insulin, which lowers it.

A barrage of sugar taken into the body in the form of refined carbohydrates produces sudden, repeated elevations in blood sugar. Eventually, this causes the pancreas to overcompensate with a surge of insulin, as if in a panic to stabilize the repeatedly high sugar levels.

When in balance, insulin helps the body store and burn sugar properly. When it is out of balance, insulin causes disharmony within the entire body because body and brain do not have the proper amount of fuel (glucose) essential for normal function. When the pancreas is oversecreting insulin, the result is low blood sugar and a variety of accompanying disorders, since both body and brain are dependent upon a stable glucose level. The interacting relationship of hypoglycemic (and other blood-sugar) disorders and allergic responses may rest largely in the pancreas. Not only hypoglycemia (low blood sugar), but allergic responses may be triggered in this way, since deviations in insulin production depress production of pancreatic enzymes.[11]

Pancreatic-enzyme insufficiency may result in absorption into the bloodstream (in the form of polypeptide—large protein—molecules) of improperly digested or undigested foods, and this may evoke an allergic response in any part of the body, including the brain, as the allergic material becomes lodged in target areas of the body.

When the pancreas fails to offer a balanced amount of hormones, other parts of the protective system try to compensate for its inadequacies.

The Drained Adrenals

The adrenal glands are located on top of each kidney. They consist of a center portion, the medulla, and an outer portion, the cortex. Through the secretion of hormones, the adrenals help the body handle stress. Adrenaline, secreted from the medulla, is the emergency hormone that stimulates the liver to reconvert glycogen (glucose stored in the liver) back into glucose so that it is immediately available for a "fight or flight" response. The cortical secretion from the cortex also works along these lines, but with a slow, steady release instead of the intensive production of adrenaline.

The adrenals struggle to raise the blood-sugar level when the pancreas overreacts and produces too much insulin (which lowers it). If insulin production is high, then there will be a magnified production of cortical hormones. Under this stress, the adrenals have been found to become enlarged. Dr. Eli Seifter at Albert Einstein Medical College in New York has linked this adrenal enlargement to the destruction of lymph cells. This in turn deprives the thymus of nourishment and causes it to atrophy. Thus repeated stress on the adrenals may lead to exhaustion which profoundly affects other members of the protective system.

The Atrophied Thymus

The thymus is centered in the middle of the chest under the breastbone. It was once thought to have no function in adulthood, since the advent of puberty causes it to shrivel. It has been found, however, that the thymus does have extremely vital functions other than growth. Its key role is stimulating defense mechanisms that prevent the body from succumbing to illness or disease. The thymus is closely involved with hypoglycemic/allergic responses, since allergic reactions are the body's attempt to defend itself from substances that threaten well-being. Furthermore, it has been observed that such stresses as severe illness, injury, trauma, chemical exposure, radiation, and other allergic insults may cause the thymus to shrink to half its size.[12]

The Insufficient Thyroid

The thyroid is a butterfly-shaped gland at the base of the neck. Like the adrenals, the thyroid influences blood-sugar levels by stimulating the release of glucose (stored as glycogen) from the liver. When the thyroid gland is underactive because of a deficiency, an allergy, or stress put upon it from another part of the body, it secretes insufficient hormones, bringing about an imbalance of the blood sugar in conjunction with nutrient disruption (especially of minerals) on a cellular level.

The Wavering Pituitary

The pituitary gland, located at the base of the brain and the size of a large pea, exerts a profound influence on the body and regulates almost all vital processes. The pituitary is referred to as the "command gland" and receives its directions from the brain. The pituitary can force the pancreas to produce more insulin. It can stimulate the adrenals and the thyroid gland to nudge the liver into releasing glucose into the bloodstream. Although the pituitary keeps a close rein on the endocrine system, its influence is futile if the other glands are exhausted and not functioning properly. Consequently, this counteracts on the pituitary gland and the protective interaction among the glands is weakened.

The Sluggish Liver

The liver, the largest gland in the body, stores and manufactures glucose. Excess sugar entering the body is picked up and stored in the liver for future use by transformation of the glucose (water-soluble) into glycogen (fat-soluble). (This prevents the water-soluble glucose from being washed out into the bloodstream.) The storage and release mechanism may be interrupted, though, since refined sugar brings about an increased need for nutrients, the B vitamins in particular. An overload of refined sugar (and refined foods) may bring about deficiencies that "inhibit the liver's control of its glucose reserves." [13]

The Responding Brain

As the body's endocrine system goes round and round trying to right itself, the brain is inevitably affected, since the brain is wholly dependent upon blood sugar as its source of energy. The impact on the brain plays a major role in the multitude of problems children experience. Blood-sugar studies conducted by Yaryura-Tobias showed that a drop in the blood-sugar-level—as may occur when an overload of refined carbohydrates or allergenic food is consumed—disrupts the level of neurotransmitters which control sleep, mood, motivation, and learning. Hyperactivity or violent behavior may result.[14] Entry into the bloodstream of incomplete protein-breakdown products due to improper digestion may induce allergic effects, as described by Hemmings,[15] on the brain. Isn't it time to take a second look at the sugary candy and cookies and cake so lovingly offered to children?

There is a problem in this country in equating sugar with an expression of love. And there is no getting around the idea that goodies are the heart's desire even if you don't reward with or encourage sweets. Goodies run riot at Grandma's, at the neighbors', at school, at the grocery store, at any get-togethers. But what establishes goodies as especially desirable is the light in the eyes of a friend who announces, "I've got candy; want some?" It looks too good to be true, and to resist is impossible, unless your children are supplied with nutritious snacks and understand (and accept) why sugar is not for them (or for that matter, for any child).

It is most upsetting to me when a little one's first word is "cookie," reflecting what is important in that developing mind. What were *your* children's first words? If "cookie" or "candy" was among them, sweets were probably an important part of their new world. One needs to realize that the word "cookie" and its significance is the result of the erroneous attitude "Sugar is nice and fun and necessary."

The most notorious idea about sugar is that it gives you energy. The number of people who still believe this is shocking. Even if they accept that sugar is bad for the teeth (it affects far more than the teeth, but this is a start), they argue that "a little bit of sugar won't hurt," or "my child receives fluoride treatments and brushes after eating sugar, so it's okay."

Goodies are here to stay, but who says they have to contain sugar, hydrogenated fats, and white flour to taste good? Snacks can contribute to your children's health and satisfy Grandma's or your need to give your children fun foods. Lots of recipes and ideas for goodies that are also nutritious can be found in the back of this book. So when relatives are appalled by your cruelty in denying your child goodies, you can explain that the goodies have remained—only the ingredients have been changed.

I know it isn't easy to deal with relatives you are especially fond of. The first time I told a relative "No sugar," she scolded me and said that I was denying my child a pleasure that all children had. She promptly offered him sugar goodies at every opportunity. I felt helpless to argue with a person I loved and respected, but I could not allow my baby to be fed food I considered harmful. I had to take a stand, and I did. With time she did understand and came to accept the fact that sugary foods are harmful. As it is for everyone, there was much relearning to be done, but seeing results in herself and in her grandchild helped considerably in her understanding of the food connection.

And Awa-a-ay We Go . . .

Most parents wouldn't even consider giving children two or three cups of coffee a day, but you may unknowingly be giving this much or even more caffeine. Chocolate, colas (even artificially sweetened ones), and cocoa hold more than an overload of refined carbohydrate—they contain a whopping dose of caffeine, which startles the body further by putting the emergency adrenal hormones into action. The combination of sugar and caffeine works in a doubly damaging way: the sugar in the cola or chocolate causes the blood-sugar level to soar while the caffeine content stimulates the adrenal glands, and therefore the liver, to release still more glucose from storage. The body desperately tires to stabilize the blood-sugar level by pouring forth insulin. Caffeine may produce symptoms of heart palpitation, trembling, depression, anxiety, nervousness, and insomnia.

The vicious up and down pull on the blood sugar perpetrated by the combined ingestion of sugar and caffeine is hard to break. Caffeine-containing foods often become addictive, for they offer an immediate—but temporary—lift. Just as coffee gives adults a lift, chocolate, cola, and tea give children a lift, which lasts only until the overtaxed pancreas produces too much insulin. This causes a drop in the blood-sugar level, often to lower than it was before the sugar/caffeine food or drink was consumed. The low blood-sugar level leads to the desire for another lift, so more sugar/ caffeine is ingested, and the damaging cycle continues.

To compound the harm, a double-blind controlled study at the University of Mainz School of Medicine in West Germany[16] implicated phosphates found in soft drinks (used as a buffering agent) in provoking hyperactive and hyperaggressive behavior in children and adolescents. An average can of a soft drink contains about 12 milligrams of phosphoric acid per ounce. High intake of soft drinks challenges magnesium reserves in the body. A book describing the effects of phosphates on behavior[17] has now been published by the West German Society for Criminology.

Good Goodies

The taste of chocolate need not be given up forever—since sugar-free carob offers the flavor yet leaves out the caffeine. Herbal teas can replace

Lipton's and come in a wide variety of tastes; but check these carefully, since some herbal teas do contain caffeine.

"Natural" cola should not be encouraged on a daily basis, because it would be better for children to drink 100-percent real fruit juices or "smoothies" you (or they) make by blending whole fruit and ice. But for some children, it may be necessary to use "natural" cola as a stepping-stone away from "soft drinks and smiles." There are several brands on the market (available in health-food stores) that offer cola sweetened with honey or fruit juice and contain no caffeine or artificial ingredients.

Holding Back the Deluge

Each child has an individual level of carbohydrates he can comfortably handle. Elimination of refined carbohydrates such as white sugar, flour, and processed foods made with these starches constitutes a giant step in balancing the carbohydrate level in the diet. Some children, especially those with severe blood-sugar problems, need a more carefully balanced natural-carbohydrate level. To find this level requires the understanding of the two basic types of carbohydrates and an awareness of the content of naturally occurring carbohydrates in foods. It is not necessary to know the exact carbohydrate content but to understand that foods such as potatoes, pasta, crackers, breads, cereals, grains, and legumes contain complex carbohydrates; and fruit (whole, dried, juice) and concentrated sweeteners like honey (and snacks sweetened with it) contain simple carbohydrates. Both types need to be adjusted in the diet so that the concentration of nutrients in the food eaten is at an optimal level. White flour contains a high level of carbohydrate with a very low level of nutrients; whole-wheat flour offers more in its nutrient/carbohydrate ratio. Honey consumed alone would create an imbalance, with a high carbohydrate-to-nutrient-level ratio; honey used sparingly in a milk eggnog drink would provide a higher nutrient-to-carbohydrate level; but using some honey in a natural cookie containing nutritional yeast and ground seeds rich in vitamins, minerals, proteins, and essential fatty acids would offer a balance at the highest level of all.

Allergy also must be taken into consideration, for it works in conjunction with the carbohydrate overload. If an individual is allergic to any food, even if it is a pure, wholesome food such as whole wheat or eggs or milk, it can cause severe blood-sugar changes and accompanying allergic responses, thus making that food inappropriate for that particular person. Natural carbohydrates should always be consumed in a dietary balance with protein, vitamins, minerals, and essential fats. You may achieve this by offering a wide variety of natural foods in your child's diet.

Breakfast is the most important meal, because it establishes the blood-sugar level for the entire day. A starchy, oversugared breakfast offers nothing but calories; a nutrient-rich breakfast free of allergenic foods ensures that it will be a good day. All the food you offer your children is important, however, and if you plan your meals to fulfill nutritional needs instead of stomachs, emotions, or pocketbooks, then your food choices can lead only to good health—Healthy Bodies, Healthy Minds.

There's Hope Yet!

It is not possible to change your child's eating habits overnight, nor is it possible to change your own immediately, either. Our compulsive consumption of large quantities of refined carbohydrates may have a strong physical and/or emotional basis. Potent withdrawal symptoms can make resisting these goodies a monumental effort.

In combating the goodie phenomenon, rest assured that with gradual but steady improvement of the diet, the desire for sugar goodies is left behind and a desire for nutritious new goodies takes over. Thankfully, there are lots of substitutes to get you over the rough spots.

Eventually you will find that natural goodies will need to be sweetened less as this (addictive) taste appeal of sweetness fades away. It is great to hear your child tell you that something is too sweet. It is the signal that things are on their way. Four-year-old Justin's mother knew she was on the right track when she offered fruit-on-the-bottom, honey-sweetened yogurt and Justin took a firm stand:

"Okay, I'll eat it, but only if I don't have to eat the down part."

Hooray for you, Justin! That's one down and millions more children to go, if only we can help to show them how!

FOUR

Ricochet Reactions

The refined, processed food offered to our children can dramatically affect their behavior. The most notorious of its effects is hyperkinesis —or hyperactivity, as it is more popularly called. It is characterized by poor coordination, a low frustration threshold, a short attention span, sleeping problems, increased perceptual speed (the mind races), fidgeting, impulsiveness, excitability, and disruption.

Parents know hyperactivity well, if not through their own children, then through children of relatives and friends. Hyperactivity afflicts an estimated 4 million children in the United States. The actual figure for the occurrence of hyperactivity is shaky, however, owing to misinterpretations of hyperactive and nonhyperactive behavior. Some school districts in California and New York report as high as 40 percent of their students have hyperkinetic learning disabilities. This is difficult to prove, however, because an over-reactive child has a unique behavior pattern, and teachers vary in their interpretations of children's behavior. One teacher may estimate one-half of a class as hyperactive while another may conclude that only a fourth of that class is truly hyperactive and the other fourth have hyperactive tendencies only under stress (such as when hungry, tired, or ill).

The varieties and intensities of hyperactivity demonstrate that 1) different areas of the brain are involved, and 2) different influences evoke hyperactive responses. Some of the responses I have observed are the following:

Benjamin is a delightful four-year-old who is friendly and happy and can express his feelings and ideas in a surprisingly mature manner. But when confronted with a situation in which he has to sit down and participate in a game, he becomes frustrated. He must control the game by sweeping the pieces off the board and throwing or chewing them. No amount of talking or threats or spanking helps—it is as if he were in another world and could not understand or hear you. Sitting still to eat is difficult for him, as is most indoor play, but outdoors he is able to get along fairly well with other children. Sleep comes easily, and he remains asleep all night. Observing Benjamin, you probably would recognize his behavior as hyperactive;

but until you sat down to play a game or teach him something, you would not realize how seriously he is affected.

Brian, at seven, far surpasses his classmates in his ability to read and write and spell, yet becomes bored very easily with school unless he is permitted to work independently. He has difficulty getting along with other children and appears to drift off into a world of his own. At home he frequently has emotional outbursts and usually overresponds in general. He is often destructive with objects, but is gentle with people and very affectionate. Brian appears to be wound up a good part of the time, but if given something to learn and concentrate on is calm and content. His sleeping patterns are very erratic; he will lie awake for hours after everyone else is asleep, but once asleep will remain so. Brian is troubled by an inability to respond calmly, just as Benjamin is, yet Benjamin has trouble concentrating and Brian does not. And while Benjamin is friendly and outgoing, Brian has great difficulty making friends. Both may be considered hyperactive although they respond in entirely different ways.

Jody, at nine, is often whiny, wiggly, and irritable. She resists cuddling, cries without reason, and is incapable of waiting for anything. Her performance at school is uneven, since she is unable to work independently without fidgeting, procrastinating, and bothering children around her. On a one-to-one basis with her teacher she does well and is capable of concentrating. At home, nothing seems to please her and she never seems to calm down. Her sleeping is fitful; she awakens intermittently during the night. Jody is different from Brian and Benjamin. Whereas Brian is capable of concentrating independently, Jody works well only with a teacher, and Benjamin is incapable of concentrating with or without help. Yet Benjamin is happy and friendly whereas Brian and Jody are not. Sleeping patterns differ also in these children—Benjamin having a normal sleeping pattern, Brian finding it hard to get to sleep (but staying asleep when he does), and Jody having great difficulty staying asleep.

Andrew, a fearless ten-year-old, is a very aggressive child who often hits and bullies other children. He cannot be diverted from an action and rarely feels remorse for what he has done. He is oblivious to the feelings of others, is extremely impatient, and goes into a rage when he doesn't get what he wants. He does poorly in school, since his attention span is short, and he frequently disrupts the class. He is clumsy and uncoordinated, and never seems to wind down. Even in sleep he is restless and frequently experiences terrifying nightmares. Bed-wetting is a major problem. Andrew's behavior is pretty constant—he responds consistently in a hyperactive, impulsive way, whereas Benjamin, Brian, and Jody all respond in an uneven way.

Sandy, a bright five-year-old, responds normally until placed under stress. When overtired, hungry, or faced with a new situation, he becomes hyperactive. His responses are not always the same. He seems to fluctuate drastically in activity, most of the time responding in a normal manner but going through cycles of irritability, short attention span, and low frustration tolerance. Although, he is quite overactive during these cycles, they seem to last only a few hours or, at the longest, a few days and then he is his normal self again. Sandy has hyperactive tendencies yet is not truly hyperactive because the effect is not lasting.

All of these children overrespond in very different ways, to different degrees, and in different situations. To unlock the causes of hyperactivity is not especially difficult, but it must be thorough, for often we must find not only the right key but the right combination of keys. Maybe one day someone will discover exactly why Jody's brain acts differently from Brian's, but the important issue now is what is causing the problem and what can be done about it. There are two choices—to search out and find the answer or to leave the problem unresolved and smother it with drugs.

The Mechanical Zombie Effect

Hyperactive children respond in unique patterns, but parental reaction is pretty much the stereotyped "Sit still and *stop wiggling!*" We feel the tenseness of their bodies, and yet we are helpless to calm what they cannot control. And that leads to the use of drugs. What other recourse is there when a child is unable to learn or even act in a normal way? When your child is driving you up the wall, smothering the symptoms often seems more important than finding the cause and curing the problem, especially when the doctor agrees. With the diagnosis that a child is hyperactive, the doctor promptly prescribes an amphetamine. The idea is to keep the child somewhere between a zombie and a robot (it isn't yet possible to drug someone into a "normal" behavioral state). Drugs slow children down by blocking the central nervous system so their behavior is more acceptable, but this does not mean drugs improve the child's ability to learn.[1] Ritalin, a stimulant, is the most commonly used drug for controlling hyperactivity, but if it fails to establish the desired effect, then Dexedrine, Mellaril, Cylert, Thorazine, Tofranil, Benadryl, or Vistaril may be tried.[2] The use of these drugs for hyperactivity is a gamble. The product-information leaflet that accompanies Ritalin states:

> Ritalin should not be used in children under six years since safety and efficacy in this age group have not been established.
> Sufficient data on safety and efficacy of long-term use of Ritalin in children with minimal brain dysfunction are not yet available.

Instead of hyperactive behavior must we choose dizziness, loss of appetite, insomnia and interrupted sleep, headaches, loss of mental alertness, nausea, upset stomach, diarrhea? Or possible rashes, depression, shakiness, rapid heartbeat, irritability, blurred vision, or confusion which may occur[3] as side effects of taking these drugs? This is *not* to say these problems will occur, but that they have been known to occur. And what are the effects on the brain of growing up on drugs? No one knows.

The very idea of giving a stimulant to calm a child down signifies that there is something seriously warped biochemically. How is it logical to suppress this profound response with drugs?—the hyperactive child is certainly not deficient in amphetamines. And yet doctors routinely smother the symptoms without bothering to question why the child is hyperactive. Since the majority of doctors fail to search out the answers, then we, as parents, *must*.

The "Obnoxious" Epidemic

We may willingly accept our child's individual personality and be prepared to handle bouts of tantrums, crying, irritability, screaming, mood swings, disregard for others, and aggression on an occasional basis. But when such behavior (and more) dominates the child's personality to the point where no one can stand being around him, you begin to fear that friends and relatives are right—the child is spoiled rotten and needs to be jerked into line.

Yet even though you may receive the brunt of the child's unprovoked anger or other unjustified emotions (you can't avoid your children even if everyone else does), you instinctively feel the outbursts are not the result of spoiling. It is as if some inner governor had gone awry and permitted a total oblivion to the feelings and needs of others. In these circumstances, even the best parent soon runs out of patience and resorts to the punishment that everyone is sure will alleviate the problem. It yields little success. It does, however, serve to reinforce the feeling that spoiling is not the core of the problem. But just try explaining that to doctors, friends, relatives, or even your spouse.

This demanding, never-satisfied ailment has become epidemic, especially among hyperactive children. Yet because they do not always exhibit overt disabilities or psychotic behavior, they are believed to be "normal" until a crisis occurs. We hear repeatedly from the doctor that "He just needs a little time" or "You are spoiling the child" or "She's looking for attention; give her some."

Even if the child receives a descriptive label, such as hyperactive, the problem remains unchanged. Nothing seems to satisfy such very difficult and unhappy children, and medication doesn't resolve their problems but merely mocks them. Their refusal to conform, their supersensitivity in non-threatening situations, their inability to respond normally to people and situations around them, and their never-ceasing demands bond them closely together as a group of children who desperately need help, even if you don't know what kind.

Wiping Out Red Mouth

I have seen it on hundreds of children's faces, and I am sure you have too—the red stain above the lips after they have drunk artificially colored, flavored, sugared drinks. These fun drinks are served in place of natural juice at parties, nursery schools, ball games, the movies, and they appear in our homes. No one objected much to these sugary chemical mixtures until a doctor in San Francisco (who *did* bother to ask why children are hyperactive) related hyperactivity to the artificial colors and flavors that are heavily laced into most of the fun foods for children.

The most popular method of controlling hyperactivity, aside from drugs, is the diet devised by the late Benjamin Feingold, M.D. Known as the Feingold Diet, it requires eliminating from the diet artificial food colorings and artificial flavorings, which are coal-tar derivatives containing salicylates, plus discontinuing the following foods containing naturally present salicylates:

Almonds	Green peppers
Apples	Gooseberries
Apricots	Nectarines
Blackberries	Oranges
Boysenberries	Peaches
Cherries	Plums/prunes
Cucumbers/pickles	Raspberries
Currants	Strawberries
Grapes/raisins	Tomatoes

In his book *Why Your Child Is Hyperactive,* Dr. Feingold describes hyperactivity due to synthetic food additives this way:

> Synthetic food additives may, in some unknown way, be tampering with the brain and nervous system by short-circuiting some functions in a particular group of children genetically predisposed to these chemicals.[4]

But isn't it possible that deficiencies, imbalances, and/or sensitivities to other foods and chemicals besides those containing salicylates (even hypoglycemia), could bring about this same phenomenon? Could it be that Feingold does not relate hyperactivity to allergy because the standard methods of testing for food allergy are at best 20 percent accurate?

Feingold's findings are a giant step forward in relating hyperactivity and diet, but it is necessary to look for other interacting forces involved in the hyperactive response. A bonus result of the Feingold Diet is an awareness of what children are eating. Sugar is not discouraged in the Feingold Diet, but sugar is less often ingested because many of the convenience foods which so often contain artificial flavors and colors are eliminated.

It is possible that this diet works because this awareness of food has decreased the consumption of sugar and improved the child's health by offering more high-quality foods. Where the Feingold Diet has failed, is it because sugar is still being consumed in large amounts, that allergens have not been eliminated, or that nutritional needs have not been met? Dr. Ronald Printz at the University of South Carolina has observed [5,6] that when additives (synthetic colors) alone were given to hyperactive children, few reacted, but when the same dose was given with refined sugar, a significant number of children became hyperactive. A study at St. John's Hospital [7] in England endeavored to correlate the multifaceted problems of behaviorally dysfunctional children. Some children were affected by food additives; others were not. Some children were affected by foods like wheat or milk. Franklin, who conducted the study, concludes that there are behaviorally dysfunctional children who by dietary control (pure foods) receive significant clinical benefits that cannot be explained by placebo.

The Wavering Curves

One candy bar, one whole-wheat cracker, and one orange all have something in common for Nathan: each gives him a severe case of the wiggles. Hyperactivity is only the first step of the response, though, since drastic mood swings may follow, manifested in the form of irritability or giddiness. Uncontrolled crying or a screaming-and-kicking jag also may occur when his blood-sugar level has taken a sharp drop (due to a skipped meal) and he eats these foods.

Sugar poses a particularly difficult problem for Nathan, as it does for many children. For the child who eats sugar only once in a while, the side effects may take hours to wear off. But for some children the side effects *don't* wear off because they are eating a great deal of sugar *every* day. In children who occasionally or rarely eat sugar (and there aren't too many of them) a pattern is apparent between the degree to which they respond and circumstances surrounding the ingestion of the sugar. Eaten after a full-protein meal, sugar has observably less effect than skipping breakfast and having candy for lunch. This is because protein and fat slow down the absorption of the sugar. For some children, the effect from sugar is always drastic even on a full stomach, but always worse on an empty stomach.

Erratic changes in blood-sugar levels may occur when children eat foods to which they are sensitive as well as when they eat refined carbohydrates. Yet it has also been observed that even without a change in the blood-sugar level, an allergic reaction may initiate hypoglycemic symptoms. [8]

There exists an interacting bond between food sensitivity, blood-sugar abnormalities, and hyperactivity. O'Shea and Porter [9] studied the behavior of five- to thirteen-year-old hyperkinetic children and demonstrated the involvement of hyperactivity and allergies. In double-blind testing of these children, the team found artificial dyes, cow's milk, peanuts, tomato, apple, cane sugar, corn, grapes, orange, chocolate, wheat, and egg most often provoking hyperactive behavior. Doris Rapp, M.D., a specialist in pediatric allergies in Buffalo, New York, has explored in depth the effects of food allergy on children's health and behavior. In her lectures, research papers,[10,11] and books about these effects, and even video tapes of these children reacting to double-blind testing materials, the information she presents is astonishingly convincing. In a videotape one may observe a small boy who is tested in a double-blind fashion. Initially the child is calm and playing with toys with his mother. On one test he begins to whine, pull on his mother, throw toys, and then actually bite his mother. Other blind doses are used and he calms down and is relaxed. When the code is broken, one sees that the child reacted to a substance he was allergic to and calmed when he finally received his treatment dose. In a study done at the New York Institute for Child Development, it was found that 75 percent of the hyperactive, learning-disabled children tested had abnormal blood-sugar levels[12] and allergies. The Institute names sugar a "critical culprit" in hyperactivity and learning disorders, but its approach also involves the eliminating of allergens, the addition of missing nutrients, and careful monitoring of the kinds and amounts of carbohydrates eaten. Superior food along with sensory-motor therapy has brought the Institute tremendous success in working with hyperactive, learning-disabled children. Recently, dietitians at Alberta Children's Hospital in Canada have used dietary and environmental intervention (improved diets, elimination of allergenic foods, supplementation, avoidance of allergens) with hyperactive preschoolers and have had rewarding results. The hospital found the children had improved sleep patterns; decreased aches, cramps, bloating, headaches, and rashes; increased attention span; decreased complaining and weepy behavior; decreased or eliminated repetitive behaviors; increased number of commands carried out; improved small motor skills; decrease or cessation of bedwetting, in addition to decreased hyperactive responses.

An important study appearing in *Lancet* examined the effects of particular foods on the behavior and health of hyperactive children.[13] Physicians from the Departments of Immunology and Child Psychiatry at the Institute of Child Health and Hospital for Sick Children in London, England, performed a rigorous study in which hyperactive children were placed on a diet of low-reactive foods. Then common allergenic foods were reintroduced, and reactions observed. Standard allergy testing verified that food allergy provoked the hyperactivity and other abnormal responses. Out of 76 children in the study, 62 improved, 21 of these children achieved *a normal range of behavior*. Foods that provoked the most symptoms were yellow food coloring (tartrazine) and benzoic acid, cow's milk, chocolate, soy, grapes, wheat, oranges, eggs (chicken), cheese (from cow's milk), peanuts, and corn. When tested on refined sugar, some children reacted to one kind (beet or cane) of sugar but not to the other; some children reacted to both. The authors conclude that "this trial indicates that the suggestion that diet may contribute to behavior disorders in children must be taken seriously."

Trouble from Above

The light to which we expose our children's bodies may have a dramatic effect on their well-being. John Ott, a pioneer researcher on the effects of different types of light on plants, animals, and humans, has found that exposure to television and fluorescent lighting has a detrimental effect on children by distorting brain and nervous-system functioning.[14] Ott believes that light—the right kind—is an essential nutrient just as vitamins and minerals are.

Full-spectrum light, sunlight, is cut off from us when we use eyeglasses, windshields, and windows, thus depriving us of the beneficial ultraviolet rays of the sun. To remedy the situation, glasses with full-spectrum plastic lenses (CR 59) and contact lenses are available to us as well as ultraviolet-transmitting plastic material for sliding doors, windows, and skylights. Full-spectrum fluorescent tubes which closely duplicate sunlight are now available, but their use is not widespread, since they are more expensive (though they do have a much longer life) than the cool-white fluorescent tubes. Ott has linked hyperactivity to the use of regular fluorescent lighting in schools. Using time-lapse photography, John Ott photographed children in classrooms exposed to both full-spectrum and fluorescent lighting and when the two were compared, he had captured startling differences in their behavior. Children who initially appeared uncooperative, irritable, hyperactive, and inattentive under fluorescent lighting became calmer and capable of sitting still and working when the lighting was changed to full-spectrum.

The flickering tube (television) also is a cause for concern. Evidence has shown that hyperactivity may be aggravated by exposure to radiation from television sets.[15] Getting children away from the television screen is no easy task, but could be well worth the effort.

The Primrose Path

Recently, research in England by the Hyperactive Children's Support Group[16] supports the position that hyperactive children who have atopic-type allergies (eczema, hives, asthma, and other various allergies)[17] may tend to be continuously thirsty and yet produce a concentrated urine. This phenomenon is "characteristic of essential fatty acid deficiency[18] states in which the skin surface becomes abnormally permeable to water leading to the loss of fluid across it."[19] Four major observations supported the testing of defective fatty-acid metabolism:

1) The majority of hyperactive children come from families with a history of atopic disorders. Atopic disorders are known to respond to essential fatty acid supplementation.
2) Thirst is a symptom consistently reported by parents of hyperactive children.

Thirst is an early feature of essential fatty acid deficiency in animals because of greatly increased water loss across the skin. Essential fatty acids are vital for maintaining the water impermeability of the skin.

3) Hyperactivity affects boys about three times more often than girls. Male animals are known to require about three times as much essential fatty acids as females to maintain growth. A partial essential fatty acid deficiency would therefore be expected to affect males much more than females.

4) A number of substances (tartrazine, salicylates, and others) have been reported to have an adverse effect on behavior in hyperactive children but not in normal children. Almost all the substances are known to be weak inhibitors of essential fatty acids to prostaglandins (local hormone-like regulating metabolism). They would not have much effect in the presence of normal amounts of essential fatty acid precursors but their influence could be critical if essential fatty acid stores were depleted.

Evidently, even though these children may consume linoleic acid (from cold-pressed safflower oil, for example), their bodies are unable to convert it into gamma-linolenic acid (precursor to prostaglandin E1) because of a defect in an enzyme (delta-6-desaturase). Therefore, it is necessary to supply the preformed essential fatty acid gamma linolenic so that the defective enzyme and subsequent deficiency state can be overcome. The two known sources of the preformed essential fatty acid are mother's milk[20] and evening primrose oil. Supplementation of evening primrose oil in hyperactive children with atopic disorders or a family history of atopic disorders[21] has yielded 80 percent positive results, yet it appears that there is no response in hyperactive children without atopic disorders in themselves or their families. This supplies another piece in the hyperactive puzzle.

Smoke Signals

A relationship between mothers who smoked during pregnancy and the occurrence of hyperkinesis has been explored by Nichols (1980) and Naeye (1979) and reported in the *Journal of the American Medical Association* *(JAMA)*. Nichols compared the smoking habits of mothers of hyperactive and normal children. He found that out of 42 variables studied as possible causes of hyperactivity, smoking during pregnancy had by far the most significant correlation with the occurrence of hyperkinesis. Cigarette smoking during pregnancy is estimated to increase the risk of having a child with hyperactivity by 9 to 12 percent.

But what effect does cigarette smoke have on a child after he or she is born? Exposure to a parent, relative, or sitter who smokes subjects children unnecessarily to many toxic substances such as pesticides that were sprayed on the tobacco plants and many additives used in the treatment of the tobacco. But one area that has been researched is the effect of lead and cadmium (cadmium gives cigarette smoke that blue color when it hangs in the air) to which children are exposed in inhaling cigarette smoke. The

Applied Neuroscience Institute at the University of Maryland[22] correlated low-level exposure to cadmium and lead with both I.Q. scores and school achievement and found a significant effect of cadmium/lead on cognitive function. Cadmium appeared to most strongly affect verbal I.Q., while lead appeared to affect performance I.Q. to a greater degree. Smoking around a child of any age is a grave mistake.

The Heavies

Elevated levels of heavy metals such as lead,[23,24] copper, mercury, and cadmium have been found in many hyperactive children. Disturbed behavior patterns due to too much lead have received the most intensive research, and it has been demonstrated that lead has a stimulating effect on the brain.[25] Carl Pfeiffer, M.D., at The Brain Bio Center in Princeton, New Jersey, attributes this effect to *any* combination of heavy metals, not just lead. It is believed the burden of these excess heavy metals interferes with and displaces such essential minerals as zinc, iron, manganese, and potassium.[26] This interference impairs the energy supply to the brain, resulting in abnormal brain function.[27]

In experiments with animals, the ingestion of lead brought about definite changes in brain chemistry which manifested as hyperactive and aggressive behavior even when there were no symptoms of lead toxicity.[28] Studies of children also have indicated that hyperactivity may appear with elevated but not toxic levels of lead.[29]

In *Zinc and Other Micro-Nutrients,* Dr. Pfeiffer explains that the reason lead (and other heavy metals) plays so much havoc with children's behavior is that:

1) A child's blood-brain barrier has not had time to mature and thus more of the poisonous lead (or other heavy metals) goes to the brain.
2) It appears that children absorb lead more easily and retain it to a greater extent than adults. In contrast to the adult, where lead is stored primarily in the bone, in children large amounts of lead remain in the soft tissues.

Another interesting observation is that lead accumulation is more evident when a child is deficient in calcium. Since the ingestion of refined sugar inhibits the absorption of calcium, the high consumption of sugar by many children would reduce their protection from exposure to lead even if enough calcium-rich foods were eaten. The sugar-calcium-lead involvement is certainly one to avoid. Assisting children to eliminate sugar from their diets and to balance the ingestion of minerals can help accomplish this.

The addition of Vitamin C, zinc, and calcium to the diet aids in mobilizing and eliminating heavy metals from the body.[30] To prevent this accumulation in the first place, it is necessary to provide a superior diet that is rich in these nutrients in addition to the avoidance of these metals as much as possible. An awareness of the sources of heavy metals is necessary in order to accomplish avoidance:

Lead. Auto exhaust contributes a very large proportion of the lead to which children are exposed, but some of the sources we don't think about are cigarette smoke or lead-containing paint on pencils that children frequently chew on. Some of the following sources of lead may surprise you:

Asphalt	Lead water pipes
Auto heaters and	Leaded glass
air conditioners	Newsprint
Batteries	Paint and enamels
Building materials	Pewter
Cement dust	Plaster
Charcoal	Putty
Cosmetics	Rain and snow
Crayons	Rubber tires
Dust	Smelters
Dyes	Smoke
Gas burners	Toys
Incinerators	Water

Obviously, some of these are impossible to avoid, but if we are aware of what contains lead, we can keep to a minimum by (for instance) not letting toddlers chew on magazines and crayons, by using the car air conditioner or heater only during extreme weather, or by making sure children have a source of pure water.

Cadmium. Coal burning, tobacco smoke, zinc smelters, paints, and water that flows through old pipes containing cadmium. A deficiency of zinc and a high intake of refined carbohydrates enhances the absorption of cadmium and can affect intelligence and school achievement in children.[31]

Copper. This is an essential mineral, but excess is more likely than deficiency, due to the widespread use of copper plumbing. Excessive copper levels have been desmonstrated to trigger aggression and other negative mental changes in children.[32] Zinc deficiency also is a factor in overburdening the body with copper. We must thus take special care to ensure that our children have an adequate balance of copper and zinc in their diets and pure water to drink.

Mercury. Children are exposed to mercury through pesticides, petroleum products, fungicides, chemicals dumped into water supplies from manufacturing plants, coal burning, and mercury-poisoned fish. Mercury competes with selenium in the body.

Ebbing the Tormenting Tide

Deficiencies, sensitivities, erratic changes in blood sugar, imbalances of minerals or toxic metals, and possibly artificial light may interfere with the balance of neurotransmitters, or communicators between the nerve cells in the brain which control sleep, mood, learning, and motivation. This phenomenon of disturbed brain chemistry can result in hyperactive behavior as well as a multitude of other disorders.

There is no single answer to hyperactivity. The pieces of the puzzle can fit together easily if we approach hyperactivity in more than one direction as a disorder that affects the *whole* child. Feeding children the best food possible that supplies all the nutrients, eliminating foods to which children are sensitive, providing them with pure water, helping them avoid toxic substances, insisting on and, if necessary, buying the proper lighting for their place of learning, and playing outside with them instead of watching television are important for the hyperactive child—and for *every* child.

FIVE

Sneeze-Scratch-Wheeze

An allergy may first be noticeable as colic or a rash or frequent vomiting or a persistent runny nose. Often these problems compound, and the result is the allergic child with classic symptoms of eczema, diarrhea, hives, asthma, recurrent ear infections, hay fever, chronic rhinitis (the runny nose), and itching. The allergic cycle often begins in infancy with bottle feeding and the advent of solid food. The stresses of deficiency, sensitivity, illness, and imbalance may all contribute and snowball into full-blown allergy.

The Obvious Signs

The symptoms we view as allergy are the obvious signs that are easy—and often unavoidable—to spot. But too often, instead of prompting a search for the cause, an allergy symptom is accepted as normal. The colic, the cradle cap, the vomiting become a part of babyhood; the ear infections, the runny nose, the rashes become normal for the preschooler; and the hives, the constipation, and the frequent colds become a part of growing up accepted with casual nonchalance, since "everyone" has them.

Continuous Congestion

The cold that doesn't want to go away has reached epidemic proportions. The runny, stuffy, encrusted, watery secretions from the nose are not always caused by a cold but may be due to or aggravated by allergy. The source of irritation may be food or an inhalant (perfume, dust, pollen) which causes swelling of the mucus membranes and produces such responses as:

Mouth breathing
Sneezing
Coughing
Nose wiggling or rubbing

Picking or itching of the nose
Enlarged tonsils and adenoids
Incessant sniffing, snorting, or clearing of the
    throat due to postnasal drip

Often "the cold" locks the body into a perpetual cycle that is merely the advance notice of worse things to come: ear infections, bronchitis, asthma, and chronic rhinitis.

Muffled Sounds

Ear infections often follow colds as a result of the increased secretion of mucus. This secretion may block and accumulate within the ear, and in some cases lead to damage because normal drainage is not accomplished. The doctor's usual course is to try to clear up the infection with drugs, but if it persists, tubes will be placed within the ear to make possible ventilation and drainage. Kelly, a patient's eighteen-month-old daughter, began such a cycle with a cold that stubbornly refused to go away. An ear infection followed and was relieved with drugs, but within a week she had another "cold" which resulted in another ear infection.

It rapidly became apparent that no sooner were Kelly's drugs discontinued than the cycle repeated—the cold, the ear infection, and then the drugs. The amount of anitbiotics and decongestants Kelly was consuming didn't seem to alarm the doctor, but it did concern Kelly's mother, and she told him so. Her worries were smoothed over with "Lots of children get recurrent ear infections." Finally, after three more visits to see him, the doctor agreed the drugs weren't working and suggested that milk be eliminated from Kelly's diet. This seemed to help a little, but the cycle continued.

A few months passed and Kelly was taken to the doctor with her newest ear infection. This time, however, the examination revealed she had a large amount of fluid behind her eardrums and her hearing was minimal. The doctor did not know if the damage would be permanent, but suggested that when Kelly was a little older tubes could be inserted into her ears.

Unusual case? No. More and *more* children become caught up in this cycle. Dr. George Shambaugh, Professor of Otolaryngology at Northwestern University and a former president of the American Academy of Otolaryngology, stated in October, 1982, at an annual meeting in New York that

> serious otitis is the largest single cause of hearing loss in children. And the operation of inserting a ventilating tube through the tympanic membrane [ear drum] to restore hearing has become *the most frequent hospital surgical procedure with anesthesia today*. There's no question of the usefulness of ventilating tubes for otitis media with effusion to equalize the air pressure on both sides of the tympanic membrane, thus allowing the fluid to resolve or to be expelled by ciliary action to the eustachian tube. Yet tubes alone aren't the answer for parents who are struggling to cope, often unsuccessfully, with the management of recurrent ear problems in their children. Neither are they an answer for their pediatricians, family physicians, and otolaryngologists who are trying to help them. Although allergies in children are often hard to identify by the usual allergy scratch tests, I've found that a program of allergic management with attention to hidden or delayed-in-onset food allergy helps me manage recurrent ear problems in children. Moreover, my results with allergy management are far

better than those obtained by putting children on prolonged courses of anti-biotics and relying on tubes to clear up the condition.

It is far simpler to prevent ear infections (and the subsequent plugged ears; ringing, popping, and cracking sounds; on-and-off hearing; and damage that can result in permanent hearing loss) by searching out the cause(s) in the first place instead of as a last resort, and a halfhearted one at that ("Maybe it's milk"). The ears are nothing to fool around with. If your child has an ear infection, use the antibiotics the doctor prescribes, but find out through testing if the child is allergic and what nutrients are lacking so that the child doesn't have to be subjected to massive amounts of drugs which could indeed be damaging.

A Gasp for Air

Asthma is a condition in which the air passages within the lungs become blocked by constriction of the muscles that involuntarily control air going in and out. The narrowing of the air passages and swelling of the mucus membranes which then may occur produce excess mucus which forms plugs.[1] Infection often triggers asthma, but it also may be triggered by food or chemical-inhalant allergy and stress (as well as nutrient deficiency and an insufficient diet). Attacks involve wheezing, choking, shortness of breath, and the feeling of suffocation, which may be mild or severe enough to require hospitalization. Asthma frequently strikes at night; we will examine this phenomenon and the cause further on in this chapter.

Tummy Blues

Colic, diarrhea, gas, and constipation are classic digestive upsets caused by sensitivities to particular foods. Cramps, nausea, vomiting, weight fluctuations, an itchy bottom, canker sores, bad breath, and a distended abdomen also occur frequently. Infancy is usually the starting point for these gastrointestinal disorders, with the milk-switching game (frantically in search of a formula the child can tolerate) the first signal of food allergy.

Bumps, Lumps, Boils, Hives

The skin's allergic response may be eczema, rash, hives, blisters, weals, pallor, dandruff, welts, itchiness, pimples, cradle cap. Oozing, crusting, scaling skin reflects a disturbance within the body that cannot be dealt with by the topical application of lotions and creams. Skin allergies are brought about by food sensitivities, exposure to chemicals (such as soap or paint), and natural materials (feather pillows, wool) or by contact, infection and other stresses, deficiencies, and imbalances. One interesting study reported in *Lancet*[2] is another addition to the mounting evidence that nutrient therapy—in this case primrose oil in the treatment of atopic eczema—is essential in the treatment of allergy.

The Allergic Face

A good look at a child's face can reveal trouble signs that are characteristic of the allergic child. These are clues to the child's state of well-being, and many will fluctuate in intensity or disappear altogether as exposure to allergens and deficiency/imbalance states are altered. When these states are exposed and under control, you will find the signs can be turned on and off by the reintroduction of the allergen or the withdrawal of nutrients that resolved the problem.

The allergic face may contain one or all of the following signs, depending upon the degree and kind of problems the child is experiencing:

The Eyes

The eyes take on a glazed, dull look and may also respond with burning, watering, heavy crusty secretions, light sensitivity, and inflammation. *Baggy eyes* are common, with puffiness directly below the eyes or on the outer edge of each eye. Singular or multiple wrinkles or deep creases also occur under the eye. The *shiners* that appear as large black, blue, or red circles under the eye are seen frequently and are caused by swelling due to an allergen which blocks drainage to the area.[3]

The Nose

Nose twitching, itching, wiggling, rubbing, snorting, and picking are common in children with swollen and congested nasal membranes. The habit of putting things up the nose is usually an attempt to scratch the inside of the nose. *Rabbit nose* is a term applied to explain the frequent twitching and wiggling of the nose which can become an irritating habit. The *allergic salute* is also common and involves rubbing and pushing the nose upward so that a crease is formed across the nose from repetition of this gesture over and over again. This gesture is usually accompanied by a zonking sound which translates into a cross between a snort and a clearing of the throat.

The Skin

The skin may become excessively pale or be dry and scaly. Rougelike patches on the cheeks may appear and sometimes be mistaken for the glow of health. The eyelids may become swollen and inflamed, and cracks may form behind the ears, or the earlobes may be flushed.

The Mouth

The congestion within the nasal passages may make it necessary for the child to breathe though the mouth, which is thus left gaping open. Dry, scaly edges on the lips and cracks in the corners of the mouth are frequent, as are canker sores.

The Cover-Up

The course of action to alleviate the symptoms of allergy is limiting. Avoidance of the allergen is difficult, because the methods used to test for allergy are not always accurate. Deficiencies and imbalances seem to be completely ignored. The cause doesn't seem to concern the conventional doctor as much as the drug that will offer temporary symptomatic relief. Allergy is an abnormal response; it signifies that something is wrong, that the body is unable to withstand a stress. It seems only logical to build up the body's defenses rather than approach the problem in a roundabout way by giving after-the-fact medicine. Medications prescribed for allergic conditions include antihistamines, antibiotics, adrenaline, expectorants, aerosol and inhalation therapy, tranquilizers, and corticosteroids. During a crisis they save lives. But prolonged use may produce side effects of which parents should have a complete understanding. Before giving any medication to your child, insist that you be informed of the side effects by your child's physician. Better yet, purchase a Physician's Desk Reference so that you will have the information close at hand. Once medication has been started, do not ever stop administering it without a doctor's permission. The use of any medication for children should be approached with extreme caution.

Consider asthma, for example: Here we find that the drugs being used to rectify the situation are actually adrenal hormones that are administered as tablets, capsules, liquid, or inhalants or by injection. Not surprisingly, these drugs raise the blood-sugar level initially by the hormones' stimulating action upon the liver (which reconverts glycogen into glucose) and by calling upon the body's reserves (which supply essential fatty acids, amino acids, vitamins, minerals, and so on). This exertion alone points out deficiency/sensitivity/imbalance along with low blood sugar as predominating factors in asthma.

With the repeated use of adrenaline the body is being drained of its reserves. It becomes involved in a tug-of-war as the adrenaline stimulates the release of glucose, which in turn stimulates the release of insulin, often in overabundance.

Glucose injections or the ingestion of sugar may also be employed in asthma attacks, but here again the protective system of the body responds with the release of insulin. In his book *New Low Blood Sugar and You* (Putnam, 1985), Dr. Carlton Fredericks relates asthma and hypoglycemia, citing that the early morning hours—when blood sugar is at its lowest level—are often the period for an asthma attack. Further supporting evidence is the indication[4] that asthma is uncommon in diabetics, whose blood-sugar level is exceedingly high.

When asthma is severely persistent—not responding to routine procedures (drugs), and if the health and development of the child is seriously affected, then corticosteroids are administered. These drugs have an even more devastating effect than the above-mentioned hormones, for they cripple the immune system with far more severity. The immune system is so deeply affected by the prolonged use of steroids that the child will not be able to receive immunizations, since the possibility of complications due to the body's inability to handle the stress is too acute. Dr. Claude Frazier, in his book *Parents' Guide to Allergy in Children* (New York: Grosset and Dunlap, 1978) describes the effects of steroids in this way:

> Steroid dosages may be increased to cope with such stressful conditions as disease, surgery, or emotional upset. When a child is on steroids for a long time, his adrenal glands may shrink and may be unable thereafter to produce enough hormones to allow the body to handle stress adequately. Even after the steroids have been discontinued, it may be necessary to begin them again when situations of stress arise.

Let me emphasize again that under no circumstances should any drug which your doctor has prescribed for your child be discontinued without his knowledge. The use of drugs, particularly those prescribed for allergy, forcefully overstimulates and overtaxes the adrenal glands (as well as the endocrine system and the entire body). A dependency may be set up whereby the body cannot function adequately without the drug. Abrupt withdrawal of the drug could be fatal.

If you wish to discontinue such drugs, first revise the child's diet and then see if the doctor is willing to gradually reduce the dosage while providing supplemental vitamins and minerals, an optimal diet, and environmental control. Many nutrients and diet modifications may be of benefit to the asthmatic child. Researchers from the USDA and Columbia University[5] found that the plasma and erythrocyte levels of asthmatic children were significantly lower in pyridoxal-5-phosphate (the active form of vitamin B_6) than those of a control group of nonasthmatic children. Asthmatic children supplemented with B_6 experienced a "uniform reduction in occurrence, severity, and duration of asthmatic attacks." It does not make sense to drain the body of its dwindling necessities when supplements may be used to supply it with what it needs and must have to function properly. Nutrients should always be administered in a balance, however, unless a physician uses special tests to determine elevated requirements of particular nutrients. A recent development in asthmatic studies is that of exposure to sulfites, which may cause severe asthmatic reactions in sensitive individuals. The Scripps Institute in La Jolla, California, estimates that half a million asthmatics are sulfite-sensitive. Among sources of exposure are produce treated in restaurants to keep it from browning, sulfured dried fruit, and wine. Symptoms may include cold sweats, dizziness, tightness in the chest, throat constriction, and tingling/burning in the mouth, and in a few cases it has triggered anaphylactic shock.

If your child's doctor is not informed as to the nutritional and ecologic aspects that may be helpful to your child, you may inquire if he would be willing to look into them and work with you. If the doctor laughs off the idea or responds with anger (don't be surprised at this—nutrition isn't taught in medical schools), then you may wish to look for another doctor who is at least open and willing to try to find the cause of your child's problems.

The Stepping-Stone Disorders

In this chapter we have examined classical allergies that doctors easily recognize. The biochemical relationship between body and mind has not yet been given a firm stamp of approval by the American Medical Association, and this is why in conversations with many doctors you will meet resistance. Even doctors specializing in allergy often fail to see the connection. There are five distinct classes (IgA, IgD, IgE, IgG, IgM) of antibodies, called immunoglobulins, produced by the body that are present in the blood and external secretions. Yet allergists tend to regard allergy as primarily IgE-mediated, and if the child's IgE levels are not elevated he is not, according to them, allergic. Each of the immunoglobulins has a specific function in immunity, but IgE is focused on because the most is known about it. As we learn more and more about the other immunoglobulins, we begin to realize how narrow a perspective it really is to limit ourselves to working with only one of them, IgE.

New syndromes are popping up, however, that may very well be the bridge that helps the larger part of the medical establishment (a small percentage of doctors recognize this already) to accept the influence of deficiency/sensitivity/imbalance within the body upon the brain. One such connection of allergy and its effect on the body and brain has been demonstrated in a double-blind study reported in *Lancet*[6] of children with severe migraine headaches. Food allergy (most commonly to milk, egg, chocolate, orange, wheat) proved to be the cause of migraine in 93 percent of the 88 children studied in London's Hospital for Sick Children. Also inadvertently found to be associated with migraine in the children were the symptoms of abdominal pain, behavior disorders, fits, asthma, and eczema, which also responded to the treatment. Interestingly, the children in the study were not found to have high levels of IgE, and the study suggests that IgE may not be as important as thought in food allergy.

A second body/brain disorder is called the tension-fatigue syndrome and is characterized by a combination of classical signs of allergy as well as disruptions in the brain and nervous system. The syndrome may include any of the following: [7]

Leg, head, tummy, back aches	Irritable, hyperactive, disruptive,
"The allergic face"	impulsive behavior
Nausea, diarrhea, vomiting,	Exhaustion, fatigue, depression
constipation	Speech problems
Loss of bladder control	Incoordination

Nasal difficulties   Sleeping difficulties
Low-grade fever   Learning problems
Ear disorders   Nervousness
Appetite problems
Oversensitivity to stress (such as sound, pain, discipline)

This list is not complete, however, because responses vary from child to child and feelings (such as fears, dysperceptions) are difficult to measure. But the recognition by the orthodox medical community of a link between mind and body will be more firmly established if acceptance of such interactions as the migraine/tension-fatigue syndromes continues to grow.

All Systems Go

As with all the syndromes children usually experience, deficiency/sensitivity/imbalance must be alleviated before results are obtained. An optimal diet that is unique for each child (dictated by what the child will eat and bodily needs) must be established, with special emphasis on those nutrients which help the adrenals handle stress—Vitamin B_6, pantothenic acid, and Vitamin C. All nutrients are needed, however, for *all* interrelate; evening primrose oil, for instance, may stimulate the immune system to handle the stress. Cerebral and classical allergies are often interrelated, but the optimal diet offers a means of overcoming allergy no matter what form it takes.

SIX

Growing Pains

The frustration and anger we express when children don't turn out the way we've planned may take the form of labeling them "bad," "spoiled rotten," "stupid," "just like his father," "hopeless," "good for nothing." We feel we have nurtured them with everything we are capable of giving and have received only disappointment in return. What we are truly feeling is failure and guilt because we are unable to reach a child we love very much while at the same time disliking or possibly even hating the uncontrollable factors the child is demonstrating.

Usually, we foresee problems in our children before they become teenagers, but it is possible for problems to present themselves with the advent of adolescence, when alcohol, drugs, and fast food are readily available and the push for independence is in full swing.

The Search for Feeling Good

When adults don't feel good physically—in other words, their nutritional needs are not being met—they reach for something to make them feel better. Most often it's alcohol, aspirin, Valium, coffee, sugary foods, or cigarettes. For many of us, the search for feeling good is a struggle. Sometimes we're tense and need to be calmed down; at other times we need something stimulating to perk us up. Children suffer from the same stresses and inadequate diets as adults, and they too search for substances to make them feel better (to fulfill their nutritional needs). The substances may take a different form, but the reason for taking them is the same.

Adults find it hard to accept the feel-good substances their children choose, mostly because they fail to recognize their own crutches. When we find a crutch that we believe makes us feel better, it often (though perhaps without our realizing it) becomes addictive. When escaping from the reality of feeling bad becomes the priority over facing problems, stresses, or boredom, it is time to find out if biochemical inadequacy is causing our children —and ourselves—to make this choice.

When the Only Way Up Is Down

Drugs have lent themselves to much experimentation among teenagers. The popularity of pills and pot exploded in the mid-sixties as a counterculture alternative to the establishment escape prop—alcohol. Drugs continue to hold irresistible mysteries for teenagers that can cause them to become caught up in a bizarre and often addictive web.

The beginning of the sweet ride may be curiosity, boredom, kicks, a dare, or the need to feel accepted. Parties, dates, and friends who are into booze or drugs escalate the "just this once to see what it's like" into once a week and then . . . ? Resistance is difficult when "everyone" is doing it; their friends take drugs, and *they* seem perfectly normal.

At first the effects are subtle, but the teenager may soon become more and more dependent on pills that can turn emotions and energy on and off. The tools of the mind-altering trade are extensive. Some bring you up, some bring you down, some mellow you out, some take you far out into the cosmos.

The use of drugs may stem from many causes: They may help cover up a feeling of being unwanted and unloved; they may produce the feeling of being included in something, regardless of whether it is negative; they may offer escape from an unbearable situation; they may make everyday stresses seem to diminish. But the root cause of reaching for drugs may be that the individual *does not feel good* (his nutritional and biochemical needs are unfulfilled, with resulting mental and physical changes such as exhaustion, depression, discontent, and so on) and *seeks to feel better*.

Teenagers often define their reasons for taking drugs as "I don't want to face my problems," "My hurt is too much to deal with," "I don't want to feel anything." Their unhappiness is real, and their antidote for discontent and disillusionment is to drown all feeling, capabilities, and control of themselves by altering the functioning of the brain. It most certainly offers an artificial and temporary feel-good response to a body and mind that are improperly nourished. But in reality, it does not touch upon the true problems that exist—dealing with the stresses of growing up and a nutritionally unfulfilled body and mind. Thus the pleasure-seeking part of the brain (limbic system) may have greater control over decisions than the self-control part of the brain (cortex) as the individual reaches out desperately to find anything that will bring about feeling "better."

TGIF!

In high schools and colleges throughout the country, alcohol and marijuana rank the highest in the celebration of "Thank God it's Friday." The consumption of alcohol by teenagers is on the rise—and goes far beyond Friday nights. Many adults aren't overly concerned about teenage use of alcohol. They are relieved it isn't experimenting with the dangerous items: *drugs*. Besides, it is hard to believe teenagers can become alcoholics (but they *can!*).

The impact alcohol has upon teenagers and ourselves has come about for many reasons, the three most important being that 1) alcohol is so widely accepted, available, and traditionally a part of our lives, 2) our inferior diets, which are highly refined and inadequate in supplying essential nutrients, and 3) genetic enzymatic weaknesses of the liver's ability to handle alcohol. Alcohol abuse is heavily bonded to allergies, blood-sugar abnormalities, and nutritional deficiencies. These problems often entrap victims in the vicious circle of having to drink more alcohol (which is 50 percent sugar) to appease the body's blood-sugar level, which responds by doing figure-8s in an effort to keep up with the turmoil (stimulation of the adrenals to release stored sugar from the liver) the alcohol produces within the body. In addition, most alcoholics are allergic to the very foods alcohol is derived from—barley, rye, yeast, grapes, corn, and so on—and they easily become addicted to alcohol which is a concentrate of these foods. Haven't you ever wondered why one person can "hold his liquor" better than another? The livers of different individuals have varying abilities to handle the consumption of alcohol, which is why alcoholism "runs in families." There is a biochemical link to helping these kids release themselves from the grip of alcoholism.

Every Good Boy Does Fine

In our culture, we expect children to be good, and when they are not we punish them moderately to severely until they conform. But some children are incapable of being good—not because they are stubborn or mean, but because their reasoning brain (the cortex) is not properly nourished, thus is unavailable to contemplate right and wrong. The irritability, sullenness, and flaring temper that mark the "bad" or "deviant" child are very often due to hypoglycemia, allergy, or nutritional deficiency—factors which may also be to blame for accompanying discontent and unhappiness.

"Bad" behavior may be manifested in stealing, cruelty, destructiveness, lying, or fire setting, and when these actions cannot be alleviated, the behavior may worsen into juvenile delinquency and often progress to adult criminal behavior. If the delinquent is caught, punishment is administered, and the fact that punishment has little rehabilitative effect on the majority of offenders is beginning to concern many people, especially now as the cost for containing offenders escalates out of control. It is against almost all odds for a child to improve morally or mentally in such an environment as a detention center or reform school when the diet there is very high in processed foods and doesn't even come close to reaching the requirements for building health. Stress in these institutions is appalling, and this further strains dietary needs.

Research led by Alexander Schauss, Ph.D. (Cand.), on the metabolic and biochemical disturbances of juvenile delinquents and criminals has overwhelmingly confirmed this view.[1] Schauss, director of the American Institute for Biosocial Research in Tacoma, Washington, and the author of the book *Diet, Crime and Delinquency* (Berkeley: Parker House, 1981), has had considerable administrative experience in correctional rehabilitation as well as fifteen years of research into the physiological and environmental factors contributing to deviant behavior. He has found that many offenders have food and environmental hypersensitivities, abnormal blood-sugar levels, nutrient deficiency/imbalances, and neurotoxic substances in their bodies in addition to the common problems of alcoholism and drug misuse. His college course Body Chemistry and Behavior has been attended by more than 20,000 professionals in the fields of mental health, medicine, education, and corrections to implement a variety of physiological and nutritionally oriented treatment options. To break the delinquent/criminal cycle, which Schauss terms "biocriminogenesis," the diet must be altered to fulfill bodily needs. Studies show that metabolic abnormalities[2] are involved in a tremendous number of cases, but as with all behavioral difficulties, there are many pieces to the puzzle. Schauss has also found heavy-metal burdens (especially lead), nutrient deficiencies, insufficient sleep, food sensitivity (especially large milk consumption has been observed in offenders), and fluorescent lighting to be contributing factors to the accepted psychosocial influences involved in criminal behavior.

The most exciting research currently is that of a blind covert series study[3] led by Dr. Stephen Schoenthaler that altered the diets of several thousand juvenile offenders confined in institutions in Virginia, Alabama, and California; the study has provided a strong correlation between diet and antisocial behavior. An improvement in behavior in male juveniles of more than 45 percent was achieved by just the removal of sugary, artificial foods in their diets. Five universities have examined Schoenthaler's findings, and no alternative explanation has been found for this phenomenal reduction in antisocial behaviors. Interestingly, no significant improvement in behavior was observed in female delinquents in this study. My own clinical experience with children who have behavior problems led me in the same direction as I observed that girls had far more complexity of health problems than boys. The removal of sugar often had significant positive effects on a boy's behavior, while a girl's behavior was not altered significantly until other avenues such as allergy were thoroughly explored. Schmidt[4] studied chronic juvenile offenders over a two-year period and found that 88 percent had hypoglycemia (low blood sugar) and 90 percent suffered from food and environmental allergies. The offenders were high in their consumption of milk (especially large quantities of), white bread, sodas, and refined sugar. The elimination of dairy products and refined sugar reduced behavioral fluctuations, hostility, aggressiveness, irritability, and depression.

If we can see this much improvement from the general approach of eliminating sugary, artificial foods and one or two possible allergens, how much more improvement in behavior would we observe with more specific measures such as eliminating more allergens, identifying nutritional deficiencies and imbalances, and so forth?

Probation officers have also had tremendous success in rehabilitating offenders outside institutions by implementing Schauss' ideas. Alexander Schauss continues to make outstanding contributions to the body/mind connection. Now, thanks to his expertise and perseverance, there is hope for the individual who responds in an aggressive manner to biochemical imbalances.

Girls Just Wanna Have Fun

Adolescent girls often become caught in the vicious grip of anorexia (self-induced starvation), bulimia (binge/purge cycle), or a combination of the two as they seek desperately to find their "true" selves. Obviously the emotional need to fit in or better oneself is a motivating factor, but some interesting physical involvements can cause the dieting situation to spiral out of control. First of all, once an individual drastically reduces food intake, she may feel better as a result of the avoidance of refined and/or allergenic foods. Reintroduction of these foods can cause strong negative symptoms (headache, nausea, spaciness, weakness, and so forth). Zinc appears to play a role in dieting complications because of the increased need for it in adolescence and its quick depletion during dieting. A zinc deficiency results in diminished taste sensations; thus food then further loses its appeal to the dieter. To determine zinc status, Bryce-Smith developed a zinc taste test for anorexics and others suffering from possible zinc deficiency.[5] The use of zinc in the treatment of anorexia has been reported in *Lancet*[6,7] to be overwhelmingly positive. Those involved in binge/vomiting tend to gorge on huge quantities of junk foods (cake, cookies, ice cream, and so on) and highly allergenic foods (bread, crackers, peanut butter, milk), only to vomit them up and experience a temporary "high." The search for feeling good is incredibly intense in adolescence as the body's increased nutrient demands go unfulfilled. Thus the lift experienced from vomiting or choosing by starvation not to subject oneself to foods that are not well tolerated can lead to frightening diet disorders.

Before a teenager starts a diet is the best time to seek the help of a professional who can offer guidance on a nutritionally balanced diet. If a dieting problem is already in existence, do not delay helping your teenager find the help she needs. An informed physician can do a complete workup to uncover blood-sugar problems, hidden allergies, and/or nutritional deficiencies that may be causing or contributing to the problem. Small, frequent allergy-free, nutrient-rich meals (six small meals a day) are often helpful, as well as zinc (and other nutrient) supplementation.

Munching Out

Part of the fun of being a teenager is enjoying newfound freedom by staying away from home as much as possible. Hamburgers, french-fries, and shakes take over for the majority of meals, with doughnuts, pizza, soft drinks, ice cream, and candy filling in the remainder of the diet. (And the use of marijuana doesn't help the situation, since it usually brings on an acute case of the munchies which is met with *more* of something sweet.) The refined food teenagers eat contributes to, compounds, and often causes some of the problems they experience such as acne, overweight, irritability, and negative attitudes. The adjustment to adolescence is often rockier than need be, bad enough for most without making it worse with a poor diet. Maybe some day the burger hangout will become the health-hut hangout —but first it will have to become an established chain, since no self-respecting teenager would place a foot in a restaurant that doesn't have an image as *the* place to be as well as a jingle ("Your kind of place") and fast, cheap food.

School Is a Drag

Peer pressure is strong at any age, but adolescence pushes it into action full force. Suddenly what children wear, how they talk, where they go, what they do, even what they eat is governed by what "everyone" is doing, although each will insist he or she is doing his or her own thing. And, of course, it is *essential* above all other things to act cool. Let's face it, it is uncool to whip out raw carrots and spinach to munch on when everyone is eating hamburgers and french-fries. Independence from parents is all-important in adolescence, and to hear ol' Mom nag, nag, nag about one more thing is often intolerable. Trying strong-arm tactics to get a child to eat better never works, and most other attempts draw a loud and disgusted "Aw, Mom!" or "Oh, *Mother!*"

School considerably adds to the problem, since it offers the perfect opportunity to indulge in junk food to the max. Most teenagers take part in the flood of candy, soft drinks, ice cream, cupcakes, and other highly refined foods aimed at them from vending machines and the lunch line where supposedly exist the only foods they will consent to eat. What actually is happening here is that the school is perpetuating teenage addiction to junk food, making available inside *and* outside the lunchroom food that does not nourish. It is true they may eat junk food someplace else anyway during the course of the day, but it is most difficult to help them relearn something after the school has given its stamp of approval.

What we need to do is approach our teenagers from a new angle! Since we have so many forces working against us—peers, advertising, the school, previous eating habits—the only way to reach them is by what they are concerned about: A girl worried about her figure, her grades, or her complexion or a boy worried about his strength, his hair, or his performance on the tennis court or football field is more likely to be receptive to a change in diet. When you get their attention, give them alternatives to their previous eating habits—where they can go for wholesome snacks, what to order if everyone decides to hit McDonald's. They need to know how to make the best of a bad situation. If they do go to a fast-food restaurant, Mexican food offers the best chance of a nutritionally fulfilling meal (tacos, beans, tostadas). If they go for pizza, it is better to eat only the topping of the pizza (especially vegetable toppings) and leave the bottom crust. Some fast-food restaurants offer salad bars, fruit salad, chili, and even baked potatoes (instead of french-fries), which are nutritious. The coating of fried chicken may be peeled off to eliminate the deep-fried white-flour coating. Hamburgers are best eaten with lots of lettuce and tomato while the bun is tossed aside and forgotten, although one popular fast-food chain offers a multigrain bun that is acceptable. Don't forget to offer to supply food for parties and snacks just as you would for younger children. This can be a great way to introduce teenagers to nutritious fun food.

Give your kids some alternatives to what they are doing!

Adolescence is a time of turmoil and stress. For teenagers to deal with these forces effectively, we must ensure that they step toward independence with strong bodies and strong minds which do not fall prey to props that only simulate feeling good.

Feeling Fine

Often we don't realize just how bad we feel until we are properly nourished and see the difference in the way we then feel for ourselves. Nutritional needs skyrocket at the advent of adolescence, requiring the teenager to consume an extremely well-balanced diet. When these expanded nutritional needs are not fulfilled, the teenager can fall prey to addictive substances in the futile attempt to feel better. As the body loosens its hold on the need for pills, alcohol, pot, sugar, chocolate, and the like, it becomes apparent that body and brain have been missing something and have been trying to compensate with stimulants and depressants in the search to feel good. When feeling good naturally really takes over, the missing pieces are supplied and put into place so that this state of ill health is replaced with truly feeling fine.

SEVEN

Night Moves

The reality of being a parent always strikes hardest at 3 A.M. when your child wakes up crying. Such moments may be a rarity for some, but for many it is a nightly occurrence. There *are* parents who use sweet reason and calming words to handle night cries, and there are those who resort to "Be quiet or I'll smack you" logic. Either way, the problem is not resolved if it continues night after night. No amount of screaming or reasoning can help when the problem lies in what the child is eating—or not eating.

Turning Out the Light

Simply getting your child into bed may leave you torn and frustrated. It is so easy for some children: They receive the inevitable glass of water, then the story, and finally the kiss good-night. But if the child spills water, wiggles through the story, and refuses to let you turn out the light, you are faced with a difficult situation. Finding a quick avenue of escape may be futile if the child kicks, screams, or in some other charming way refuses to go to sleep.

The storm will prevail until a snap decision is made on your part whether you should spank or reason, but let's face it—either way you lose. If you spank, the child will scream for an hour until he finally wears down enough to sleep, and if you reason, the wheeling and dealing involved ends up making you feel inadequate, angry, guilty, or all of the above. Then, to top it all off, you may sit down to hate stares from your spouse.

Exhaustion Takes Over

The child who is unable to relax does not calmly drift off to sleep but drops from utter exhaustion. This moment of repose, when all is calm, may be a good time for rationalizing and sorting out what has happened. Was it your fault? Your reactions have an effect on the severity of children's behavior, but what caused the child to act so strongly in the first place?

A stressful situation during the day may be a factor in the child's inability to relax at night, but the body's inability to handle the stress is the root of the problem. Stress may originate as an emotional upset, but it is quite often accompanied by a drop in blood sugar (or other blood-sugar abnormalities), an allergic reaction, a lack of essential nutrients, or any combination of these.

Sadly for some children, their problems at night do not end here. Sleeping as a result of exhaustion often gives way to the struggle of staying asleep; thus we move on to . . .

Night Cries

Difficulties in sleeping usually show up early in childhood. A child with recurrent sleeping problems may awaken once or intermittently throughout the night. There are lots of ways the little buggers like to awaken us, but the most frequent approaches are:

"Mommmm-e-e-e-e-!"
A tickling of the toes. Yours.
Noises as the child roams about the house.
A piercing scream or hysterical crying (take your pick).
Wheezing, coughing, sneezing, or (heaven forbid) vomiting.

The excuses for waking us are always the same:

"I'm so-o-o hungry!"
"Can I sleep with you?"
"I need a glass of water."
"A monster grabbed me!"
"I have to go to the bathroom."
"I didn't make it to the bathroom."
"Mom, I threw up."

These requests can usually be handled with some degree of patience. But the screaming that won't stop, the refusal to return to sleep, hyperactive or terrified behavior, bed-wetting, and night tantrums are unnerving because you are at a loss as to how to handle these situations.

In night tantrums (a frequent problem) the child is half in and half out of sleep, thus is not conscious enough to respond to comfort, and in fact, may fight it vehemently. Amid screams and crying, you are dealing not with a rational child but with a child whose brain is not functioning properly (the emotional brain is in full charge), most probably owing to a drop in blood sugar, a lack of some vital nutrient, or an allergic (withdrawal) reaction.

What is going on during these night cries is similar to what happens during the day to a child with a brain sensitivity. The waking response may be anything from nausea to daytime tantrums, but during sleep the brain continues to dysfunction and respond as it did during the day. Allergies that have manifested themselves as addictive may cause a child to awaken in the middle of the night from withdrawal symptoms produced when food is not eaten frequently. This in turn may bring about fluctuations in the blood-sugar level, although a drop in blood sugar may occur without allergic withdrawal symptoms.

Fluctuation in the blood-sugar level is one of the most frequent causes of sleep disturbance. With a fall in blood sugar, the body desperately tries to balance itself by pouring forth adrenaline, which in turn stimulates the liver to release stored sugar. The release of adrenaline, however, brings about disturbances in sleep just as it does during the waking hours with the "fight or flight" response. Dr. Lendon Smith describes this condition in his book *Improving Your Child's Behavior Chemistry:*

> Everyone secretes adrenaline in response to fear, anger, or tension. In the dream state the fear, anger, or tension may be the *result* of adrenaline secretion. The dream may not be as bad as the feeling accompanying it. This would produce the manifestations of fear that the parents observe: dilated pupils, rapid heartbeat, sweaty palms, and readiness for flight.

Not every night cry is the result of a drop in blood-sugar level or addictive withdrawal symptoms or nutritional deficiency. Emotional trauma may be involved in sleeping problems; but when a child's abnormal sleeping patterns cannot be attributed to anything in the life situation, one should explore the nutritional/allergic connection. Nightmares do occur as a result of emotional stress, but responses of overreactive, sensitive children are more than just nightmares. They are frightening, reoccurring responses that are simply an extension of what goes on during the day.

The Morning After

The demand for food "right now!" by children in the middle of the night may be followed, surprisingly, by a refusal to eat breakfast. This phenomenon often is due to the body's needing a constant energy source (glucose) to function. In the absence of glucose, fat will be burned instead. This process is termed keto acidosis and may result in nausea, headache, irritability, and sometimes vomiting which, of course, depresses the appetite. Sugary foods before bedtime often set the child up for this no-breakfast acidosis cycle, since the blood sugar drops (causing depressed glucose levels) and food is not eaten again for a prolonged period of time.

Bed Food

Munching on food before bed is a common practice in many homes, including ours. What is offered children, however, is of vital importance in preventing night moves. The traditional bed food is usually a carbohydrate one:

cocoa and cookies	chips and cola
sugared cereal and milk	bread and jam
ice cream and chocolate syrup	popcorn and Kool-Aid

Refined sugary-starchy bed food has an overwhelming effect on how a child sleeps at night or whether sleep arrives before midnight. A refined-carbohydrate overload (and the threshold is unique to each child) brings on a drop in the blood-sugar level, which in turn releases adrenal hormones as the body struggles to balance itself. Sensitive children react with their usual hyperactive response, and parents are faced with some pretty wild nights.

Night cries also may be caused by the ingestion of a particular food to which the child is addicted (and thus sensitive), and when it isn't eaten in time to keep up the addictive cycle, the blood sugar may likewise drop, bringing on the allergic response.

Often, the older child learns to simply get up and eat in the middle of the night when his blood-sugar level falls below normal, but most young children are usually unable to wake up soon enough or completely enough to say what their body urgently needs. In this state the child responds with crying, screaming, moaning, and the like.

Bed food needs to be in the form of high-quality protein along with a generous amount of vitamins and minerals so that a restful sleep can be assured. Nutritional yeast meets these requirements superbly (unless your child is sensitive to yeast, and in that case there are replacement supplements) and can be used in a milkshake or in such goodies as gingerbread or cupcakes (see recipes).

The addition of fat (preferably an unrefined oil) to the protein accomplishes two things: first, it slows down the absorption of the natural carbohydrates used and helps keep the blood sugar stable, and secondly, the fat aids in the absorption of fat-soluble vitamins.

The child with an extremely low tolerance for any type of carbohydrate or severe food allergies should be fed primarily simple protein foods such as nuts, seeds, chicken, and so on along with raw vegetables (avocado, broccoli, celery, and the like) and natural dip. Should your child prove allergic to milk or yeast, chewable multi-minerals may be used along with high-protein foods. Bed foods can still be fun foods, but the ingredients must be chosen with care.

The Soggy Bed

For some, the reality of the soggy bed is a highly emotional issue. Besides the stigma of shame associated with it, the continual washing of sheets and blankets can be a never-ending chore. Various methods have been used in attempts to alleviate the problem: spanking, restricting fluids before bedtime, a trip to the psychologist, yelling, embarrassing the child in front of others, making the child wash the wet sheets, putting diapers on the child, and getting the child up at night. All without much success.

Dr. William Crook, a pediatric allergist, has linked many cases of bed-wetting to allergy. He explains that eating allergenic foods may cause spasms in the bladder muscle, so that the ability to hold urine is severely diminished and bed-wetting results. A proper choice of bed food with special emphasis on the nutrients magnesium and Vitamin B_6 (which help the bladder muscle function normally) is needed, as well as a search for food sensitivities.

For little ones, it is important to determine that they are physically capable of being toilet-trained by waiting until they can stay dry for a few hours at a time. With a belief that it was best to withhold training until the time was right, Sheilah did not push her son Zachary into bathroom warfare until, by circumstance, the heat of summer one day forced him to remove his diaper. Nudity at the pool did not bother his mother, but urinating did, so she escorted him to the toilet earlier than intended. Twenty-four months is not especially early to begin training, but Sheilah was determined not to force her child until he was physically ready.

Obviously Zach was ready, for one week later he was a graduate—taking himself to the toilet. Since that time, on only one occasion has he ever wet the bed: the evening some relatives gave him some cola and sugary dessert before Sheilah was aware of what he was eating. Being only 29 months old at the time, Zach was not always asking whether foods had sugar in them or not. Thus we can all learn that:

1) Children need prompting about acceptable foods until they are old enough to make the right choices. The child needs to learn to be concerned and responsible for his or her own diet. This can be done at a surprisingly young age.
2) The ingestion of refined carbohydrates can bring about a drop in blood-sugar level which can affect the body in many ways, including loss of urinary control.

If your child is not physically ready for toilet training, please do not force the issue. If the child is trained during the day yet continues to wet at night, check the diet carefully, and use nutritious foods (especially those rich in magnesium and Vitamin B_6) for all meals including bed food.

Bed-wetting has been known to continue through puberty, especially in adolescent boys who manifest hyperactivity and/or learning disabilities, if not addressed through diet and nutrient therapy. This is not a signal to use shaming or threats, but a very important message from the body that something is wrong and must be taken care of.

A Good Good-Night

Enjoying bedtime is impossible for many children and their parents, but it need not be this way. Yelling and even reasoning don't contribute much to solving the problem, but proper nourishment of the body can and *does*.

Food to which a child is allergic can evoke a response that involves loss of urinary control. Nutrient deficiency also plays a role, especially deficiencies of magnesium and pyridoxine. If night cries are to be quieted, it is crucial that we understand what the problem is and do something about it.

Bedtime is a time for a story, a glass of water, and a kiss good-night—but don't forget the vital nutrients!

EIGHT

Silent Screams

I t may seem unusual to discuss learning disabilities and emotional disturbances in the same chapter and equate these two seemingly different disorders. But both involve dysfunctions of the brain, often caused or complicated by biochemical imbalances within the body. The impact of schizophrenia is far more intense than that of learning disorders, but the effect upon children in either case often leaves them unable to explain what is wrong—their screams for help turn inward and are silent. The realization that many of these children are reacting to psychochemical and not psychological stimuli has come slowly, but the beginning of an understanding of psychochemical responses has arrived with the advent of orthomolecular (nutritional) medicine.

The "Emotionally Disturbed" Deception

Treatment of emotional disorders once was solely limited to the use of drugs and behavioral and talk therapy. It was (and largely still is) thought that these measures would change the emotional well-being of patients, since it was believed the problems originated from faulty environment. This theory often pointed an accusing finger at parents, who were said to be negligent in nurturing their children. The guilt produced by this supposedly conscious (or unconscious) rejection of the child is heart-wrenching, since the parent searches desperately to learn what he or she has done to produce such a devastating effect upon the child.

The most disturbing component of this guilt-based belief is that it continues to hold its own as *the* explanation for mental illness. Though environment may well be a contributing factor in triggering an emotional crisis, and in some instances may be a major part of the problem, to use it to account for all emotional illness is a grave mistake.

We have only to look in the back wards of our mental institutions to see the tragic failures resulting from mishandling of mental illness. My own visit to a children's ward in a state mental institution is one I will never forget. As I entered the ward, there before me sat a small child, his head hanging. The aura of pain and hoplessness surrounding him was so over-powering I felt I must first comfort him before attempting to find a bio-chemical involvement. But how do you comfort someone whose mind is so clouded with drugs it is virtually impossible to get to the real person?

Turning children into zombies is *not* the answer to reaching them—it only drives them further away. The mistaken idea that mind and body have no biochemical connection has become riveted in the minds of many psychologists and psychiatrists. But as more and more failures of standard-treatment procedures are compiled, the more daring doctors are looking toward a new approach based on the overlooked link between body and mind.

Into the Realm of Depression

Delving into the biological dysfunction of mental illness, researchers have struggled to provide the essential nutrients required to allow the brain and nervous system to function at peak efficiency; but of course, for this to be established the body must also be at optimal performance. Dr. Linus Pauling, the originator of the term "orthomolecular psychiatry," describes this approach as

A treatment of illness by the provision of the optimum molecular composition of the brain, especially the optimum concentration of substances normally present in the human body.[1]

The mind does not respond in a simple way, nor does dysfunction have a simple explanation. Thus schizophrenia, one of the most disturbing mental illnesses, is more appropriate in the plural form—schizophrenia*s*. These are prime examples of psychochemical mental illnesses, as there is conclusive evidence that altered function expresses an alteration in biochemical relationships between the interacting body and mind. Attempting to find the right molecules is not an easy task when we realize there is a diversity of symptoms and causes unique to each individual.

The starting point for treating mental illness biochemically was the pioneering work of Dr. Abram Hoffer and Dr. Humphrey Osmond, who administered niacin to schizophrenic patients. Niacin proved useful (and continues to be) in alleviating emotional responses, and the individual uniqueness factor caused many researchers to try other avenues of the biochemical connection.

As more and more research was conducted, it was discovered that schizophrenias had a tendency to fall into distinct patterns. Some of the most intense work has been performed at the Brain Bio Center in Princeton, New Jersey, and their findings to date point to five major categories or combinations of categories as factors in schizophrenias:

1) Blood-sugar abnormalities
2) Cerebral allergy (and therefore nutritional deficiencies)

3) Low blood-histamine level (histapenia)
4) High blood-histamine level (histadelia)
5) Pyroluria or malvaria due to the urinary mauve factor, kryptopyrrole.[2]

Dr. Carl Pfeiffer, the Brain Bio Center's director, names 23 possible combinations for these biochemical imbalances and estimates they account for 95 percent of the schizophrenias.[3]

The connection of hypoglycemia and cerebral allergy to schizophrenias is not surprising. It has been previously noted in this book how severely the brain's function is altered (impaired) when allergens are introduced into the body and when dramatic fluctuations in blood sugar occur. Dr. William Philpott and Dr. Marshall Mandell, conducting research at Fuller Memorial Sanitarium in Massachusetts, found that 90 percent of the patients had a significant degree of cerebral (brain) allergy.[4] The late Dr. Harry Salzer, a Cincinnati, Ohio, psychiatrist, found that hypoglycemia *unquestionably* is an important cause in an estimated 40 percent of neuropsychiatric illnesses. More recently, the Brain Bio Center reported hypoglycemia was involved in 60 percent of schizophrenias.[5] We know that blood-sugar abnormalities, metabolic errors, nutritional deficiencies, digestive dysfunction, and cerebral allergies are closely intertwined in their action upon the brain and may even evoke a schizophrenic condition. Thus one cause is not always the answer; a combination of causes may easily develop.

One of the ways in which a biochemical imbalance may be involved in causing a schizophrenic condition is through dysregulation of the histamine level in the brain. Histamine is a biochemical which is normally present in all soft tissues in the body and can be made, by the removal of an acid group, from the amino acid histidine. Dr. Pfeiffer believes that histamine is released in the brain from the bloodstream and is involved in the transmission of neuronal (brain-cell) impulses. The indication that imbalances of the histamine level were a factor in schizophrenias came about when analysis of the blood of schizophrenic patients revealed abnormally high and low levels of histamine in two-thirds of the patients.[6] (Remember that these five major imbalances overlap.) Normal levels of histamine would occur when the illness had been arrested.[7,8] Dr. Pfeiffer, a leader in the search for answers to schizophrenias, states that "the biochemical leads now appear to be with the storage of histamine and the use of histamine as a neurotransmitter in the brain."[9]

Because it is believed the level of histamine in the blood is a reflection of the level of histamine in the brain, the blood-histamine level may be used as a key to treatment.

The patient with low blood histamine is classified as histapenic, and this imbalance is estimated to occur in 50 percent of schizophrenias. Histapenia is characterized by severe dysperceptions, paranoia, and hallucinations. The patient tends to be overstimulated and may manifest hyperactivity and sleeping difficulties.[10] Histadelia, high blood histamine, has resemblances to histapenia in the *degree* of thought disorder and overarousal suffered by both types of patients. But the histapenic is disturbed by hallucinations and paranoia, while the histadelic is plagued with suicidal depression, compulsive-obsessive behavior, high pain sense, headaches, dysperceptions (but not accompanied by paranoia), and loss of contact with reality (but with a blank mind rather than hallucinations.)[10] Histadelia is estimated to occur in 20 percent of the schizophrenias.

Dr. Pfeiffer found that the remaining 30 percent of the schizophrenics had a condition called pyroluria, which depleted their bodies of zinc and Vitamin B_6. This condition is detected by something called the mauve factor, which is a discoloration of the urine caused by the excretion of pyrroles. The depletion of zinc and B_6 in this condition is believed to bring about many of the classic symptoms of schizophrenics (dysperceptions, depression) as well as other characteristic signs and symptoms—morning nausea, white spots on nails, inability to tan, itching in sunlight, constipation, china-doll complexion, muscle spasms, shaking, inability to remember dreams, unexplained fever, hypoglycemia, irregular menstrual periods, malformation of knee cartilage, the characteristic smell of schizophrenics, and a distinctive, sweetish breath odor.[11]

The Brain Bio Center has extensively and successfully treated these biochemical imbalances with nutrient therapy. Its approach is to improve the diet and to supplement it with those nutrients needed in large amounts to alleviate the patient's individual problems. In therapy with histapenic patients, the Bio Brain Center elevates the level of histamine available to the brain by supplying supplemental niacin, folic acid, Vitamin B_{12}, pantothenic acid, zinc, manganese, and Vitamin C. By lowering the level of the copper-containing enzymes that were destroying histamine, the use of these supplements reestablishes histamine in the blood and tissues and thus appears to eliminate the problems in the brain chemistry. In the case of histadelic patients, calcium, methionine (an amino acid), zinc, and manganese are administered to depress the histamine level. The patient with pyroluria is treated with B_6 zinc, and Vitamin E. The Brain Bio Center has had tremendous successes, but it does not have all the answers to the phenomenon of the schizophrenias. As other biochemical imbalances and metabolic errors come to light, it relies on the belief that "adequate nutrition for prevention is the best medicine."[12]

More recently, William Philpott, M.D. (Philpott Bio-Ecologic Medical Center, St. Petersburg, Florida), has opened up new therapies[13] in resolving the schizophrenias, as well as many other disorders. Philpott, a brilliant physician, performs a comprehensive assessment (chemical sensitivity, bioecologic allergy, infectious sensitivity, nutritional-medical evaluation) to determine inbalances, deficiencies, sensitivities (inhalant, food, chemical) and metabolic errors that are causing the individual condition. New information concerning schizophrenia and disturbed essential fatty acid[14,15] and amino acid metabolism has led Philpott (and many other orthomolecular physicians) to begin testing for these phenomena. Imbalances in fatty acid metabolism, caused or aggravated by dramatic changes in the types of fat (trans, or man-made, fats such as margarine) consumed in the American diet, can be corrected by a balancing of essential fatty acids in the diet and supplying of appropriate supplemental nutrients. The brain is predominantly lipid, and specific fatty acid requirements must be met by the diet for normal brain function.[16,17] The results of Philpott's program on mental and physical disorders are astonishingly positive because he believes (like all orthomolecular physicians) in searching for the root cause of a patient's problems and solving it.

Lost in a World of Their Own

Autism is hallmarked by isolation and withdrawal, thus is often termed the aloneness syndrome. It usually is apparent before age two, afflicts more boys than girls, and occurs in one in every 2,500 children. Autistic children portray a profound inability to relate to other people [18] along with varied symptoms such as prolonged rocking, lack of interest in surroundings, head banging, odd responses to strangers, obsessive interest in certain toys or mechanical appliances, unusual lack of fear, repetitive ritualistic behavior, abnormal perceptual responses, and the need to preserve sameness in the environment.

Speech is often absent; or when it is used the child is usually unable to employ it as a means of communication; instead, it occurs as mirror speech —"Are you hungry?" may be answered with "Are you hungry?" or simply "Hungry?"

Diagnosis of autism is often obscure, since to measure the function or dysfunction of the mind is often beyond our grasp. Thus, autistic children may be labeled retarded, schizophrenic, deaf, or learning-disabled, among other things. When the ability to comprehend and communicate is severed it is difficult to establish cause and effect. And since the autistic child portrays uneven abilities and behavior patterns, there are indications in a large percentage of cases that dysfunction rather than permanent damage is involved. For instance, the child may appear not to hear certain sounds, but may respond to those sounds at another time.

In his book *Psycho-Nutrition* (New York: Grosset and Dunlap, 1976) Dr. Carlton Fredericks describes other symptoms of autistic children that "bespeak a twisting of reality": their poor balance, frequent falling, walking in zigzag fashion, bumping into objects, walking on tiptoe while peering anxiously at the floor; and that they have "strange aberrations in perception of time, space, depth, vision, hearing, and their images of their own bodies" such as "lifting his foot very high when stepping from the bare floor to a carpeted area, as though he perceived the carpet as being a foot high."

Research at Yale, led by Dr. Donald J. Cohan, has indicated that answers to autism lie in the imbalance of neurotransmitters (between-nerve-cell communicators) within the brain. Since brain scans (as well as other tests) reveal no brain injury in many autistic children and parental blame has been ruled out, the researchers at Yale philosophically describe autism as both a biological and a psychological disease.

Researchers at the U.C.L.A. Medical Center have found that some autistic children have elevated levels in the brain of the neurotransmitter serotonin. Their approach was to lower the serotonin level with the drug fenfluramine. The autistic children in the study did show some improvement in I.Q. levels and language skill; however, the children were also in a new therapeutic environment during the study.

Further testing[19] of fenfluramine on 200 children in twenty-one centers across the country was then undertaken in a double-blind fashion and is still in progress. However, some weaknesses appear in this study:

1) Dietary tryptophan, niacin, and pyridoxine (B₆) levels are not being measured, all of which have an impact on serotonin levels.
2) The drug may have side effects of lethargy, loss of balance, insomnia, loss of appetite, and regression.
3) The cause of the elevated or altered serotonin levels is not being examined. Administration of fenfluramine at best may only suppress—not solve—the autistic phenomenon.

Preliminary results of the study have not been what the researchers had hoped for. They did not find significant improvements in behavior. One child in the study was a patient of mine whose behavior deteriorated sharply while she was on fenfluramine and improved while off the drug.

Research at Stanford has also indicated that some autistics may have an autoimmune response (an attack by the body against its own tissues) in which antibodies against serotonin receptors are present in the brain. Thus this response would "short-circuit" the availability of serotonin.

Another interesting area of research is that of infection with the intestinal fungus *Candida albicans* whereby the toxin (acetaldehyde) released by the fungus into the bloodstream may unite with neurotransmitters to form false neurotransmitters termed tetrahydroisoquinlins (TIQ). The story of an autistic six-year-old, Duffy Mayo, suffering from *Candida albicans* infection received quite a bit of media coverage in San Francisco when treatment for the infection resulted in disappearance of his autistic symptoms. Cecil Bradley, M.D., is presently working with autistic children who have *Candida albicans* infection, and although he has seen no "cures," he has seen some dramatic improvement in behavior.[20]

There is an answer for autism, but it does not lie in drugs or the standard bribery treatment ("behavior modification") with M&Ms candy.

These researchers have taken a giant step toward equating autism with dysfunction of the brain; but why not go a step further and ask why this imbalance exists and, more important, what is to be done about it? Must the course of action be the same for dysfunction as it is for injury? Something must be causing the dysfunction, and treating the autistic child with drugs or shoving the child into a mold with behavior modification will not wipe away the problem.

Autism, like schizophrenias, does not have a single cause or a single remedy, which is why it is so difficult to pinpoint the problem(s). Because injury to the brain *may* be present in some cases of autism, the approach to dealing with it may need to be altered somewhat from that of dysfunction.

A nationwide study[21] by Dr. Bernard Rimland, director of the Child Behavior Institute in San Diego, demonstrated that well over 50 percent of the autistic children improved significantly in behavioral responses with the use of large doses of five nutrients—Vitamin B$_6$ (pyridoxine), Vitamin C, niacinamide, pantothenic acid, and magnesium. But when we realize that in many instances the basic diet remained unchanged, cerebral (brain) allergies were not taken into account, errors in metabolism were not studied, and only a few nutrients were used in the study, it is quite possible that a combined investigation of all these factors may yield even more improvement or complete absence of symptoms.

The Brain Bio Center in New Jersey has found the accumulation of heavy metals to be an important factor in autism, as may occur in hyperactivity. Dr. Carl Pfeiffer, the Center's director, writes in *Zinc and Other Micro-Nutrients* that a deficiency of zinc may render direct vision painful for the autistic child, which may be why direct eye contact is often shunned. Concentrations of lead and copper also are believed to be major factors of autism, since studies indicate that characteristic symptoms include perceptual and behavioral dysfunction.[22] Many doctors have reported beneficial results from the use of d,d,dimethylglycine in stimulating speech in autistic children, while others have found Vitamin C, niacinamide, pantothenic acid, B$_6$, magnesium, and the amino acid cystine (and other amino acids) to be effective in helping some autistic children.

The effects of particular foods on an eight-year-old autistic boy were studied by O'Banion,[23] who found a direct correlation between particular foods consumed and levels of hyperactivity, uncontrolled laughter, and disruptive behaviors.

As a consultant for the Kaplan Foundation, a residential school for children with autism in Orangevale, California, I set up a nutrition program that implements the approaches found within this book. Wholesome foods, elimination of allergenic foods, rotation diet, supplementation, and environmental control have proved to be important factors in helping to improve the behavior of these children. The school's director, Karen Kaplan Fitzgerald, has done a phenomenal job of reaching these children with a diverse range of modalities in addition to the nutrition program. Children often enter the school in a sad state: screaming, crying, no bladder control, severe aggression, hyperactivity, and so on. The transformation is breathtaking to me when I observe these same children a few months later—calm, more aware, more responsive, and toilet-trained. These children are often heavily medicated with Mellaril and Thorazine when they enter the school, and slowly but steadily these are eliminated entirely. The Kaplan Foundation gets rewarding results with these children without drugs. It is the opinion of the director that without the nutritional program this would not be feasible. She also reports that with the nutrition program their attention skills, attitudes, behavior, and self-concepts improve.

One child in particular was extremely allergic and upon the ingestion of particular foods would fly into a rage and tear at her skin. With the elimination of these foods the outbursts almost disappeared completely; their reintroduction into her diet provoked these outbursts once again. The same child was taken off supplements temporarily and within the first week there was severe regression—her outbursts increased sharply, she cried and began to constantly suck her thumb, she tore at her feet and hands, she was uncoordinated (would fall out of chairs) and laughed inappropriately. With the reintroduction of supplements these symptoms faded away. Another child was completely out of control when he entered the school. He was so destructive that he would literally "tear the house apart." Milk was isolated as a triggering factor in this child's aggression. Amazing, isn't it? Milk! His parents could not believe the difference in their now calm, happy child. The Kaplan Foundation is the only facility in the country at the present time to follow through with such intensity and dedication in helping children with autism.[24]

Autism has many aspects; the total answer is not with one nutrient or a select few. Dr. William Philpott[25] and Dr. Alan Cott have treated many autistic children. Many improve and a few are symptom-free in response to the combined efforts of eliminating allergens, supplying all essential nutrients, improving digestion, controlling metabolic errors, and helping the child adhere to a nutritious diet. Any disorder children have *must* be approached wholly. To try one vitamin or to eliminate one allergen may lead to failure in the child's complete response, which in turn may cause parents to become disillusioned with the orthomolecular approach. Autsim must be observed from all angles if we are to find the pieces of the puzzle for each unique child.

The Upside-Down Perception

A learning disability causes difficulty in listening, talking, reading, writing, spelling, or arithmetic[26] through subtle nervous-system dysfunction. Learning difficulties often occur simultaneously with hyperactivity and are termed minimal brain dysfunction, whereas a learning disability that is not accompanied by hyperactivity is called a specific learning disability. Whether the child's brain is dysfunctioning as a result of allergy, imbalance, or nutritional deficiency or has sustained injury is a problem of great complexity. The mind is an elusive organ, one that is difficult to effectively evaluate. This is especially true with children because they are often unable to describe, fearfully silent, or unaware of their learning disability.

The degree of the child's learning problem may fluctuate in intensity or remain fixed at a certain level, but first we must eliminate allergens and correct the deficiencies and imbalances.[27,28,29] A controlled double-blind study by Kershner and Hawke[30] demonstrated dramatic changes in learning-disabled children placed on a high-protein/no-sugar diet. Dr. Marshall Mandell relates in *Dr. Mandell's 5-Day Allergy Relief System* that most of the children diagnosed as having learning disabilities were "suffering from reversible allergic and nutritional disorders whose causes can be identified and eliminated or controlled."

Mandell and others have found that the variable intensities of learning problems may be expressed through such visual evidence as deterioration of handwriting and spelling during testing for cerebral allergy. Clear, legible writing may become scribbled and inconsistent and manifest omission or reversal of letters with the testing of various foods.[31]

The current theory is that children with learning disabilities have experienced minimal brain injury or were genetically predisposed to learning difficulties, both conditions considered to be permanent. Injury and heredity surely are involved in some cases of learning disability, but impressive evidence exists that dysfunction is due to allergy, deficiency, or imbalances. A combination of causes—brain injury and brain dysfunction—may also occur. Evidence indicates that the brain-injured child may be greatly improved through a combined effort of superior nutrition and patterning.[32]

When techniques are employed to eliminate allergens from the diet, we may see fixed learning responses reappear with the reintroduction of allergens. Handwriting is, of course, only one of a multitude of aspects of disabilities, just as allergens are only one facet of the orthomolecular approach. Powers[33] examined the effects of dietary factors on children classified as learning-disabled and found that their conditions aggravated by diets high in sugary, processed foods which triggered unstable blood-sugar levels. Improvement in both behavior and achievement was observed with the elimination of refined foods. The learning-disabled child often suffers from nutritional deficiencies intertwined with unstable blood-sugar levels and cerebral allergy. In *Psycho-Nutrition* (New York: Grosset and Dunlap, 1976), Dr. Carlton Fredericks cites an example of deficiency in which "the delusion of moving letters and numbers is a common symptom of an unsatisfied need for niacin (and other nutrients)." Even chronic iron deficiency has been shown to cause impairment of cognitive function and memory, apathy, low responsiveness, and functional hyperactivity in young children.[34,35,36,37]

We have much more to learn about the effects of specific nutrients on learning, but we have made a tremendous start in the right direction when we look toward what the body and brain require to function optimally, not toward a drug to repress symptoms or an excuse to wish them away. Certainly the place to begin is revising the diet to include a wide variety of whole foods and general supplementation with a multivitamin, multi-mineral tablet. If success is not complete, then that is the time to explore a child's specific biochemical needs with a physician concerned about the cause of the child's problems.

Light at the End of the Tunnel

Mental disorders may have many different root causes: cerebral allergy to foods, chemicals, and/or inhalants, *Candida albicans* infection, heavy-metal toxicity (especially that of copper, lead, cadmium), nutrient insufficiencies and imbalances, blood-sugar abnormalities, elevated nutrient needs for particular nutrients like zinc, pyridoxine, or niacinamide (to name a few), digestive difficulties, disturbed essential fatty acid and amino acid metabolism, and even diets that fail to offer a borderline level of commonly known nutrients like iron. All of these can play critical roles in mental health and the function of the brain.

Once we sat back and helplessly watched while our children struggled to escape the effects of the "hungry mind." No longer. Instead of wishing the child to grow out of the problem, or smothering the problem with drugs, or using guilt as a basis for therapy or special teaching to try to force the brain to work differently, we can now approach the disorder from a completely new direction: the cause.

PART II

Discovering

No longer can we be content merely to treat symptoms. We must direct our attention towards the prevention and treatment of degenerative disease by studying and using those substances that normally occur in the human body. Then and only then will we be able to understand the total disease process.

DR. WILLIAM PHILPOTT

NINE

The Biochemical Clues

Pursuing the reasons behind children's mind/body difficulties involves the piecing together of many clues which should converge to form the answers. Some clues are obscure and require close attention to minute details; others are quite obvious although they may never have been interpreted nutritionally. These clues need to be examined at different angles with respect to interrelationships of cause—are they of nutrient, ecologic (allergenic or environmental), or of injury origin?

Ideally, the search begins with a thorough evaluation of the child so that the possibility of such problems as anemia, parasites, visual/hearing impairment, or infection may be ruled out. Neurological and intelligence tests also may be performed as indicated. Depending on the severity of the child's difficulties, help may be needed from an orthomolecular physician —a nutritionally oriented doctor—to evaluate the child's nutritional status.

Orthomolecular medicine grasps the entirety of prevention and treatment of illness by providing and balancing the natural constituents of the body ("the right molecules") rather than introducing foreign chemicals (drugs) into the body. Drugs act as alien chemicals, which mask symptoms rather than eliminate them, alter the chemistry of cells rather than support or nourish them, and often precipitate side effects far more severe than the original symptom. In crisis intervention, drugs are often necessary and crucial to helping the patient, but they are by no means a panacea.

Orthomolecular medicine is respectful that each person is biochemically unique and has a wide variance of nutritional requirements. Thus orthomolecular physicians resolve their patients' symptoms by fulfilling these unique needs and in doing so uncover the true cause of the disorder. To determine the cause or contributing factors, various laboratory and diagnostic testing may be used, such as:

Amino acid assay—to search for metabolic errors in amino acid patterns that are disturbing the mental and physical health of the patient

Membrane lipid analysis and essential fatty acid profile—to search for errors in fatty acid metabolism that also may be disturbing the mental and physical health of the patient

Blood analysis—whole-blood vitamin panel (protazol or erythrocyte), broad-spectrum chemistry screen

Immune competency testing—immune testing for T and B cells, immunoglobulins, complements, immune complexes, null cells, PGF_2A, and T helper/suppressor ratios, which offer information regarding the strengths and weaknesses of the patient's immune system

Glucose-tolerance test and insulin levels—blood-sugar/insulin evaluation

Hair analysis—to screen for the presence of heavy (toxic) metals and mineral imbalances

Heidelberg gastrogram—for an assessment of gastrointestinal function

Hormone evaluations—to check for endocrine dysfunction

Cytoscan—intracellular mineral evaluation to measure mineral deficiencies or imbalances on cellular level

Lactose-tolerance test—to test for an individual's ability to handle milk sugar (lactose)

Infectious assessment—to determine if *Candida albicans* or other fungi or bacteria are interfering with the health of the individual through infection

Enzyme studies—erythrocyte transketolase, erythrocyte glutathione reductase, and so on for coenzyme activities

Urinalysis—for evidence of the mauve factor indicating pyroluria, glucose, ketones, and other abnormalities

These and other indicated tests, as well as a comprehensive history and physical examination, enable the physician to determine the cause of abnormal responses and symptoms a child is portraying. For example, the glucose-tolerance test (GTT) is used when a blood-sugar problem is suspected. This test involves the recording of the body's ability to handle glucose, beginning with a fasting blood-sugar level (the usual procedure is for the patient to fast after dinner and on the following morning so that the test begins on a fasting blood-sugar level), the ingestion of glucose, and the measuring (from blood specimens) of the blood-sugar level at half-hour intervals. The glucose solution (which may consist of refined sugar or fruit juices and honey) offers evidence of the patient's ability to handle the stress of the glucose in relation to the release of insulin and therefore the responding blood-sugar level. Problems in evaluation of the GTT may develop, however, because:

1) Some patients do not show abnormal blood-sugar fluctuations until the fourth or later hour, and the test often is discontinued before abnormalities appear.

2) The blood sugar may be measured at hourly rather than half-hour intervals, and thus declines (and other deviations) may be missed.

3) Some patients exhibit strong reactions (dizziness, convulsions, crying, mood swings, trembling, cold sweats, fainting) but fail to show abnormal blood-sugar curves; when this occurs, different glucose derivatives (other than corn) should be tried.

4) The botanical source of sugar must be considered during a GTT, because an allergy to a particular food brings on a variety of blood-sugar responses; glucose derived from corn is the standard used in this test, but different foods produce varied results if the patient is sensitive to them.

5) A flat curve (no wide fluctuations but an abnormally depressed, flat response), as well as many other blood-sugar curves, are often mistakenly thought, by untrained physicians, to be normal.

Children with hyperactive behavior and/or learning disabilities often have a flat curve (overproduction of insulin) or a sawtooth curve (characterized by an erratic production of insulin) as observed by the New York Institute for Child Development.[1] It is essential to determine the type of glucose intolerance a child has so that it may be assessed when the rise and fall of the blood-sugar abnormality occurs. For some it is delayed; for others, immediate.

William Philpott, M.D., records the blood-sugar changes of every food that is suspect of an allergic response. It is the optimal comprehensive testing for receiving a complete picture of a patient's glucose response in relation to any ingested food. However, not all physicians are able to incorporate such time and effort in their testing; in those cases a wide variety of whole, natural foods and avoidance of all refined carbohydrates would be adhered to.

The expertise of an orthomolecular physician is of utmost importance in evaluating and solving a child's unique biochemical imbalances and inadequacies. The guidance, however, is incomplete without parental involvement.

Of Vital Concern

As the causes of dysfunction unfold, parents become instrumental in a child's recovery, for they will be working to help achieve an optimal health level. Close contact with the child offers an awareness of positive and negative effects of manipulation of diet. The food offered is of vital concern because it fulfills the child's unique nutritional needs.

But just what is an optimal diet?

We are bombarded with contradictory information about nutrition. Sifting through books on the subject can be frustrating indeed. One book glorifies a vegetarian diet, another a low-fat diet, and still another a high-natural-carbohydrate diet. Unfortunately, no one carbon-copy diet applies to everyone. A diet that is nourishing for one person may evoke profound difficulties for another.

An optimal diet is one that supplies the body with the entire spectrum of nutrients—vitamins, minerals, amino acids, fatty acids, water, glucose—necessary for growth and repair. The body *is* capable of repairing itself, but it can do so only if the proper quantity and balance of essential nutrients are made available to it. Interferences such as metabolic errors, severe nutrient deficiencies and imbalances, glandular imbalances, blood-sugar abnormalities, biochemical defects, immune dysregulation, allergic manifestations, and digestive disorders will require the use of supplements to fulfill the child's nutritional needs. Supplying nutrients in quantities necessary to overcome biochemical disorders has opened up a new area of treating patients called nutritional pharmacology.[2] However, a wide variety of whole, natural food forms the basis of optimal nutrition.

The most common mistake in nutrition is concluding that one vitamin or mineral or food is more important to health than another. *Every* nutrient is an essential component of well-being, and all must be supplied in a specific balance that respects biochemical individuality.

The Individual Factor

In order to supply children's bodies and minds with nutrients vital to their well-being, the individuality of their inherent needs must be understood. How simple it would be if we could use one magic formula to dissolve every child's nutritional difficulties! Many fail to realize this individual makeup of humankind, but cookie-cutter people (stamped-out people without a wide variance of biochemical/nutritional individuality) we are not. Just as no two fingerprints are alike, our biochemical makeup also is unique. It is a uniqueness that "pervades every part of the body," according to Dr. Roger J. Williams,[3] a pioneer medical researcher. He writes:

> From birth, human beings are highly distinctive in both microscopic and gross anatomy, in the functioning of their organs, the composition of body fluids, and in their nutritional requirements.

Deficiencies may occur that are due to an unbalanced diet or assimilation or metabolic factors or an allergic manifestation (immune dysregulation) or fluctuations in nutritional needs, or an individual may be predisposed to them by any form of stress or by an inordinate hereditary need (sometimes magnified a hundred or a thousand times) which a "normal" diet cannot possibly fulfill.

This hereditary/nutritional concept is an interesting one also brought forth by Dr. Williams. He describes this condition as genetotrophic, which means it "is predisposed by heredity and precipitated by nutritional factors."[4] Thus, when we fail to meet "distinctive patterns of our nutritional needs," deficiency results. Supplementation along with an optimal diet is crucial to overcoming these deficiencies and ultimately serves to prevent nutritional difficulties.

The Interacting Factor

To isolate specific nutrients as all-important has been pointed out as a common misunderstanding in nutrition. There are no wonder nutrients; every nutrient has a profound purpose and is necessary for the function of all other nutrients. No single one acts independently of another or is more essential than another. However, some nutrients are harder than others to obtain in a standard American diet.

Dietary interrelationships, Harte and Chow[5] have concluded, are so closely interlocked that

> the shortage of a single essential vitamin/mineral element, amino acid, or fatty acid will create a shock wave that spreads to affect the utilization and/or function of every other essential nutrient.

This shortage, however, does not occur abruptly, as the body may draw upon its reserves when the diet supplies inadequate amounts of nutrients. This draining effect caused by a borderline deficiency cannot go on indefinitely, for the reserves will be used up and full-blown deficiency will occur. Before this happens, though, the deficiency may bring on symptoms somewhat less intense.

The severity of deficiency involves the intensity as well as the various kinds of symptoms. A severe niacin deficiency, for instance, would result in pellegra, but long before the deficiency reached that severity, the victim might experience such symptoms as a delusion of moving letters and numbers.

To determine the exact symptoms resulting from a particular degree of deficiency is not possible, for invariably a deficiency in one nutrient is associated with a deficiency in others. In essence, the interaction of *all* nutrients must be observed in the search for a child's unique nutritional needs.

The Quality Factor

The quality of the food a child ingests is of utmost importance. Pure, whole foods offer the highest quality of nutrients without interference of chemical preservatives, additives, flavorings, and colorings. Denatured foods (those containing chemicals, white flour, white sugar, white rice, all processed foods) are cause for concern because they are without appreciable nutrient value, and their empty calories exert a negative effect on the body.

The avoidance of denatured foods is primary in an optimal diet. Among widely sold denatured foods are the following:

breads, muffins	canned soup	cookies
cakes	cereals	crackers
candy	chips	doughnuts

drink mixes	ketchup	Pop-Tarts
frozen dinners	luncheon meats	processed cheese
fruit drinks (*not*	mini casseroles	soft drinks
juice)	pasta	syrup
ice cream, Popsicles	pizza	and so on
jam, jelly		

Whole, natural foods will replace the negative foods in the diet. In most of the above items, the undesirable ingredients can be exchanged for wholesome ingredients in home food preparation, or pure ready-made products can be purchased. Optimal foods would include any of the following natural foods:

Animal protein—Include fresh poultry (duck, chicken, turkey), fish (fresh- and saltwater), meat (venison, rabbit, beef, lamb, pork), eggs, and pure dairy products.

Fresh fruit—Any fresh, whole fruit may be used; use unsulfured dried fruit and fresh-squeezed juices (in moderation).

Fresh vegetables—Any fresh green or yellow vegetables or fresh-pressed juice; stress raw vegetables in the diet; when cooking, either steam, bake, or stir-fry.

Legumes—Any beans or peas may be used, as in soups (navy, lentil); baked beans (soy, kidney, pinto); as a flour in baking (soy, lima, or garbanzo flour); or as a snack (roasted peanuts, toasted soybeans).

Natural seasoning—Use natural flavorings such as herbs, spices, cold-pressed oils, natural sweetening (maple syrup, honey, dried fruit), apple-cider vinegar, sea salt, and the like.

Nuts/seeds—Consume nuts and seeds in their raw state; try almonds, cashews, filberts, brazils, walnuts, pine, macadamia, pecans, and pistachio nuts, and sunflower, chia, pumpkin, sesame, and flax seeds.

Pure water—Pure, spring water bottled in glass (avoid plastic bottles, as plastic molecules end up in the water).

Sprouts—Grains, seeds, and legumes may be sprouted at home or purchased. Use in salads, in casseroles, in place of lettuce in sandwiches, or as a snack.

Supplement foods—Lecithin, nutritional yeast, fiber, garlic, kelp, aloe vera, and the like.

Whole grains—Try millet, brown rice, buckwheat, oats, rye, barley, triticale; wheat and corn are overconsumed in the American diet.

The Utilization Factor

An awareness of not only what a child eats but what is utilized is a crucial factor in optimizing the diet. It is possible for *any* pure, natural food to be inappropriate for a child's body and to cause profound difficulties. It matters little how nutritious a food is if it cannot be utilized. Therefore, if a child is allergic to milk (as one example of a food that can become inappropriate), the ability to utilize nutrients from that food is considerably diminished. In fact, more harm than good may result from continued ingestion of the milk. If an allergic manifestation is in progress, it often is necessary to eliminate the stress factors (the allergy-evoking foods, for example) to give the body a chance to recover from the allergic insult as well as to provide an overall optimal molecular environment through a nutritious diet, nutrient supplementation, and digestive support.

The Metabolic Factor

Underlying metabolic problems must be identified and treated, not smothered with medication; their symptoms are urgent signals that must not be brushed aside and ignored. Errors in metabolism may occur that cause severe impairment of nutrient availability to the cells of the body. Even if a wholesome diet is consumed, an individual may be incapable of proper digestion (of food), absorption (of nutrients), distribution (to sites of need), uptake (of nutrients at the site), utilization (in the cells in need), or excretion (of waste products). There may be interference due to genetic predisposition, infections (such as with *Candida albicans*), unavailability of nutrient cofactors, or severe environmental stresses on the body.

Although essential fatty acids, for example, are available in a wholesome diet, an individual may have an impaired enzyme structure that does not allow ingested essential fats to be converted into other essential fats and prostaglandins. A high-protein diet may be consumed but an individual lacking the ability to digest, or break down, the protein into its component parts—amino acids—may become deficient in certain of these acids. A nutrient such as pyridoxine (Vitamin B_6) may be plentiful in the diet, but a metabolic error may impair the ability to convert pyridoxine into the coenzyme form, pyridoxal-5-phosphate, the active form of B_6 which the body can utilize.

Such metabolic errors must be identified and essential nutrient support supplied if we are to rectify the root causes of children's biochemical difficulties.

The Diversity Factor

A wide variety of wholesome foods must be included in an optimal diet. When you stop to think about it, the American diet is really quite restrictive:

beef	corn	milk	pork	tomatoes
chocolate	egg	oats	potatoes	wheat
citrus	lettuce	peanuts	sugar	yeast

Inappropriate foods tend to be those a child consumes again and again. Yet when an inappropriate food is identified and removed from the diet, there is often a tendency to exchange it for another and use it in an inappropriate manner. For example, there are infants who are allergic to cow's milk, but when soy milk is substituted, they become allergic to that too. A cycle may be set up in which the infant becomes allergic to each new milk that is introduced. This is due to the element of frequency and also is riveted in nutrient deficiency.

There is a threshold for each food an individual consumes. Some of us can consume a gallon of milk a day and tolerate it quite well. Others can handle a pint, others a cup, and still others may have a threshold of one tablespoon or less. To ingest any more than that causes trouble.

To protect a child from going over the threshold of particular foods, it is wise to diversify the diet to reduce the chance of allergic complications. In addition, a wide spectrum of foods will contain many different nutrients and therefore optimize nutrient availability.

The Enjoyment Factor

Food is to be enjoyed! New food choices will undoubtedly be necessary to fulfill unique nutritional needs, but the diet may be optimized within the realm of *your* child's acceptance.

TEN

The Immune Clues

The hallmarks of an allergic state are watery eyes, runny nose, hives, itching, wheezing, and sneezing. Allergy, however, covers a far broader range than asthma, hay fever, and eczema, in that it may affect any system of the body, including the brain.

Where Orthodox Medicine Leaves Off and Orthomolecular Takes Over

Conventional allergists approach the allergic condition in a very narrow scope. They consider only one type of allergic response—atopic—which encompasses effects on the skin and mucous membranes: eczema, hay fever, asthma, and related disorders. Their testing consists primarily of multiple scratch and prick techniques to determine inhalant allergies (referred to as IgE-mediated allergic disorders) and is followed by desensitization injections adminstered in the office. Months or years may pass before relief or even partial relief of symptoms occurs. Testing for food allergy is largely avoided by conventional allergists because the results by their methods are so unreliable—20 percent accurate at best. Conventional methods of treating allergic manifestations merely touch upon the tip of the iceberg of allergy.

Clinical ecologists, on the other hand, not only seek to uncover all allergenic substances through precise testing, but are concerned with systemic reactions occurring *anywhere* within the body. Clinical ecology is the study of an individual's reactions to his/her environment. Disturbances (allergic reactions) may be mediated by foods, inhalants, or chemicals the body is unable to tolerate. Thus allergy (or more specifically, the clinical-ecologic or bioecologic illness) is treated not by "scratching the surface" of the illness, but by 1) determining the root causes, 2) investigating the interrelationship of environmental factors and the health of the individual, including all systems of the body, and 3) treating the illness by strengthening the immune system.

Allergy Times Two

An allergy is an adverse response to substances that do not cause adverse responses in most people. The traditional concept of allergy has led us to believe that symptoms of allergy are limited to wheezing, sneezing, itching, and hives. There are, in fact, two different kinds of allergic manifestations, each mediated by disturbed mechanisms in the immune system. Alan Levin, M.D., a prominent immunologist in San Francisco, labels these two different kinds of allergy as Type 1 and Type 2.

Type 1, or classical, allergy we know well by the inflammation it provokes in the respiratory tract and nose, the skin, the eyes, the ears, and the gastrointestinal tract. Hay fever (allergic rhinitis), asthma, nasal stuffiness, wheezing, chronic sore throat, postnasal drip, laryngitis, sneezing, eczema, rashes, hives, insect-sting reactions, itchy/watery/inflamed eyes, stomach cramps, nausea, vomiting, heartburn, indigestion, diarrhea, bloating, and constipation are the predominant symptoms. Factors triggering an allergic response in Type 1 include dust; animal dander; molds; insect stings; tree, grass, and weed pollens; wool; feathers; and a few foods like milk, wheat, egg, strawberry, shellfish, corn, and yeast.

Type 2 allergy is often referred to as immune-system dysregulation and, in contrast to Type 1, involves a much wider range of symptoms that may occur anywhere and everywhere in the body but especially in the nervous system and the brain, evoking disturbances of mood, perception, behavior, thought, or emotion. Any number of foods, inhalants, and chemicals may trigger these allergic Type 2 responses.

There isn't always a firm, straight line that separates these two types of allergies, as it is possible that both are present, with their symptoms overlapping. However, one type of allergy usually predominates, so that an individual is classified as suffering primarily from Type 1 or Type 2 allergy.

To understand how these two allergies differ, let's look at some of the interacting components of the immune system that make it work. Two very important kinds of white blood cells are involved in immune reactions—T cells and B cells. T cells tell the B cells what to do. B cells make antibodies to fight off foreign substances. They start and stop the production of antibodies under the direction of the T cells. Individuals with Type 1 allergy inherit overactive B cells (which make antibodies) and "confused" T cells that are unable to tell the B cells which foreign substances are safe (pollen) and which are dangerous (bacteria). So the B cells manufacture an uncontrolled overabundance of antibodies. When too much of one antibody in particular is produced, IgE, a classical allergic reaction, occurs—for example, hay fever. The more IgE produced, the worse the reaction.

In Type 2 allergies, a different kind of antibody is formed by the B cells, which is called immunoglobulin G, or IgG. Problems with the T and B cells that occur in Type 1 allergy also occur in Type 2, but in Type 1 the problems are inherited. In Type 2 the T-cell dysfunction is usually acquired through outside factors that weaken the immune system such as chemicals, nutrient deficiency, stress, radiation, and infectious disease.

Elevation of IgE levels found in Type 1 allergy is usually not found in Type 2. And most doctors specializing in allergy do not even recognize an allergic condition unless there is an overabundance of IgE. Type 1 allergy may be treated with immunotherapy (allergy shots) as well as medication. Type 2 allergy often remains undiagnosed. This is because not all the different components of the immune system have been considered before the doctor rules out allergy. Medication is often prescribed to suppress the symptoms of Type 2 allergy somewhat, and the condition is explained as "stress-related" or "psychosomatic"—yet the underlying disease process remains.

The Immune Constellation

The material that follows is a more detailed description of the immune system. If you wish, you may skip this material and resume reading with the section called "Immune Insults."

How the immune system works as the primary defense mechanism in the body is easily related, for a clearer understanding, in terms of warfare. The *thymus gland* heads the immune system as the commander-in-chief. Lymphocytes (white blood cells) pass through the thymus gland and are converted into three kinds of T cells: killer, suppressor, and helper. *Killer T cells* work independently by directly attacking abnormal cells in hand-to-hand combat and may be thought of as the "Green Berets." *Helper T cells* act as the strategic air command which "alarms" (stimulates) B cells in the bone marrow. The B cells act as the air force, by forming and sending out antibodies (missiles) that "seek out and destroy" the invaders (antigens). *Suppressor T cells* act as the field commanders which bark out commands to control the formation of antibodies in B cells and oversee everything with "radar." Left on their own, the air force (or B cells) would just keep on sending out missiles (antibodies), and therefore must have the order of the field commanders (suppressor T cells) to halt the attack (antibody production).

When an invader, or antigen (a foreign substance like wheat), enters the bloodstream, a scout sneaks up on the invader, tags it, and signals the T suppressor cells. These field commanders then tell the air force (B cells) to start making missiles (antibodies) to seek out the invader (antigen). The missiles then zero in on the invader and make contact by binding themselves to the antigen with complements to form an *immune complex* (captured prisoners). The immune complexes (prisoners) may be put to death or may escape, depending on the strength of the *macrophage* regiment, which are big white blood cells that chew up the immune complexes and spit them out in their component parts so that they are no longer harmful to the body. The macrophage regiment works like "Pac-Man" tanks which cruise through the bloodstream grabbing and gobbling the immune complexes. But the ability and strength of the macrophage regiment is determined by heredity and may not be able to handle all the immune complexes (prisoners). If the invaders (antigens entering the body) are too heavy in number, the prisoners (immune complexes) are released and lodge in target organs (take up residence) throughout the body and even the brain. Symptoms are then observed as this allergic insult (losing battle) continues. In other words, the bad guys win.

Immune Responses

The commander-in-chief of the immune system is the thymus gland, a flat, pinkish-gray, two-lobed organ centered in the middle of the chest under the breastbone. Working in unison with the thymus are the spleen, bone marrow, lymph, and liver. Constituents of the immune system include:

T cells—white blood cells (lymphocytes) which arise from the thymus and regulate the immune system. T cells cannot produce antibodies, but stimulate and suppress antibody formation through B cells. There are suppressor T cells (which inhibit antibody formation), helper T cells (which stimulate antibody formation), and killer T cells (which directly attack abnormal cells). Suppressor T cells regulate reactions that move too far in either direction and in doing so help the body maintain immune homeostasis, so that neither reduced immunity nor hypersensitivity occurs. Unfortunately, suppressor T cells are acutely sensitive and may succumb to insult such as exposure to chemicals, flu, radiation, deficiency states, or other agents. This destruction of suppressor T cells provokes runaway helper T cells to stimulate B cells in the overproduction of antibodies. Thus immune dysregulation (the allergic state) flares, and an inappropriate immunological reaction occurs.

B cells—white blood cells which arise from the bone marrow and function in the production of antibodies. T and B cells work closely in regulating the immune system. Helper T cells activate B cells to stimulate plasma cells to produce antibodies.

Null cells—the population of cells which are precursors to many immune modulators. Elevation of null cells indicates a block of maturation of the helper/suppressor immune population.

Mast cells—control the activity of the inflammatory process by releasing fast- or slow-acting substances—leukotrienes (one thousand times as inflammatory-evoking as histamine).

Immunoglobulins—circulating proteins (antibodies) matched specifically against foods, pollens, bacteria, and the like. Currently identified immunoglobulins—IgA, IgG, IgE, IgM, IgD—protect different areas of the

THE IMMUNE SYSTEM

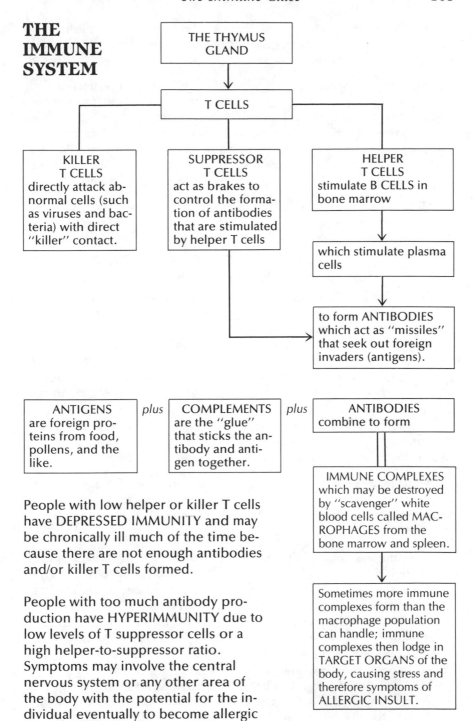

```
                    THE THYMUS
                      GLAND
                         │
                         ▼
                      T CELLS
        ┌────────────────┼────────────────┐
        ▼                ▼                 ▼
```

KILLER T CELLS	SUPPRESSOR T CELLS	HELPER T CELLS
directly attack abnormal cells (such as viruses and bacteria) with direct "killer" contact.	act as brakes to control the formation of antibodies that are stimulated by helper T cells	stimulate B CELLS in bone marrow

which stimulate plasma cells

to form ANTIBODIES which act as "missiles" that seek out foreign invaders (antigens).

ANTIGENS are foreign proteins from food, pollens, and the like.	*plus*	COMPLEMENTS are the "glue" that sticks the antibody and antigen together.	*plus*	ANTIBODIES combine to form

IMMUNE COMPLEXES which may be destroyed by "scavenger" white blood cells called MACROPHAGES from the bone marrow and spleen.

Sometimes more immune complexes form than the macrophage population can handle; immune complexes then lodge in TARGET ORGANS of the body, causing stress and therefore symptoms of ALLERGIC INSULT.

People with low helper or killer T cells have DEPRESSED IMMUNITY and may be chronically ill much of the time because there are not enough antibodies and/or killer T cells formed.

People with too much antibody production have HYPERIMMUNITY due to low levels of T suppressor cells or a high helper-to-suppressor ratio. Symptoms may involve the central nervous system or any other area of the body with the potential for the individual eventually to become allergic to "everything."

body. Whereas the conventional allergist observes only IgE-mediated — atopic—disorders, the clinical ecologist recognizes the importance of all the components of the immune system.

Immune complexes—the merging of antibodies and antigens, along with complements (enzymatic proteins which "glue" together the antigen and antibody), which under normal conditions are cleared from the body by the action of special scavenger white blood cells termed macrophages (they digest and guide in the elimination of immune complexes). When an allergic manifestation occurs, the body is unable to rid itself of this allergic material and it lodges in key areas, producing systemic reactions.

Histamine—a substance released during allergic reactions that involve inflammation and swelling. Histamine causes an increase in the permeability of cellular walls, which results in inflammation and swelling as plasma (the fluid part of the blood) moves into surrounding tissues. Hives, wheals, and swellings result from this release.

Prostaglandins—local hormonelike chemicals which are generated in tissues and organs from essential fatty acids. Approximately thirty prostaglandins have been identified and are crucial in immune regulation as well as being essential messengers in relating metabolism throughout the entire body. Some prostaglandins initiate immune function (inflammation, smooth-muscle control, constriction/dilation of blood vessels, and similar bodily actions), while others suppress it. Formation of prostaglandins is dependent on dietary fatty acids. Unfortunately, the American diet contains high quantities of saturated and man-made fats (margarine, hydrogenated fats, fried foods), which can cause a prostaglandin imbalance, in turn giving rise to allergic manifestations.[1]

Macrophages—special large white blood cells from the bone marrow and spleen that filter the immune complexes (formed by the combination of foreign antigens with antibodies) from the blood and digest them into their component parts.

By examining the constituents of the immune system through specialized testing a clinical ecologist may be able to isolate faulty, missing, or overactive parts. People with too much antibody production have hyperimmunity due to low levels of suppressor T cells or to high helper-to-suppressor-T-cell ratios. These individuals can become allergic to "everything." Others with a low level of helper or killer T cells have depressed immunity and may be chronically ill much of the time because there are not enough antibodies and/or killer T cells to protect the body.

The immune system is now being recognized as far more than just the defense system of the body. It really serves as a network of biological regulation that is intertwined with the endocrine and neurologic systems. This is why we see so much of an overlap in children's health problems when we seek out their underlying causes. A child may manifest, for example, severe aggressive behavior that is riveted in an allergy to milk (immune), blood-sugar difficulties (endocrine), and imbalances of neurotransmitters in the brain (neurologic). The effects on our health of the immune network are so far-reaching that we should examine it closely to be able to protect our children from those factors which can damage or alter it.

The strength of an individual's immune system dictates his ability to handle environmental stress factors (foods, inhalants, or chemicals). If the immune system is defective, immune dysregulation takes place, which results in allergic responses within any system of the body.

Immune Insults

The immune system is subject to failure under genetic or acquired[2] conditions. Individual susceptibility is riveted in the threshold to which the immune system can withstand insult and the person's nutritional status. Acquired damage to the immune system may occur through such factors as:

1) Chemical poisoning (example: pesticide exposure)
2) Physical or emotional trauma (example: death of a loved one)
3) Radiation exposure (example: X rays)
4) Severe viral/fungal/bacterial illness (example: mononucleosis)
5) Severe nutritional deficiencies (example: inadequate diet)
6) Metabolic dysfunctions (example: hormonal imbalances)
7) Unresolved digestive disorders (example: pancreatic enzyme deficiency)

Acquired damage may occur slowly through an accumulation of stress factors, a combination of many factors, or massive exposure to a single stress factor. The primary target of acquired damage appears to be the crippling of suppressor T cells which, in turn, influences the dysfunction of the entire immune system.

Genetic errors in the immune system may involve such defects as missing, undersupplied, or inoperative components. Genetically predisposed immune dysregulation (allergic states) may occur in combination with acquired damage.

Blood tests can be performed to determine immunological competence. These tests involve analysis of immune variables (T cells, B cells, immunoglobulins, complements, and so on) and offer clinical ecologists information on the severity of the allergic manifestation and the areas of immune abnormality.

Nutritional Aspects of Immunity

Many nutrients are involved in keeping the immune system healthy. Vitamin A; pyridoxine; Vitamins C and E; folic acid; pantothenic acid; the minerals zinc, selenium, and magnesium; the essential fatty acids; and amino acids are especially important to immune function.

The enhancement of immune function by the administration of specific nutrients has begun to appear more and more frequently in the medical literature. An article appeared in the *Journal of the American Medical Association* on the involvement of nutrients in immunity in 1981, and in 1982 an entire supplement volume by the same author was dedicated to single nutrients and immunity in the *American Journal of Clinical Nutrition.*[3]

Vitamin C is especially effective in activating T-lymphocytes,[4] but is needed in much higher levels than the Recommended Dietary Allowance to accomplish this action. The most exciting new application of enhancing immune function is that of specific essential fatty acids and their impact on immunity.[5,6,7,8,9] The predominant ingestion of partially hydrogenated fats (as found in margarine and processed foods), severe restriction of all fat intake, or an imbalance of fat intake (such as a high intake of saturated fats like meat, cream, and butter) can alter the availability of essential fatty acids (found in fish, cold-pressed oils, whole grains, and raw seeds) to the body. Supplementation is the best defense against the onslaught of "invaders."

The Missing Link

Immune dysfunction can proceed from many different causes, yet the most perplexing is the involvement of the fungus *Candida albicans,* which inhabits the mucous membrane of the intestinal tract. This fungus probably lives within everyone and may remain entirely compatible for an individual's lifetime; yet it can at any time establish itself in the tissues and release its by-products chronically into the bloodstream.[10] As the physician who has researched and presented a tremendous contribution on *Candida albicans,* Dr. Orian Truss states in his book *The Missing Diagnosis*[11] that "the very existence of *Candida albicans* in the tissues on a chronic basis reveals an immune system at least partially "paralyzed" and "unresponsive" to its antigens (79 at latest count), an immune system that is tolerating the continued presence in the tissues of this foreign invader. Functionally, a state of immunologic tolerance exists, since *Candida albicans* is tolerated rather than rejected." Up to this time, Dr. Truss has linked the suspected by-product of *Candida albicans* acetaldehyde with crippling effects on the immune, endocrine, and nervous systems as well as protein, fat, and carbohydrate metabolism. *Candida* appears to be a complicating factor in many allergic manifestations. Some allergic conditions are wholly due to *Candida* infection, and once the infection is treated the allergic state will disappear.[12] Many clinical ecologists have made this observation in their patients. The number of people suffering with *Candida* infection is staggering. Reversal of the *Candida* infection is crucial, as it can seriously disturb metabolic functions in the body. If you suspect this infection, immediately seek out a physician who can diagnose and treat the illness.

The most prominent cause of *Candida albicans* infection is the administration of antibiotics—especially broad-spectrum antibiotics. An infant's first infection that is treated with antibiotics may trigger the *Candida* infection, with persistent initial symptoms of oral thrush, clear nasal discharge, diarrhea, and diaper rash. Evidence now points to the *Candida albicans* infection[13] as the cause of epidemic recurrent illnesses, especially ear infections, in infants and young children (usual treatment being broad-spectrum antibiotics, decongestants, tubes in ears). As the child grows, many other symptoms may occur and persist into adulthood:

fatigue, drowsiness	gastrointestinal disorders
irritability	bloating, gas, belching
mood swings	constipation, diarrhea
incoordination	poor appetite
inability to concentrate	postnasal drip
autistic symptoms[14]	retarded growth and development
headaches	muscle aches
itching, rashes	athlete's foot
fungus under nails	chronic infections

Treatment of the *Candida albicans* infection requires aggressive action. Prevention is far easier. If an antibiotic is necessary because of illness, use an acidophilus (a friendly bacterium that exists in the intestine but is killed by antibiotics) supplement along with it and for two to three weeks after the drug is discontinued. Breast-feeding an infant and using pure, wholesome foods at the appropriate age (no refined, starchy cereals!) are also preventive measures. When *Candida albicans* is diagnosed by a physician, the following measures may be suggested in addition to antifungal yeast-killing medications (Niastatin powder):

1) Avoid foods that promote yeast growth:

refined sugar	malt (in cereal, milk drinks, candy)
natural sweeteners	peanuts, peanut butter
refined flours	smoked and dried meat and fish
all cheese	processed meats (luncheon meat
mushrooms	and the like)
melon	dried fruit
brewer's yeast	gluten grains (wheat, oat, rye,
alcohol	barley)

    yeast and yeast-containing foods (bread, crackers, rolls), vinegar, pickles, sauerkraut, and condiments containing vinegar (such as salad dressing, relish, mustard, ketchup, soy sauce, mayonnaise) supplements—B complex and chromium should be obtained yeast-free

2) Optimize diet, reduce carbohydrate intake

3) Digestive support—pancreatic enzymes and Megadophilus (concentrated acidophilus) supplement to support friendly intestinal flora

4) Nutrient supplementation—especially antioxidant nutrients

5) Control of allergic manifestations—avoidance of environmental chemicals and molds (damp basements, hampers, bathrooms, humidifiers, carpets, plants)

6) Ingestion of foods that inhibit yeast growth—garlic, onion, turnips, cabbage, broccoli

The Intertwined Regulatory System

The immune system closely interacts with the nervous and endocrine systems to maintain bodily homeostasis (stability). The allergic state can be triggered or worsened by many factors or a combination of factors such as infections, errors in metabolism, nutritional deficiencies, environmental stress factors, and digestive disorders. Blood-sugar abnormalities and digestive disturbances (pancreas) frequently accompany allergic manifestations. Hormonal imbalance is common, as the thyroid gland may be underactive and the adrenals overactive in allergic states. The brain and nervous system are acutely sensitive to allergenic materials, and a diverse range of symptoms may occur. Interestingly, Philpott has observed that with the elimination or rotation of allergens the function of the endocrine glands usually returns to normal.[15]

The Realm of Sensitivity

An allergic response due to exposure to food, inhalants, or chemicals may provoke adverse reactions within any system of the body. Reactions are specific to allergic stress factors. If the target organ for an allergic manifestation is the brain, a child may experience hyperactivity when drinking milk, unprovoked anger when ingesting peanuts, or dizziness when smelling perfume. Allergic manifestations, however, may involve one or multiple systems of the body and result in such responses as the following:

1) *Nervous system and brain*—hostility, hyperactivity, mood/personality changes, forgetfulness, confusion, lack of concentration, dizziness, light-headedness, insomnia, nightmares (recurrent), sleepiness, headaches, un-coordination, depression, nervousness, irritability, obnoxiousness, anxiety, cloudiness, stammering or stuttering speech, restlessness, learning problems, unprovoked panic/fear/crying, hallucinations, exhaustion, indecisiveness, lethargy, convulsions, fainting, trembling, apathy, short attention span, marked shyness/timidity

2) *Gastrointestinal tract*—bloating, indigestion, cold sores, nausea, vomiting, cramps, bad breath, diarrhea, abdominal pain, belching, mouth dryness, coated tongue, constipation, ravenous hunger, loss of appetite, flatulence

3) *Musculoskeletal system*—muscle stiffness/pains/cramps, backache, spasm ("growing pains"), arthritis, muscular weakness, twitching muscles (tics), joint pain, poor posture

4) *Genitourinary tract*—itching, frequent/urgent/painful urination, bed-wetting, discharge

5) *Skin*—hives, eczema, wheals, itching, acne, rash, pimply skin, white spots on the fingernails, sweating (including night sweats), blisters, burning, tingling, rough/bumpy areas, hot or cold flashes

6) *Eye, ear, nose, throat*—blurring, painful, spots before, watery, swollen, dark circles under, itchy eyes, double or distorted vision (eyes); aches, recurrent infections, itching, ringing, popping, fullness, intermittent deafness, fluid behind eardrum, dizziness, imbalance (ears); sneezing, itching, dripping, snorting, bleeding, stuffiness (nose); coughing, clearing, sore, dry, tickling, swelling, hoarseness, itching palate, difficulty swallowing (throat)

7) *Cardiovascular system*—heart palpitations, rapid beat, fluttering, chest pain, numbness

8) *Respiratory system*—asthma, bronchitis, respiratory infections, shortness of breath (smothering spells), wheezing, tightness in chest, hay fever, sinusitis, rhinitis

Allergic Cycles

Allergic reactions typically are identified as eating strawberries and breaking out in hives or eating shellfish and having an asthmatic attack. Most allergic reactions, however, are hidden under a cloak of addiction and are uncovered only when they are revealed by manipulation of the diet (avoidance of the food breaks the addiction). Hidden allergenic foods are epidemically prevalent in the American diet.

The Big Three are *sugar, wheat,* and *cow's milk.* These staples often are ingested three or more time per day and cause profound problems in sensitive children. Some other common allergens are

apple	citrus	oats	potato
beans	corn	onion	strawberries
beef	egg	peanut	tomato
chicken	fish	pepper	walnut
chocolate	melons	pork	yeast

Any food a child craves or eats in large amounts should be suspect as causing allergic responses, for it is the nature of allergy for the body to develop an addiction to any food it cannot handle. Thus frequency is an important factor to be considered in allergic manifestations. This is not to say that eating large amounts of a particular food is the root cause of allergy, but it does increase the possibility of an individual's reaction to a food. Each of us possesses a unique ability to handle particular foods in particular amounts. Take milk, for example. If we lined up one hundred people, we might find that some people could drink a gallon of milk a day without any allergic problems occurring, some people may be able to drink a quart, others a cup, and still others only a few teaspoons before an allergic or intolerance difficulty would appear. If an individual goes over his own specific limit of tolerated amounts, allergy (with or without addiction) or intolerance problems may result from the stress imposed upon the body. Therefore, large amounts in the diet of single foods, such as wheat and milk, are not recommended. The human body constantly attempts to adapt to its environment. When exposed to a substance that exerts a stress, such as food the body is unequipped to handle because of insufficient pancreatic enzymes, the body tries to reach metabolic homeostasis by first adapting and then developing a dependence on that substance as it is reintroduced again and again. Typically, we think of an allergy to a food as eating a food and then experiencing an allergic reaction to it within a short period of time. But once an allergic addiction is established, allergic withdrawal symptoms are experienced when the food is *not* eaten, not when it *is* eaten. For example, a hyperactive child who is allergic to milk might drink milk all throughout the day and not exhibit any reactions to milk. Yet if you withdrew the milk in all forms from his diet, in a few hours to a few days you would observe negative responses in health and behavior as the milk feeding the child's allergic addiction was not permitted. Reintroduction of the milk may actually make the child feel better because it feeds the addiction. However, the symptoms of the food allergy persist and will occur sporadically throughout the day. Perhaps we can best understand this phenomenon by the analogy of drug or alcohol addiction in adults. These substances at first are rejected by the body, but may become addictive in susceptible individuals as more and more is ingested and the body struggles to deal with the alcohol or drug stress factors. The body becomes addicted to these substances. Removal of the drug or alcohol produces withdrawal symptoms just as in addictive forms of food allergy or intolerance.

Symptoms may occur in the very young in response to allergenic foods, but often these go unrecognized as parents do not attribute irritability or constant crying to allergic reactions. When allergy *is* recognized by such symptoms as a rash or diarrhea, the offending food is withdrawn. But often is it reinstated at a later time when the child supposedly has outgrown the milk or other allergy. What is happening when the child no longer exhibits typical allergic symptoms? The response has changed as the child grew older and the symptoms just became masked. The infant who responds to drinking milk with diarrhea later may appear to have outgrown a milk allergy because there is a new response at age two of a constant runny nose and dark circles under the eyes and at age four there are hyperactivity and bed-wetting. By that time, other foods, inhalants, or chemicals often have complicated the original milk allergy to a great degree.

The very foods the child is allergic to often are favorites or an integral part of the diet. Many parents insist their child does not seem to crave particular foods, but they have not considered the many forms in which food is available. Wheat, for example, is nearly impossible to avoid as it is in breads, cakes, cookies, sauces, pasta, cereals, soup, casseroles, and so on. Even when a food (such as milk) is suspect, an attempt to eliminate it from a diet to see if symptoms diminish often fails because:

1) There is usually the involvement of more than just one food, and the withdrawal of one allergen may not make a significant difference if other allergens remain in the diet.

2) Milk, corn, wheat, and sugar are extremely difficult to avoid since they are so prevalent and hidden in so many food combinations. An accidental or unknown intake of a "little bit" of the allergen may precipitate the child's response.

3) Initially, the child's symptoms will worsen if addictive/withdrawal allergies are involved; the child not only will not improve after a few days without the allergen but actually will appear worse by exhibiting withdrawal symptoms. Responses may continue if the allergen being tested is not eliminated entirely; it thus remains hidden and masked.

4) An inadequate diet may overshadow sensitivities because of the existence of deficiencies or an overload of refined carbohydrates.

5) Adequate information and guidance are often unavailable.

Picture an allergic threshold as a raging fire (full-blown symptoms such as asthma, hyperactivity, learning problems) that subsides only when the allergic stress factors (chemicals, foods, or inhalants) are removed. If one allergic substance is removed, the blaze may be reduced a little, but it won't make a tremendous difference. If most or all of the allergic stress factors are removed, then the fire will die down to a glow because the allergic load has been decreased.

The allergic response may take on different forms and intensities. Relating these responses to a specific substance can be difficult because so many kinds of food in so many combinations are eaten. There are various types of allergic responses, and they may take on different cycles.

1) *Addictive/masked/withdrawal*—Occurs when the body becomes addicted to the very substance to which it is allergic; thus the symptoms are masked. Symptoms reoccur (withdrawal) when there has been a time lapse (three to four days) between exposures to the addictive/allergic substance.

2) *Hyperactive*—Occurs when an individual eats an uncommon food (or is exposed to another allergic substance) which provokes a severe reaction that may require medical attention (such as an asthmatic attack).

3) *Cumulative*—Occurs when an individual is exposed to two or more substances at the same time and experiences symptoms, but does not have symptoms if exposed to each substance individually.

4) *Fixed*—Most allergic substances and the subsequent reactions may be controlled, but a few substances may exist that provoke reactions no matter what attempts are used to help overcome them; these fixed allergens must be eliminated for an indeterminate period of time to avoid reactions—no amount of avoidance increases tolerance to them.

5) *Acute*—When an addiction is broken to a specific substance (by avoidance of that substance for four to ten days), the hidden reaction is exposed on reintroduction of the food.

6) *Cross-sensitive*—Foods may be categorized into families. An allergy to one member of a food family may cause or predispose an individual to react to other members of that family.

7) *Cyclic*—This describes a variable state in which a small or medium portion of food (or exposure to an allergic substance) is tolerated, but if a large portion is eaten or the food is eaten two or three days in a row, a reaction occurs.

8) *Delayed*—Some reactions occur immediately (in seconds) after exposure to the offending substance, whereas others take hours or even days to surface.

Allergy Within the Brain

We recognize that an allergy to specific substances can cause the tissues to become inflamed, with resulting swelling and tenderness. This is visibly evident in hay fever as a person's nasal passages become red and swollen owing to exposure to an inhalant (pollen) allergen. When an allergic reaction occurs in the brain [16,17] this same inflammation and swelling may take place, but now it occurs within the rigid confines of the skull. We cannot see the inflammation and swelling, but doctors have observed this phenomenon during brain surgery. Brain, or cerebral, allergy can seriously disturb brain chemistry,[18] leading to abnormal behavior, mood, thought, emotion, and perception.

Marshall Mandell was the first physician to suggest and then demonstrate that learning and behavior disorders were linked to allergy. Mandell recognized the existence of cerebral (brain) allergy in the 1960s and in 1972 developed the term "bioecologic mental illness" to describe how cerebral allergy and nutritional difficulties were linked in causing learning the behavior disorders.

The first bioecologic (allergy) mental-illness program in a mental institution was established in 1971 at the Fuller Memorial Sanitarium in South Attleboro, Massachusetts, by Drs. Mandell and William Philpott. These doctors found that 90 percent of the patients admitted to the institution had cerebral allergies. Wheat and milk proved to be major factors triggering allergic brain responses, but various other foods, inhalants, and environmental chemicals also provoked the severe mental symptoms that these patients suffered. When Abram Hoffer, the pioneering orthomolecular psychiatrist, learned of the ecologic (allergy) involvement in schizophrenia, he found that 50 percent of his schizophrenic patients who had not responded well to meganutrient therapy did in fact have cerebral allergy that blocked their progress in getting well. Research continues to support the involvement of wheat and milk as sensitizing agents in the schizophrenias.[20,21,22]

We now understand that cerebral allergy is not involved just in schizo-

PENMANSHIP CHANGES (DETERIORATION) AND SYMPTOMS INDUCED BY
SUBLINGUAL TESTING FOODS AND MOLDS

LAURA BELANGER   AGE 7

PRESENTING COMPLAINTS: LEARNING DISABILITIES, LOSS OF EQUILIBRIUM, ENURESIS.
INTERMITTENT HYPERACTIVITY AND HYPOACTIVITY

PATIENT'S USUAL PENMANSHIP Laura Belanger

POTATO PATIENT WAS UNABLE TO REMEMBER HER MIDDLE NAME. SHE EXPERIENCED
PHARYNGEAL PAIN AND ABDOMINAL PAIN.

Laura Belanger

MILK PATIENT HICCUPED FREQUENTLY.

Jaura Belahger

REVERSAL OF "L" AND "B," OMISSION OF "n"

Jaura Belanger

REVERSAL OF "L," "B," AND "e"

PEANUT PATIENT BECAME SILLY WITH UNCONTROLLED LAUGHTER.

Laura 'Belanger

FUSARIUM PATIENT EXPERIENCED EXTREME HYPERACTIVITY. "THIS
mold IS WHY WE ARE HERE" WAS THE MOTHER'S COMMENT.

Laura Belbnger

REVERSAL OF "a" IN LAST NAME

Belang gr

REVERSAL OF "e"

ASPERGILLUS PATIENT BECAME CRANKY, UNCOOPERATIVE, AND FRUSTRATED
mold HER TONGUE AND NECK BECAME EXTREMELY ITCHY.

Lautanger

PATIENT COMBINED HER FIRST AND SECOND NAMES

Sample handwriting changes occurring when a child is exposed to substances to which she is allergic. From *Dr. Mandell's 5-Day Allergy Relief System* by Marshall Mandell, M.D. (Thomas F. Crowell, 1979).

phrenia, but in a very wide spectrum of mental disorders and symptoms. Allergic factors triggering responses within the brain—foods, inhalants, chemicals—can be isolated through testing and treated by avoidance of these antigens and nutritional support.[23]

Unveiling the Allergenic Offenders

Various tests can be employed to uncover allergenic food, inhalant, or chemical offenders. Some tests can be performed only in a physician's office, but others can be conducted at home.

Conventional scratch and prick techniques offer little information about a child's allergic condition. An orthomolecular physician or clinical ecologist may perform one or more of the following tests to help identify offending substances:

Cytotoxic test—a blood test that measures the degree to which white blood cells are damaged or destroyed when mixed with different food extracts. The accuracy of this test is limited, but it is more accurate than scratch and prick techniques. This test falls short of supplying adequate information, but used in conjunction with other testing may offer additional information because the results are obtained in a relatively short time.

RAST (Radio-Allergy-Sorbent Test)—This is also a blood test which delivers results in a short time. It measures the quantity of IgE antibodies in the blood as they relate to specific allergens by using radioactive isotopes as markers. The RAST alone does not supply adequate information, since many food reactions are not IgE-mediated, but may be used in conjunction with other testing.

FAST (Fluorescent Antigen Absorbent Test)—This new test is a monoclonal antibody—IgE only—measurement that is less expensive and has better specificity and reproducibility than RAST. Nonradioactive materials are used. This test for IgE-mediated allergens has a high potential for success, as it is more accurate than RAST.

Provocative Neutralization Tests[24,25]—This type of testing is an intricate method that determines the degree of allergenicity, the particular antigens provoking symptoms, identification of symptoms, and neutralizing which can turn off allergic reactions and stimulate immune function. Provocative neutralization tests of foods and inhalants may be performed by injection of a dilution of an antigen under the skin (the *intradermal* method) or by the dropping of a dilution under the tongue (the *sublingual* method). Although costly in time and money, this testing provides accurate information that will help in treatment of the allergy. (If your child is acutely sensitive, be sure that the dilutant used in the test is free of chemicals such as phenol or glycerine, which may provoke a reaction.)

Deliberate Food Test—In this type of testing, the patient avoids all foods commonly eaten or fasts for a short period of time (don't *ever* put a child on a fast except under instructions of a physician). Foods are then challenged (reintroduced) one at a time and symptoms, blood-sugar changes, pulse rate, and saliva pH are recorded. The patient is then instructed on how to establish a strict rotation diet and how to avoid provocative foods. This method is the most accurate in determining food allergy and food intolerance but is quite time-consuming.

Nasal Inhalation—This is a sniff test to determine inhalant and chemical sensitivities. This test should be performed only under a physician's guidance.

Some of the groundwork for determining food allergy, however, can be performed at home.

The basis of establishing what is causing allergic response, regardless of the test used to point to allergens, is the actual process of eliminating foods from the child's diet and then reintroducing them. In this way, we learn how intense a response may be and under what circumstances as well as what form it may take. This process of trial and error is quite generalized, however, and if no methods were available to reduce the odds of potential allergens, it would be far too time-consuming to carry out.

The very fact that the most commonly eaten foods are the most likely to cause allergic responses in an important clue in narrowing down potential allergenic substances. Food habits are established early as children are bombarded with the American mainstays—wheat, sugar, milk, corn, eggs, citrus, chocolate, potatoes, beef, oats, peanuts—and children may eat them to the point of addiction. A masked addictive state is the major characteristic of cerebral and many other allergies; thus the favorite foods children eat most frequently are often the allergenic culprits.

In *Tracking Down Hidden Food Allergy* (Jackson, Tenn.: Professional Books, 1978), Dr. William Crook describes an elimination method of pinpointing allergens by using what he calls the rare-food diet. This approach eliminates the most common allergenic foods. Dr. Crook recommends foods in their natural state that children may not ordinarily eat frequently (for example, pineapple and blueberries instead of apple and orange; rice and millet instead of wheat).

Withdrawal symptoms usually appear between several hours and two days after elimination from the diet of the frequently eaten allergenic foods. Watch for a flaring of responses (hyperactivity, nausea, extreme irritability, and so on shortly (several hours to four days) after allergens are eliminated, but then a leveling off as the addictive cycle is broken. After a few "clear" days (symptoms do not necessarily have to be completely gone, but significant improvement should be evident), begin introducing suspected allergens into the child's diet *one at a time* in their pure form. A pure form would be a glass of milk, for instance, not milk in a mixture such as custard or ice cream, because other ingredients could cause a response rather than the milk. Individual foods are systematically reintroduced into the diet and the symptoms are noted.

One must be very careful to connect individual allergens to individual symptoms. A short period of avoidance usually causes exaggerated symptoms when allergens are reintroduced. This reaction can wear off in two to three weeks, so it is necessary to complete testing during this period before the acute reaction diminishes. If the testing is long, symptoms may not appear at all unless the food is eaten in large quantities. A prolonged period of avoidance (this varies from a few weeks to many months for minor or unfixed allergens) increases the child's tolerance of foods to which he normally is sensitive. However, if these foods are eaten in large quantities the symptoms may show up again.

An additional tool for monitoring symptoms is the pulse rate. Some elusive symptoms can be caught this way. The relationship between allergic responses and the rate of pulse was discovered by Dr. Arthur F. Coca in the 1930s. Coca developed a pulse test based on the observation that ingestion of allergenic foods causes a rapid increase in blood sugar followed by a sharp decline in blood sugar that provokes the release of adrenaline. This in turn causes the pulse rate to rise.

To check for an increased pulse rate, the range of the pulse must be established a few days prior to the beginning of any manipulation of the diet. To do this, measure the pulse rate for a full 60 seconds and record its highs and lows to establish its baseline:

1) Just before the child gets out of bed in the morning
2) Just before each meal
3) Three times, at half-hour intervals, after each meal and snack
4) Just before the child goes to sleep

After recording this information for two or three days, arrange the child's diet so that meals and snacks consist of only one or two foods. Continue to record the pulse-rate information. Note the lowest pulse rates, and compare them with higher pulse rates. A pulse rate elevated six or more beats after a suspected meal is eaten in an indication that allergy may be present. The pulse rate should stabilize when allergenic foods are eliminated.

Milk, wheat, and sugar are the most frequent major allergens—which is, of course, because they are the most heavily consumed in our diet. I have observed that either milk *or* wheat is a major allergen; for both to occur simultaneously as major allergens in children with mild allergies is infrequent. Children with severe allergies may be allergic to both wheat and milk, but one or the other usually predominates.

Refined sugar is almost always a major sensitizing agent when a child has food allergies. Some types of refined sugar seem to cause more of a reaction than others, as sugar may be derived from beets, corn, or cane.

The sugar sensitivity comes into play with allergy because the pancreas has a dual purpose—it releases digestive enzymes which ultimately make possible the proper digestion of food and it controls the supply of glucose (blood sugar) through the release of insulin. We know that if food is not digested properly the undigested particles may trigger allergic reactions. We also know that when the pancreas fails to release enzymes properly, it usually fails to regulate glucose properly. Thus food allergies and the ability to digest and metabolize sugar are closely linked.

Major allergens tend to be fixed (permanent), whereas minor allergens may be eaten on a rotation basis after a period of withdrawal. The rotation of foods can prevent, isolate, and treat food sensitivities, and if this manipulation of the diet is not used, new sensitivities will invariably appear. This is because children who have established some food sensitivities are extremely vulnerable to establishing others. For instance, if wheat and oats were determined to be allergens and those foods were replaced with rice as the exclusive grain in the diet, then the element of frequency would be established for rice just as it previously was for wheat and oats. There could soon be a dependence on rice and a withdrawal reaction when it was not eaten. Thus a rotation diet eliminates the frequency factor which stresses the immune system.

Stimulating the Immune System

Resolving ecologic illness, regardless of where it is manifested in the human body, requires a total look at the health of the individual child. Stress factors such as chemical interference, infection, insufficient sleep, emotional turmoil, and so on which strain "the expenditure of mental or physical effort beyond one's biochemical limits"[26] must be removed. Yet paramount to every child's recovery is the isolation and treatment of those factors causing the symptoms. The next step is to supply an optimal molecular environment for the recovery of the immune system.

ELEVEN

A Time to Heal

For many of us in the field of orthomolecular medicine there is A Story. Something that happened in our lives which altered it so sharply that for me, and perhaps for you, the parent or professional reading this, the world stood still, if only for a moment, and our view of it changed. In my case, I watched a story of horror unfold as my child's condition was diagnosed as hopeless. "Hopeless" is a devastating word. It provokes a stream of uncontrollable emotion—guilt, anger, denial, frustration—and, of course, the inevitable question "Why my child?" "Hopeless" occurs to many different degrees in many different health problems children experience. But it doesn't have to be accepted.

Shawn

My two-year-old son lay in intensive care with tubes connected to his small body as I sat riveted beside him waiting for a diagnosis. This was the second hospital my son had been in, as the area and extent of damage deep within his brain required special testing. The day before, Shawn had fallen from a tall slide onto cement and within hours lapsed into a coma.

Shawn was an extremely agile child who climbed playground equipment like a little monkey, which quickly earned him the nickname. His physical and mental development had always been far above the norm, which I attributed to an optimal diet (breast milk, wholesome food, and supplements) and environmental stimulation. At eighteen months he would take his plastic bat and ball out to play and surprised us all with his ability (after watching older children) to throw the ball up in the air with one hand and hit the ball with the bat in the other as it came down. At this age he also learned to read and could draw triangles, circles, and squares on demand. He was a bright, happy child who was determined to try anything and everything new.

Now he lay before me beyond my reach. It's odd how in the face of tragedy we pull ourselves together and we see ourselves and others for who they truly are. The seven-year-old in the bed next to Shawn's was dying of cancer, and in the last few days of his life his concern was not for himself but for Shawn; it nearly broke my heart. After three days and three nights at my son's side the diagnosis came: he was hopelessly brain-damaged and would be "a vegetable the rest of his life." Hopeless . . . the word that rips people apart.

As the days passed, I realized that I must find an answer—that waiting and hoping was not enough.

I began a broad-spectrum nutrient program for Shawn, the emphasis on nutrients that stimulate brain function. For two weeks although he began to seem more alert, there was no apparent physical change. I would prop Shawn up with pillows, as his muscular control was that of a rag doll. If not watched constantly, he would flop forward on his face or to the side. After two weeks in intensive care, Shawn was transferred to the rehabilitation area of the hospital. The head neurologist was opposed to this move, as he felt the child belonged in an institution; however, he allowed us time in rehabilitation until we could "decide in what institution we would place the child."

The new environment was much more stimulating, with bright colors and toys; and Shawn appeared more alert than ever after the move to rehabilitation. We didn't know how alert until we propped him up in a chair and he scooted himself off the chair and stood up! I couldn't believe it—he stood up! The nurse insisted he be tied down, because she said he would hurt himself. But she wasn't prepared for the event that took place the next day, for Shawn not only stood up: he *ran*. His movements were horribly crippled, but he did in fact run. This caused a fury of excitement among the nurses and a visit from the head neurologist one hour later. Shawn's relationship with the head neurologist was an intense one—he hated him with a passion. The minute Shawn spotted this particular doctor he would scream in terror, and he kept on screaming until the doctor left. I'm afraid I shared my son's opinion of the head neurologist, who had the gross insensitivity to tell me flatly that "your child will be a vegetable the rest of his life; put him in an institution and forget him" and then turn on his heel and joke with the nurse in the adjoining room. This time he was utterly disgusted that Shawn had dared to defy his "hopeless" diagnosis. He stomped off in a huff mumbling about physical therapy.

Shawn was seen by a physical therapist the very next day. Lynn was a really sweet lady who tried very hard to make the therapy fun with games, songs, and puppets. Shawn lasted five minutes and then he was off and running (and falling). We couldn't catch him—at two, he had a will of iron, and no amount of kindness, bribery, ordering, or yelling (last resort) could get him to do the required exercises. But every day that passed, Shawn got *better*. I continued his nutrient program vigorously—much to the distress of the nurses, who lectured me on the dangers of vitamins.

Two weeks later, the only visible sign of the brain injury was a slight limp involving the left leg. The miracle child was escorted into a room filled with residents, interns, and neurologists for examination of this most un-usual phenomenon. Mothers were excluded; therapists were not, so Lynn went in with Shawn. When Lynn emerged with Shawn forty-five minutes later, I asked what had happened. Lynn was excited because for the first time Shawn had cooperated totally (the kid needed an audience to per-form!), and she had put him through the entire therapy program that had been designed for him. She then said that the doctors attributed Shawn's recovery to . . . physical therapy. I asked Lynn if she had explained that Shawn had refused to do the therapy. She looked at me as if I had totally lost my mind and said, "I can't tell them that; they're doctors!"

Shawn was released from the hospital a few days later. The resident who spoke to me before Shawn's release shrugged his shoulders in response to my questions concerning the supplements' contributing to Shawn's re-covery, but he did say that he and the other doctors in this hospital had never seen such a profound recovery and we were very, very lucky.

After being cooped up in the hospital for five weeks, I felt that visiting some friends with young children in northern California would give us a chance to breathe clean air and relax. After a few days of romping with the other children, my friend turned to me and said, "I don't see any signs of Shawn having had a brain injury—look, he doesn't even limp anymore." Sure enough, he didn't! Again, I was plagued with why Shawn had re-covered: was it his age, the nutrient therapy, or his "I'll do it myself" attitude that had produced this unbelievable return to normal? I continued the nutrient program, for whatever it was that had induced Shawn's recov-ery, I didn't want to change anything. What I didn't foresee, however, was that one of the nutrients I was using—a wheat-germ-oil concentrate high in octacosanol—would be unavailable in the city we were visiting.

Three days after we ran out of the wheat-germ-oil concentrate, Shawn began limping, then falling. The nightmare had begun again. At first I did not link Shawn's regression to the absence from his diet of the wheat-germ-oil concentrate. In fact, I did not see the connection until we returned home (at once) and I purchased more of the supplement. Within three days on the supplement there was an improvement; within one week he had regained all he had lost.

In the months that followed I was careful never to run out of the wheat-germ-oil concentrate, because I was terrified of the deterioration that had occurred before. But as the months slipped by, there were days when the supplement was forgotten. Five months after the accident, Shawn's pre-school teacher called me extremely upset. She had noticed that Shawn had been clumsy the last day or two, but on this day he had taken a drastic turn for the worse. I realized as she was talking that it had been four or five days since he had received his supplement. Reversal of the symptoms took three days with the supplement. Similar events occurred over the next year when-ever the supplement was forgotten. Was the fact that when my son received octacosanol he was free of symptoms and when it was stopped the paralysis and uncoordination returned absolute proof that octacosanol resolved my son's "hopeless" condition? Perhaps not; but this case history and many more like it (especially of two well-known individuals) opened the door, as case histories so often do, to further exploration and formal studies. The trial of a harmless nutrient (*now* being used successfully on many coma patients in hospitals) resulted in healthy, active, bright child with no evidence of the brain injury.

Every child deserves the chance to soar above the "answers" we so often hear from professionals about the child's difficulties:

1) You'll just have to learn to live with it.
2) Maybe he'll outgrow it.
3) Let's give him a little medication.
4) It's hopeless.
5) It's all in his mind; he needs therapy.
6) You don't really love the child.
7) He's spoiled.
8) It's stress-related.

Answers to painful questions usually aren't available until long after the crisis is behind us. Why my child? My child's crisis led me to find answers for many other "hopeless" children. My position as Chief of Nutrition in the Preventive Medicine/Clinical Ecology Center in Sacramento, California, offered a clinical setting where children's health problems were *resolved* through orthomolecular testing and treatment. The following case histories are of children who were my patients. Some had severe health problems requiring extensive testing; others required only a simple evaluation and general health suggestions. Yet each suffered needlessly because of previous failure of recognition of the intimate relationship of diet and health.

Eric

Eric appeared a well-mannered ten-year-old when he and his mother entered our clinic for evaluation just after school had let out for the summer. Eric's mother's primary concern was his schoolwork, as he tried very hard in school but was unable to retain information. He would learn something on Monday and have no memory of it on Tuesday. A special-education teacher had been assigned to him to help with this short-term memory defect, but she had gotten nowhere in the previous school year. Eric also had difficulty reading and writing, but continued in regular classes, as a C-D student, with one period of special help.

Eric also experienced quite an array of other problems determined through an extensive health questionnaire and interview. He was exhausted most of the time, with bouts of nervousness, anxiety, moodiness, irritability, confusion, and forgetfulness. He was often clumsy and had muscle aches. Headaches occurred daily; he was subject to gas, bloating, and excessive hunger and thirst; he craved sugar. He sniffed constantly and was plagued with sneezing, itching, wheezing, puffiness around the eyes, and occasionally hives.

Testing revealed that Eric had immune dysregulation (elevated IgM, IgE, C_4, and null cells), dysinsulinism (a blood sugar that rose and fell dramatically twice during the test), and indications of mineral deficiencies (manganese, chromium, selenium, and especially magnesium).

Eric's diet wasn't too bad at mealtimes, but because of his cravings for sugar he gorged on ice cream, candy, cookies, and soda pop between meals. His favorite foods were corn, bacon, sugar, peanuts, soda pop, cashew butter, and ice cream. After Eric's mother and I discussed with him why changes in his diet were necessary, he agreed to finding replacements for processed and sugary foods, trying new foods to add more variety, and a general multivitamin-mineral supplement.

Allergy testing proved that Eric was indeed a very allergic child. He was allergic to every inhalant tested and most of the foods. Foods that provoked symptoms (provocative) were peanut, corn, white potato, barley, and wheat, which induced primarily central-nervous-system symptoms.

Treatment with allergy-neutralization drops was administered after testing. Further treatment included a rotation diet with avoidance of provocative foods and avoidance of chemicals in the home environment. Supplements included free-form amino acids, multimineral complex, GTF (Glucose Tolerance Factor) chromium, buffered Vitamin C, evening primrose oil, pancreas compound, magnesium, pyridoxal-5-phosphate, pantothenic acid, manganese, selenium, glutathione, phosphatidyl choline, bromelain, Vitamin E, B complex, and Vitamin A.

One month later, Eric's mother reported that Eric's fatigue, itching, sneezing, sniffling, wheezing, puffiness around the eyes, digestive problems, and excessive thirst were greatly improved. He appeared happier and more confident.

School began again in the fall, and Eric returned to the clinic for his September follow-up. Eric's mother was ecstatic as she entered my office. The special-education teacher could not believe the difference in Eric. When told of the health program Eric was on, she agreed that the program must be the reason for the dramatic turnaround in Eric's memory recall. This was to be Eric's first good year in school—his grades escalated to A's and B's, and he began to see challenges as fun. The real Eric had emerged.

One year later, Eric continues to remain free of symptoms unless he slips on his diet and supplements (now at a maintenance dose).

Gregory

Gregory suffered from eczema on his face and extremities. At eighteen months he was also a whiny baby who was pale and listless. Gregory was on a fairly wholesome diet that contained predominantly egg, oatmeal, whole-wheat bread, apples, orange juice, banana, chicken, milk, beef, various vegetables, and so on. Initially, we began with suggestions of an elimination diet (eliminating commonly eaten foods, rotating and adding remaining and new food choices), general checkup testing, hair analysis, and general supplements (inclusion of cold-pressed oil with Vitamin E in the diet, B complex, Vitamin C, and Vitamin A–rich foods).

At the follow-up two weeks later, Gregory had experienced no improvement whatsoever. The test results explained why. Gregory was anemic, but what concerned us most was the results of the hair analysis. The cadmium level was so high it was off the scale. It had to be a mistake! We took another hair sample to recheck the results. In addition, I questioned Gregory's mother about possible exposure to cadmium. No clues until she told me that they used well water and that Gregory seemed to crave the water, especially the last six months. He drank seven to eight (and more) glasses of the water daily! We suggested she have the water tested for its cadmium content and waited for the results of the second hair analysis. On researching cadmium poisoning, I found that it may cause an anemic condition as well as disturbing the central nervous system. Cadmium is antagonistic to zinc, which was also grossly abnormal in the hair analysis.

The second hair analysis returned the same results as the first. Gregory's mother had had their well water tested, and it was found to be contaminated with high levels of cadmium. Along with a wholesome diet and pure water, supplements (zinc, Vitamin C, garlic) were used to help pull the cadmium out, in addition to iron, folic acid, and B_{12} supplementation. In ten days Gregory's eczema was improved; in three weeks it was gone. The anemic condition was also soon corrected.

Hair analysis has been abused by many people who think they can evaluate an individual's complete health status with one test. Hair analysis is a screening tool that gives us one piece of the puzzle. But it can at times give us urgent information—especially where toxic metals are concerned—that would otherwise be missed. What would have happened to Gregory if we hadn't used this important screening tool?

Nicole

Nicole, at nine, was a nervous child who suffered frequent bouts of colds and flu. She was tired all the time; had heart palpitations; was spacey, depressed, and tearful. She had eczema on her hands, hay fever, and digestive problems. A glucose-tolerance test revealed hypoglycemia (a dip down to 50), allergy testing showed sensitivities to many inhalants and foods, and her blood workup indicated anemia. Nicole achieved some improvement on allergy-neutralization therapy and general supplementation, but not enough to attain the results she and her mother expected. We began a rotation diet (strict) with complete avoidance of provocative foods and a more aggressive supplement program which included pyridoxine, zinc, evening primrose oil, buffered Vitamin C, pancreas compound, bromelain, multiminerals, Vitamins A, E, and B$_{12}$, B complex, and iron.

Within one month the hoped-for results occurred: her schoolwork improved, cerebral symptoms subsided so that she could think clearly, digestive problems disappeared, the eczema cleared up, and her fatigue vanished.

Ian

Nine-year-old Ian had been fully informed by the other children in the clinic's waiting area that I would make him stop eating sugar. Thus when he entered my office, he was ready to fight me tooth and nail, flatly informing me that under no circumstances would I stop him from eating sugar. "I love sugar," he announced, "and you can't make me stop eating it!" I agreed! I couldn't make him stop eating sugar, but I could listen to some of the problems he was having and might be able to help. He reluctantly agreed.

Ian's mother had come to our clinic first for help with her own overwhelming health problems. A severely allergic woman with cerebral symptoms (exhaustion, depression, spaciness), she had seen her problems clear up with treatment of her *Candida albicans* infection, chemical avoidance, allergy-neutralization therapy, and supplementation. Ian was brought in because of the success she had had with our program.

Ian's mother had already attempted some changes in Ian's diet, but without too much success in the area of his craving for sugar, milk, cheese, ice cream, white bread, chocolate, peanuts, carrots, celery, and barley cereal.

Ian had been breast-fed for the first six months of life. His mother remembers that he screamed continuously during his waking hours (sleeping very little) and that the pediatrician could not find anything wrong with him. He had developed recurrent ear infections starting at five months of age, with subsequent antibiotic treatment. He had had bronchitis and pneumonia twice before his third birthday and had bed-wet until age four.

Ian had erratic grades in school that ranged from A to F and tended to retrace his handwriting. He cleared his throat constantly; he had a dry cough, itching throat and palate, and contact dermatitis. He was exhausted, withdrawn, nervous, forgetful, irritable, and restless and had periods of hyperactivity, feelings of rage, headaches (severe, four a week), dizziness, and confusion. He had muscle cramps and joint and muscle aches and pains and was clumsy. He experienced nausea, indigestion, gas, stomachaches, and abnormal thirst. He had fungus under his nails and often suffered anal itching. But most frightening of all was that Ian had contemplated and then attempted suicide. At age nine, this child was so depressed over his condition that he wanted to die.

Ian's dietary intake was as follows:

Breakfast:	Barley cereal, sugar, milk—five days a week
	Bacon, eggs, whole-wheat pancakes, real maple syrup—once a week
	Doughnuts—Sunday
	Occasionally orange juice
Lunch:	Whole-wheat-bread sandwich with a filling of peanut butter, beef, or leftover chicken (mayo, tomato)
	Chemical-free, natural chicken or beef hot dogs, ketchup
	Carrots, celery
	Peanuts, cheese
	Milk—1 pint
	Cookies (both natural and processed)
	Fast food—once a week (Saturday)
Snack:	(Always ravenous at this time in the afternoon)
	Peanuts, apple, banana, corn chips, sugary ice cream with chocolate syrup, natural or sugary cookies, cola
Dinner:	Beef, pork, chicken, lamb, fish (mother tries to rotate)
	White or sweet potato, whole-grain pasta
	Vegetables—broccoli, squash, brussels sprouts, carrots, cauliflower, asparagus, string beans, tomato
	Dessert—sugary ice cream with chocolate syrup (loves this and sneaks ice cream and chocolate syrup whenever he can get away with it), fruit (banana, orange, apple)

Testing revealed that Ian had a flat-curve glucose-tolerance test; hyperimmune state (B cells, lymphocytes, null cells all elevated); indications of low levels of magnesium, zinc, calcium, and manganese; too much acid produced in his stomach, influencing the pH of the small intestine and therefore digestion; and suspected *Candida albicans* infection. Ian was sensitive to molds, weeds, and many foods during allergy testing. Foods produced the following symptoms:

Headache was provoked by corn, milk, yeast, vanilla, wheat, chicken, celery, malt, barley
Tiredness was provoked by carrots, peanut, wheat, tomato
Hyperactivity was provoked by maple syrup, pumpkin, banana, cola
Runny nose was provoked by pork, corn, milk
Depression was provoked by black pepper, soy

His worst reaction was to almond, which provoked violence, black circles under his eyes, double vision, restlessness, and deep depression. Interestingly, Ian's mother also had such a response to almond.

Ian received allergy-neutralization drops, supplements (beta carotene, multimineral complex, Vitamin E, octacosanol, evening primrose oil, pyridoxal-5-phosphate, free-form amino acids, buffered Vitamin C, bromelain, pancreas compound, phosphatidyl choline, B complex, magnesium, pantothenic acid, manganese, glutathione), and consideration of nystatin therapy to treat *Candida albicans* infection; chemical exposures were to be avoided;

he was to be put on a rotation diet with avoidance of provocative foods; and that left the sugar question besides! Would he cooperate? Sometimes we must feel things to believe them, and the frightening reaction to almond that Ian had experienced in the allergy-testing room had shaken him up— he had felt cause and effect firsthand. We decided to make a deal on the sugar. I bet him that if he took the supplements every day for two weeks he wouldn't crave sugar nearly as much. He consented, if the free-form amino acid supplement could be taken in capsule form instead of in powder form (it has a bad taste). We agreed. He caught me in the hall long before the two weeks were up and told me excitedly, "I don't eat sugar anymore. I feel great!"

As time went on I asked more of Ian, and his compliance was infectious. All the adult patients in the allergy-testing room heard about his success in giving up sugar and his continued progress with his diet; they felt that if a child could change his diet so quickly, then they certainly could too.

Ian's digestive problems, cerebral symptoms, muscle/joint aches and pains, schoolwork, and atopic (itching, coughing, dermatitis) allergy problems all dramatically improved within the next six weeks. But most important of all was that the little boy with suicidal depression found peace within himself.

Brandon

Brandon's parents were at their wit's end when they brought their five-year-old son into our clinic. For four years of his young life Brandon had suffered from asthma, and now it was uncontrollable—even by Brandon's daily doses of potent steroid drugs.

Brandon had been a fussy infant who was breast-fed for six months, then switched to cow's milk. About the time he was weaned from the breast he developed his first ear infection and cold, which were treated with antibiotics and decongestant. It became a pattern, however. Every six weeks Brandon had another ear infection and cold followed by antibiotics. Then at a little over a year of age, Brandon developed asthma. The illnesses continued, but now Brandon developed dark circles under his eyes, wheezing, and spasmas of coughing, especially at night. Sleep was difficult for everyone in the family because of the coughing and Brandon's parents' helpless attempts to stop it.

The pediatric allergist Brandon was taken to between the ages of two and three tried scratch allergy tests, allergy treatment, and stronger drugs (steroids). Brandon's asthma got worse. His parents were frightened over the large doses of steroids their child was taking every day which were intended to be used occasionally. So at age four Brandon was taken to an ear-nose-throat specialist who recommended tubes be put in the child's ears and his tonsils removed. The surgeries were performed. Brandon did not get better; in fact, his mother told us that one week after coming out of the hospital Brandon had had the worst asthma attack ever and ended up in the emergency room once again.

Brandon appeared an easygoing, shy child who was very well behaved. In the past his parents had tried eliminating milk and sugar from his diet, but had not seen much difference in his asthmatic condition. Our clinic was their last resort.

Immune-competency tests revealed abnormalities (low IgA, low CH_{100}, high B cells, high null cells, and total WBC and lymphocytes elevated). A glucose-tolerance test showed hypoglycemia, and indications of very low levels of zinc and selenium were present, with calcium, magnesium, and manganese depressed to a lesser degree.

We began with an elimination diet and general supplementation due to Brandon's age. Wheat proved to be a major trigger of wheezing, so it was completely eliminated from the diet. Brandon's parents also found that buffered Vitamin C would stop the coughing at night and wheezing during the day. Brandon got better, so much better that he was gradually taken off the steroid medication.

Eight months went by and Brandon was free of asthmatic symptoms! But mold season hit in the fall, and the wheezing began again. We decided to test Brandon in the allergy department even though he was only five. Most little children respond well enough to environmental control, general supplementation, and change in diet, but Brandon now needed special help.

Brandon proved to be allergic to virtually every inhalant and food tested. He had provocative wheezing reactions to beef, grape, peas, walnut, egg, milk, wheat, vanilla, pineapple, soy, pork, honey, malt, yeast, cheeses.

Brandon was placed on a strict rotation diet with avoidance of provocative foods, allergy neutralization drops, and more aggressive supplementation—beta carotene, free-form amino acids, zinc, multimineral complex, Vitamin E, evening primrose oil, buffered Vitamin C, selenium, B complex, pantothenic acid, pyridoxal-5-phosphate, B_{12}, pancreas compound, glutathione.

Brandon's asthma disappeared, the recurrent illnesses ceased, and Brandon's mother entered the clinic to clear up *her* allergies!

One year later Brandon's mother reports that he looks great, is doing well in school, loves sports—especially soccer—and does not cough or wheeze! Occasionally, during mold season or in the spring, a slight wheeze will begin, and the allergy/nutrient program is intensified to handle the stress of the additional allergy load.

Eddie

Eddie's "hopeless" condition began before he was born; it was due to his mother's alcoholism. Fetal alcohol syndrome refers to birth defects occurring together (severely impaired brain development, abnormal facial appearance, growth abnormalities) induced by the effect of alcohol on an unborn child. Eddie's foster mother knew the prognosis for Eddie's growth and development, yet she was determined that he receive the best care possible. But it hadn't been easy. Eddie's gains were tiny steps, with regression around every corner.

When Eddie's foster mother brought him into the clinic at age three, her expectations were only that we optimize his diet. We were not optimistic, but felt that guidance in improving Eddie's diet could do no harm. Eddie's foster mother fed her family a completely natural vegetarian diet, and she had already determined that cow's milk caused diarrhea. His diet included the following foods:

Breakfast:	Millet, buckwheat cereal
	Goat's milk
	Fruit—pear, apple, banana
Lunch:	Rice bread (contained yeast)
	Almond butter, avocado, carrot, alfalfa sprouts
	Tofu, steamed vegetables (broccoli, squash, spinach)
Dinner:	Tofu, beans
	Potato, grains (corn, wheat, oat, rice)
	Vegetables, avocado

Eddie's difficulties at this time included severe retardation; wild play; fatigue; screaming outbursts; no bladder control; loose bowels; no eye contact; dullness; parrot speech or one-word answers (Yes, No, Mama); hyperactivity; dry, itchy skin; restless legs; insomnia; clumsiness; uncoordination.

We discovered that Eddie was very sensitive to grains, and this made sense because the alcohol he was flooded with before he was born is derived from grains. Soy, goat's milk, apple, broccoli, and almond also proved to cause problems. Eddie was placed on a strict rotation diet with avoidance of all allergenic foods. Liver was supplemented in his diet. Other supplementation included B complex, Vitamin E, octacosanol, evening primrose oil, dimethyglycine, buffered Vitamin C, multimineral complex, zinc, Vitamin A, and free-form amino acids. Later glutathione, phosphatidyl choline, and pancreas compound were added.

Over the next month Eddie's foster mother kept in contact with the clinic by phone, as they lived two hours away. She informed me that he was talking more, alert, and now potty-trained completely. However, when the evening primrose supplement ran out and was not refilled for six days, Eddie had slipped back dramatically (reverted to parrot speech and mental dullness).

Four months after the start of Eddie's nutrient/diet program, his foster mother brought him in for a follow-up. I had not spoken to Eddie's mother in the last few months and was pleased when Eddie's name appeared on my appointment list. It was a wild day when Eddie came in and I was running in twelve directions. I rushed out into the waiting area to photocopy papers the secretary couldn't get to and that I needed immediately. As I placed the paper on the machine and was about to push the start button, a clear voice piped up: "Can I push the button?" I looked down and there was Eddie. I blinked and looked again. How could this be Eddie? Four months before, he had been dull, without expression or interest in anything. He wouldn't have known what a button was, let alone verbally ask to push it. Now he was smiling up at me! I was confused, and I looked around for his foster mother. Yes, there she was, her eyes dancing with excitement. "He's just been retested by psychologists at the testing center, and they said he is *no longer retarded!*" He was in the low-normal range of intelligence but out of the retarded range, which surprised the psychologists, as they had never seen a child with fetal alcohol syndrome who was not retarded. Previously, they had determined that Eddie was severely retarded; thus the new evaluation caused a stir of interest and excitement. Eddie was speaking in complete sentences, he was bright and alert, his coordination had improved, his skin had softened, and the outbursts had ceased. I couldn't believe it, his foster mother couldn't believe it—but there was Eddie smiling up at us.

One year later, Eddie continued to soar with improvement. Today, at five, Eddie has attended preschool and can print his name, knows the letters of the alphabet, counts, and has begun to read. He's on his way! I applaud you, Eddie, and your very special family who adopted you so that all your needs could be fulfilled and you would always be accepted, understood, and loved.

Brian

Brian, also an adopted child, displayed severe hyperactivity when his parents took him into their home at sixteen months of age. The agency had suggested that the parents keep Brian in a playpen or crib at all times because the hyperactivity was so intense. Brian's adoptive mother didn't listen, as she had waited a long time for a baby and was willing to give him all her attention and energy. From age two until his present eight years of age, Brian's parents had taken him to a long string of doctors for help. Of all the evaluations, tests, diets, and drugs that had been attempted, none seemed to improve Brian's hyperactivity, which was complicated as he grew older with unprovoked violent behavior. His fist would go through a wall, he would kick someone, he would scream obscenities without apparent cause—it would occur out of the blue. Yet during my interview with Brian and his parents, I was deeply impressed by the warmth and love that obviously flowed from parents to child and from child to parents. I was shocked later when Brian's mother told me privately that the last doctor had told her that Brian's problems were all due to her because she "really didn't love Brian." Nothing could have been further from the truth! Besides, the child's hyperactivity had begun before she had any contact with Brian.

For some doctors, it is impossible to say, "I don't know the answer to your child's problem." It's as if it were a sign of weakness not to know the answer. And thus the blame is tranferred to the parent ("You don't really love him").

Brian had previously been through scratch allergy testing and elimination diets to no avail. But not once had any doctor suggested that sugar be eliminated from his diet! Brian's diet had always included many sugary, processed foods, so the first course of action was to eliminate those foods.

Testing revealed that Brian was prediabetic, with a blood-sugar reading one hour after drinking the glucose solution of 280! Mineral testing indicated deficiencies of chromium and zinc. Food-allergy testing of commonly eaten foods showed no allergy whatsoever.

Brian's testing results did not follow the usual pattern that is seen when professionals work with similar health problems. And Brian's symptoms did not follow the usual pattern either. He was clearheaded and alert, warm and affectionate with his parents, and was as much confused about his violent outbursts as his parents were. He wanted help!

We began a supplement program (Vitamin A, B complex, pancreas compound, Vitamin E, multimineral complex, buffered Vitamin C, pyridoxal-5-phosphate, phosphatidyl choline, zinc, magnesium, GTF chromium, octacosanol, free-form amino acids) and suggested a natural-foods diet that restricted concentrated natural sweeteners such as honey and dried fruit.

After one month there was some improvement in Brian's hyperactivity, but he continued to have violent outbursts.

Finally we solved the problem of Brian's unprovoked outbursts with a careful diet diary. Every time Brian ingested simple carbohydrates—juice, fruit, milk, honey, and especially sugar when it was experimentally introduced—he would go into an uncontrollable rage. With careful monitoring of Brian's diet, the violent outbursts disappeared altogether, as did his hyperactivity. As long as Brian's diet is maintained, peace reigns in Brian's world.

Lindsey and Lance

Lindsey and Lance were twelve-year-old fraternal twins who came to our clinic after their mother's severe allergic condition was resolved. Lindsey and Lance had very different health problems that required general suggestions with minimal testing.

Lindsey was troubled with recurrent infections (colds and sore throats), fatigue, nervousness, diarrhea, constipation, abdominal bloating, sensitive skin, and acne. Her diet was relatively good, since their mother had changed the family's diet when she had changed her own, but it did contain a lot of wheat. Lindsey's glucose-tolerance test was slightly abnormal, and her blood test revealed iron-deficiency anemia.

A more varied diet and supplementation (B complex; pancreas compound; Vitamins A, E, C, and B$_{12}$; zinc; iron; free-form amino acids; and multimineral complex) was suggested. All symptoms cleared up except for the acne. With the suggestion of the total elimination of wheat from her diet, the acne cleared up beautifully.

Lance was troubled with symptoms only when traveling in the car and during the spring season. In the spring, when baseball season started, Lance became, according to his mother, tense, irritable, and "antsy, with a negative attitude." His eyes were itchy, crusty, watery, swollen, and painful. He became "unglued" over little things and was very difficult to live with. The rest of the year he was an active, bright, easygoing boy except during long rides in the car, when he would fall apart emotionally and get sick to his stomach.

Lance's blood-sugar test was in the normal range, but allergy testing revealed that there were problems with trees, grasses, and chemicals. Grasses provoked crying and feelings of rage (Lance would sit and clench and unclench his fists trying to control himself), trees provoked itchy, watery eyes, and ethanol (in car exhaust) provoked irritability and black circles under his eyes.

Treatment with allergy-neutralization drops and general supplementation (buffered Vitamin C, multivitamin-mineral complex) cleared up Lance's springtime and travel difficulties completely.

One year later the twins and their mother are "feeling great" and symptom-free.

Austin

Austin was brought into our clinic for help with his hyperactive condition. At eight he was plagued not only with hyperactivity but with bed-wetting, hay fever, stomachaches, excessive thrist, inability to concentrate, short attention span, mood swings, fungus on his feet, sleeping difficulties, nasal congestion, and recurrent infections.

Testing revealed that the recurrent ear infections and colds Austin had suffered since infancy had impaired his hearing. He was anemic; had indications of deficiencies of zinc, chromium, magnesium, and calcium; and was hypoglycemic.

Austin had been on a completely natural-foods diet with total avoidance of sugar. The Feingold diet had also been attempted, without success. Ritalin was used to control his hyperactivity but did not improve his poor grades (C's and D's), his moodiness, and his generally depressed attitude.

Allergy testing showed malt, pepper, yeast, cinnamon, cheese, cola, grape, mint, spinach, wheat, beef, milk, and orange as provoking hyperactivity. Everyone in the testing room was quite aware of his reactions to particular foods. Often Austin brought his schoolwork, and dramatic changes in handwriting and learning performance would occur when he reacted to something for which he was being tested.

Treatment included a rotation diet, avoidance of provocative foods, supplementation (beta carotene, buffered Vitamin C, pyridoxal-5-phosphate, Vitamin E, octacosanol, phosphatidyl choline, multimineral complex, iron, B_{12}, zinc, chromium, selenium, magnesium, pantothenic acid, pancreas compound, free-form amino acids), and allergy-neutralization drops.

In the three-month follow-up, Austin's mother reported that Austin's schoolwork had improved, his attention span was much longer, his hyperactivity a little better, he seemed happier, and his congestion, bed-wetting, and stomachaches had disappeared. The fungus on his feet persisted, however, and nystatin therapy was added to his program.

Retesting and reevaluation at the six-month checkup revealed that Austin's glucose-tolerance test was now normal, his anemia was resolved, and his hearing was greatly improved. Austin's grades had gone from C's and D's to straight A's, and he was happy and content. Austin's mother then reluctantly asked if she could speak with me alone. She began, "I know I shouldn't complain because Austin is so much better. He's happy now, whereas before he seemed so lost and unhappy. He feels good, and he tries so hard to follow the diet and take his supplements at the right time; but the truth is, he is still hyperactive. Oh, it's better, but it's still there."

We decided to try a strict rotation diet of rare foods for one week to see if there was a change in the hyperactivity. One long week for Austin that took a lot of willpower even most adults don't have! But the hyperactivity persisted. Next we tried evening primrose oil as a supplement. Within *three days* Austin's mother called, ecstatic, to tell the news that Austin's hyperactivity was gone! "I can't believe it," she said. "I can sit down to a relaxing evening with him and no more wiggling!"

Two years later, Austin's mother reports that Austin's schoolwork is excellent, he gets along great with other children, and he didn't miss one day of school all last year. His hyperactivity begins to resurface when the evening primrose dosage is reduced. Austin no longer lives under the shroud of a clouded mind but is free to experience life to the very fullest degree.

PART III

Solving

Now that it is clear that everyone has a metabolic pattern all his or her own, it becomes more obvious that disease may occur in selected individuals simply because they have genetic nutrient needs that are difficult to meet. Likewise, genetically derived individuality causes people to react very differently to potentially deleterious substances.

DR. ROGER WILLIAMS

TWELVE

A Fresh Start

Upon learning that you or your child (or children) have food sensitivities, you may vow that the next child will be fed properly to prevent allergic manifestations and other nutrition-related difficulties. To understand the influences that may affect a child, however, one must go back before conception, to the time when the groundwork for the child's health really began.

The Genetic Reflection

Classical allergies, which are commonly recognized allergies like eczema and asthma, have a tendency to run in families. If one member has sensitivities, others may have them as well. Cerebral (brain) allergies also may follow a genetic (family) pattern, predisposing the child's nervous system enzymatically and chemically to allergic (or other nutritional) insult. Children with cerebral allergies often have a history of diabetes, heart disease, schizophrenia, and alcoholism in their families. This is a sign that the child has probably inherited familial metabolic weakness, such as an inability to properly metabolize sugars, fats, and so on. Knowledge of such a history enables you to improve your health before conception and during the prenatal period, so that your children enter the world strong and healthy, better able to withstand genetic (family) weaknesses which we all have in one form or another. An inordinate need for particular nutrients can (and does) occur, causing one child to develop deficiencies/imbalances more easily than others. Yet if you liberally supply yourself and your children with all the essential nutrients along with an optimal diet, the likelihood of their experiencing nutritional inadequacies or allergy problems is considerably diminished.

To ensure a child's health, both parents should participate in gaining an optimal health level before conception. The earlier parents begin fulfilling their nutritional needs, the better prepared they will be to fulfill the nutritional needs of their children. If one or both parents have nutritional deficiencies, allergies, or other health problems, these diffculties should be brought under control as much as possible before children are conceived with a superior diet, supplements, pure water, proper exercise, clean environment, and a relaxing, loving atmosphere. By overcoming their own nutritional problems, parents can help prevent them from becoming their offspring's nutritional problems.

Growing Together

The food that nourishes mother and baby during pregnancy needs to be chosen carefully, as all nutrients are crucial to the development of the fetus. The phenomenon of severe nutrient deficiencies/imbalances may cause profound disturbances in the formation of the fetus if they occur during the first three months, but other profound problems also may arise if the fetus is improperly nourished after that time. Drugs and medications also may interfere with the development and health of the fetus; they include such common but potentially troublemaking items as aspirin and cough syrup. All drugs and medications should be strictly avoided unless absolutely essential and prescribed by a physician who is aware of the pregnancy. Better yet, have the doctor's nurse look up and photocopy any information on the drug prescribed in the Physician's Desk Reference and discuss with your doctor any potential harm it could have on the fetus.

Exposure to chemical contactants and inhalants should also be avoided. Such activity as oven cleaning, painting, spraying or insecticides, cigarette smoking, and the like should never be attempted during pregnancy. If someone else must do these things, the house should be thoroughly aired before the pregnant mother returns to it.

The diet plan must, of course, be designed to each mother's unique needs, but primarily it should contain:

1) Fish (use as much as possible), fowl, eggs, and meat (use organically grown organ meats)
2) Dairy products such as pure milk, plain yogurt, natural cheeses, non-instant low heat powdered milk (if milk is tolerated), butter
3) Whole grains and legumes
4) Fresh fruits and vegetables (as many as possible eaten raw or steamed gently)
5) Sprouts (sprouted seeds, legumes, grains)
6) Raw seeds and nuts
7) Freshly squeezed juices (fruit and vegetable)
8) Unsaturated, unrefined oils (a variety)
9) Supplement foods—desiccated liver, nutritional yeast, wheat germ, lecithin, kelp, aloe vera, garlic, fiber (wheat, oat, rice bran) as tolerated
10) Pure water
11) Allergy-free vitamin/mineral supplements (free of derivatives or additions of milk, soy, wheat, corn, and so on), which should include:

Cod-liver oil, wheat-germ oil, evening primrose oil
Vitamin E, mixed tocopherols
B complex
Vitamin C with bioflavinoids
Mineral complex with trace minerals
Digestive aid—pancreatic enzymes—if needed

The ingestion of high-quality allergy-free food will keep a steady flow of nutrients to the fetus and also will keep the blood-sugar level stabilized. Carbohydrate, protein, and fat will need balancing in the diet, but with special attention to the quality and variety of the chosen foods.

It is a good idea to keep food choices as varied as possible. If you discover a sensitivity to a particular food, avoid it as much as possible. Rotating your foods will minimize allergic complications. Supplementation of allergy-free vitamins and minerals when allergic interference occurs is an important consideration to ensure mother's and child's well-being.

Looking back with guilt at what you unknowingly provoked during previous pregnancies can bring on a painful case of the if-onlies: "If only I had known." Often as I look back at my pregnancy with my firstborn, I am overcome with the feeling that I antagonized and perhaps caused my child's sensitivites, even though I ate what I believed to be a superior diet. My son is sensitive to wheat and oranges, two foods that I consumed in great quantity when I was pregnant. Whole wheat and oranges are nutritious foods, but if you are allergic to them and eat them to excess they are not useful to the body and may even result in harm.

A fresh start does not have to begin before conception (although this is the ideal) but may occur when we have the knowledge to begin. If you possess knowledge of how to overcome your child's difficulties and fail to respond to it, that is the time to feel guilty.

Your Babe Is Born

Birth brings about a physical separation of mother and child, but the mother's continued link, bonding her closely, is her loving care of her newborn. Nourishing this new being is as important after birth as it was before, and because this is so, nature provides the perfect nourishment—mother's milk.

Nursing an infant usually continues throughout the first year, sometimes two, with the introduction of solid food occurring between the fifth and seventh months of life. It may be offered first in the form of a ripe banana or papaya or pear or avocado in tiny pureed or finely mashed portions.

The addition of one food at a time and the rotation of these foods is easily accomplished, since you have complete control over what the infant is ingesting, and a tug-of-war with the child's food preferences is not present to inhibit your efforts. The manipulation of the infant's diet offers the best circumstances to test, and even prevent, allergic manifestations. When foods are introduced one at a time, it is easier to isolate the allergenic offenders. Food mixtures (a stew, for example) can confuse the issue and should be avoided until every food you intend to mix has been individually tested. Simplicity is the key to an infant's diet. It isn't necessary or practical to prepare casseroles or other such dishes, since the baby is perfectly satisfied and really better off with a meal consisting of two to four foods. The introduction of solids too soon can predispose the infant to allergies. The order in which foods are added is at the parents' discretion, but the following pattern is suggested:

1) Fruits and vegetables (fresh only) pureed and in freshly squeezed, diluted juice form (Use caution with the addition of citrus until after age one year.)
2) Seeds and nuts finely ground (add to pureed vegetables and fruit)
3) Nutritional yeast (a pinch to ⅛ tsp to begin)
4) Fish (use this frequently), poultry, organically grown organ meats, eggs (Muscle meats may be used, but they are not as nutritious as organ meats; salty or preserved protein foods like bacon, ham, and luncheon meat should be strictly avoided; use eggs with caution, since they may provoke allergy.)
5) Milk products (The child's milk supply will be from breast milk; later when milk products are cautiously introduced use plain yogurt, goat's milk and goat's-milk cheese before introducing the harder-to-digest cow's milk and cheeses.)
6) Grains and legumes (These foods should be the last added to the diet; cereals are commonly added first because they are said to "stick to the ribs"—which comes from the attitude "never mind what the food offers nutritionally, just so it fills them up." Stuffing cereal into babies does not make them stop crying, nor does it help them to sleep through the night. It does, however, sit like a lump in their stomachs, since before the age of ten months to one year their bodies are too immature to digest this starchy mass of refined cereal.)

All foods should be rotated as much as possible. Variety is essential. Milk products, grains, legumes, eggs, and citrus are best avoided until after the age of ten to twelve months, as these are often major allergenic offenders. If food sensitivities do not exist in your family, you may add citrus and egg yolk a little sooner.

One food sensitivity that might be easily overlooked is the mother's sensitivity to particular foods which may in turn affect the infant through her milk supply. Research by a prominent immunologist, Dr. W. A. Hemmings of the University College of North Wales, has indicated that polypeptide proteins (from improperly broken-down foods) can pass into the mother's milk. Evidence also has shown that these proteins can cross the placenta into the unborn fetus. Therefore, an infant can be sensitized very early in life, even before birth!

Allergic responses may be evoked from more evasive sources such as exposure to inhalants and contactants; thus care should be taken as to what is put on the baby's skin and what the baby inhales. Perfumed powders, lotions, premoistened cloths, and the like should be avoided. If an irritation should occur, rubbing with the contents of a Vitamin E capsule or pure aloe vera gel is usually all that is needed. The healthy baby who is breast-fed, is offered only natural, highly nutritious foods, and is changed and bathed frequently has beautiful skin that does not need oils and powders, especially those containing substances that may cause irritation.

Supplements for infants will be first supplied through breast milk, but when solid food is well situated in the diet, wheat-germ oil, evening primrose oil, and Norwegian cod-liver oil may be used to supply vitamins A-D-E; nutritional yeast, finely ground seeds, and organically grown desiccated (dried) or fresh liver for minerals and B vitamins; and fresh fruits and rosehip powder to meet Vitamin C needs.

Preventing nutrition-related problems is much easier than trying to overcome them after they have taken hold. Every child deserves a fresh start so he or she will not be held back by a body and mind that are nutritionally unfulfilled.

THIRTEEN

Cafeteria Capers

Efforts to establish wholesome food in children's diets is often complicated by what is offered where they spend a large portion of their day—in school. What a child eats and drinks there is governed by what is available, which, nutritionally speaking, usually isn't much. Not only is the school lunch a nutritional disaster, but all the extras within easy reach in vending machines further challenge the children's brains to function normally.

Finally, though, the push toward improving food available to school-children is gaining wider acceptance now that many teachers and parents are realizing that the effect of nonnutritive food reaches far beyond the school lunchroom—it boldly enters the classroom.

Teachers Who Cannot Teach

How can a teacher instruct a class when the functioning of the cortex, or thinking part, of the pupils' brains is limited by inadequate nourishment? Instead of teaching, the teacher ends up trying to gain control of a roomful of children who not only are unequipped to learn, but are not in full control of themselves. Frustration and anger build up on both sides—a situation that makes learning a difficult experience indeed.

For children to be alert and ready to learn, they must be fed food that fulfills nutritional needs. And to ensure that teaching and learning proceed without disruptions, the entire class must have nutritious food available. All the children are involved in the learning experience together; one child who comes to school with a properly nourished brain cannot benefit or enjoy school as much if other children in the class cause disruptions due to inadequately nourished brains. And it would be so much easier for children to make the transition to eating wholesome food if good nutrition were discussed and encouraged in the classroom and natural food were available in the lunchroom.

The Great Sugar Escape

Now that more and more children are exhibiting subtle and not-so-subtle behavior and learning difficulties, we are realizing the necessity of removing refined foods from menus at school as well as at home. Some parents supply their children with a nutritious lunch and snacks to take to school, while other parents go a step further and demand that candy and pop vending machines be done away with and replaced with wholesome snacks. It hasn't been smooth sailing, however, as even with strong support by parents, two negative forces prevail:

1) The resistance of students to the removal or reduction of junk food which they "can't live without" and will buy at candy stores or fast-food restaurants (both invariably nearby) if unavailable at school
2) The inability of school boards to handle the loss of income the junk food in vending machines brings in

These forces, we are told, have set up an impenetrable barrier to the removal of junk food and make any revision of school lunches an impossibility. Private schools can be worse still, as they may offer only junk. In exploring private schools in the area where I live, I was shocked to see the "menu" offering hot dogs, pizza, potato chips, pretzels, soft drinks, candy, Popsicles, and ice cream. The children in one school I visited were wandering around munching on this "lunch." When I talked with the children about what they were having for lunch, one child proudly announced that he was having a Popsicle and a Coke, then promptly dipped the Popsicle into the Coke and said, "See, it's yummy!" Private schools whose programs are not subsidized by the government have no criteria to guide them in the food they offer to the children. In public schools, with some guidance, the food offered is better, but far from adequate fare. Yet molding the school lunch into something that tastes good and is good for you can be and *is* being done with great success.

The Nutra Lunch

In Atlanta, Georgia, an innovative program called the Nutra Lunch has established truly nutritious food throughout an entire school system. Sara Sloan leads this exciting food program, which grew by leaps and bounds as children at these schools became interested in eating natural food. The aptly termed Nutra Lunch includes only wholesome food while complying with all state and federal standards *and* costing exactly the same amount of money as regular school-lunch programs.

Nutra Lunch offers food that is especially appealing to goodie-craving students, as these inventive sample menus from *A Guide for Nutra Lunches and Natural Foods* by Sara Sloan demonstrate:

LUNCH I

Reuben sandwich with
   whole-wheat bread,
   natural corned
   beef, cheese,
   sauerkraut, pickle
Natural potato chips
Fresh green salad
Honey-date cake

LUNCH II

Nutra chili
Toasted cheese
   sandwich on
   whole-wheat bread
Lettuce, tomato,
   cucumber salad
Banana
Oatmeal cookie

LUNCH III

Sesame chicken
Brown rice with wheat-
   germ gravy
Waldorf salad
Whole-wheat roll/butter
Carob ice cream sundae

LUNCH IV

Nutra taco with meat
   sauce, cheese, lettuce,
   sprouts, tomato
Steamed vegetables
Whole-wheat roll
Fresh fruit cup
Nut cup

LUNCH V

Tuna fish salad on crisp
   lettuce and tomato
Baked potato/butter
Cracked-wheat roll
Carob devil's food cake

The Nutra Program also offers alternatives to the standard tray-type lunches for older students who are dieting, would like to eat outside, or are in a hurry:

1) Trim-A-Pound (chef's salad with 3 ounces of protein)
2) Karry-Out Lunch (a sandwich on whole-wheat bread, natural chips, fresh fruit)
3) Salad Bar (variety of fresh items for a salad)

Getting students interested in and actually eating nutritious food didn't happen automatically at Fulton County schools. Using the classroom as an extension of the lunchroom for the introduction of new foods and good nutrition opened the way for the Nutra Lunch.

What's Going On in the Classroom?

The interlocking process of learning about nutrition and eating nutritious food makes the classroom the perfect place to experiment with growing, making, and eating natural food. Baking bread, taking field trips making ethnic dishes, doing food comparisons, and creating fun snacks are just a few ways of contributing to a child's nutritional knowledge.

In the participating Fulton County schools, students are given the opportunity to organize health-and-nutrition clubs, teachers are encouraged to schedule a mini-nutrition time each day, and announcements are made over the school intercom a few times each week concerning nutrition. To acquaint parents with new food information, suggestions on how to prepare natural food are sent home.

Bring On the Real Food

The very basis of establishing nutritious food at your school is to spark an interest among parents, school-board members, administrators, teachers, the food-service director, the school nurse, and the local media. The support of a local physician interested in nutrition would also be helpful. Pass out samples of "Nutra" food at school functions and meetings to emphasize your point.

Once you have aroused interest you are ready for the next step. The changeover to natural foods in the cafeteria requires an exploration of how others succeeded at it. Sara Sloan covers most of the planning for you in her book *A Guide for Nutra Lunches and Natural Foods.*[1] Suggestions on how to persuade schools to revise lunch programs and how other schools carried it through can be obtained from NUTRA.[2]

Attempts to remold the food offered at school may require extreme gradualism and will be marked with a sprinkling (often a great deal) of frustration at first. But it is more important to help ensure that all the children are offered food which meets their nutritional needs than to give in to a few stubborn people who don't want to change. Changing others' minds is not easy, nor can it be done alone. It is something each of us needs to think about though, and join with others to do something about.

The food offered at school, even the Nutra Lunch, does not supply for the sensitive child the rotation and elimination that may be needed, so lunches from home will be necessary. But on a wide scale, children whose problems revolve primarily around the desperate need to eliminate empty foods from their diets (and this includes every child) can make tremendous nutritional strides in such programs as the Nutra Lunch. It is hoped this influence will extend into the home.

FOURTEEN

Untangling
the Food Maze

Remolding a child's diet to fit particular needs can be accomplished easily if the transition is gradual. An extended period of adjustment may be possible for the child who does not portray any profound difficulties, but for overresponsive, sensitive children, the urgency of their problems does not allow this vestibule of time—the changes must occur immediately. If we choose a gradual transition, the results may be so slow that parent and child quickly become discouraged. An unresolved situation is difficult to live with; to prolong it is often impossible.

The only way to effectively deal with an immediate change is to approach it openly. Children are well aware what their problems are, even more than adults, because they feel everything, while those around them just see the outward results.

Begin by talking over what is troubling the child and what can be done about it. Usually the child wants to be rid of problems just as intensely as the parents, and with their combined efforts—and those of the entire family —the transition to an optimal diet will be accepted. Perhaps not whole-heartedly, but the child may be encouraged to give it a try and determine the results personally.

Children tend to be their own most perceptive critics and often will herald improvements with "I don't feel all wild inside anymore" or "I am filled up with happiness" or "The words don't run all over the page now!" Some dysperceptions, however, may be perceived by the child to be normal or "a part of me that's secret" because they have been present for an extended period of time or the child is fearful others will find out about them.

The lessening of these dysperceptions as the diet is improved will give way to the child's realization they were not normal or inescapable, and the child may begin to talk about what was previously experienced.

A thorough but simple explanation of the diet (varying considerably depending on age of the child) should be outlined, so that the child clearly understands the modifications in food choices. It also should be stressed that cravings for sugar, chocolate, wheat, milk, or other allergens may be extremely hard to ignore, and the responses that accompany this addictive phase may get worse before they get better.

The diet will be the most rigid in the first few weeks, as that is the crucial testing time, but afterward will be extended to include food mixtures such as cakes or cookies made with nutritious ingredients. These are difficult to include at first during the testing for sensitivities because they contain so many ingredients that are possible allergens. Evenutally most whole foods that were removed on a temporary basis will be reinstated on a rotation basis.

Although most allergens (termed unfixed allergens) can be put back into the diet after a few weeks to several months of avoidance, the child should be made aware that fixed (permanent) allergens (as wheat, milk, or citrus sometimes are) may require years or possibly will never be safely returned. In all likelihood, six to twelve months' avoidance of a fixed allergen will take care of intense responses as long as the food is then rotated very carefully, but the child needs to know that the avoidance time is different for every child and for every food.

Mistakes may occur at first, as the child may find resisting certain foods difficult. Assurance should be given that the addictive nature of some foods (sugar especially) makes it hard for almost anyone to give them up initially, yourself included. But these cravings will calm down and gradually disappear as those foods the body is unequipped to handle are consistently avoided.

A Head Start

The time to begin a new diet is during a relatively calm period. Starting the diet just before or during a holiday, illness, or vacation or while moving to another home is especially difficult. Stressful situations such as these can be effectively dealt with later, but in the beginning are usually too much to handle in the initial attempt at a new diet.

Teachers, friends, and relatives should be informed of the modifications in the child's diet, but an issue should not be made of it. Some people will be interested in what you are doing and will ask lots of questions, while others will remain skeptical. It is best not to push, but to let results speak for themselves. In the meantime, though, ask them to cooperate so the food transition will be easier for your child.

Ideally, the diet should be started when the child will be at home for the first few days—on a weekend perhaps. It might be a good idea to plan special activities such as a trip to a park, a walk in the woods, or an art project to help keep the child's mind off foods that can't be handled. Don't plan anything too strenuous; a trip to an amusement park may result in a child who is tired, irritable, and frustrated. Besides, zoos and amusement parks seem to have ice cream or candy vendors lurking around every corner. If outbursts do occur, try to be as patient as possible. At least now you know why they occur, that they will not last long, and that gradually they will disappear altogether.

The Diet Diary

Menus need to be planned ahead to simplify shopping and to aid in spacing foods so the same ones are not eaten in overabundance. Older children can help with menu planning so that the food you prepare has maximum appeal.

If you will be eliminating suspected allergens and adding them back to establish which foods cause which responses, a diet diary should be kept. So that you can easily refer to which foods cause problems, it should record:

1) What was eaten
2) When it was eaten
3) How much (approximately) was eaten
4) What responses occurred

This diet record is necessary for only about a month; after that you will be an expert on what foods cause what problems.

Some parents become so ecstatic when they see improvement in their children due to the elimination of allergens and refined food that they do not bother adding back the allergens to specifically identify the effect each food was causing. For example, the parents may know that removal of beans, milk, and sugar diminishes irritability, hyperactivity, and congestion, but they cannot relate beans to the irritability, sugar to the hyperactivity, or milk to the congestion.

It really isn't necessary to purposely add allergens back immediately into the diet to relate a response to a particular food. You will have all the proof you need just from watching the intense responses disappear. But being able to relate specific responses to specific foods is helpful when you try to add allergens (but not ever refined foods) back into the diet on a rotation basis many weeks or months later. Sometimes this information occurs spontaneously if a child accidentally ingests a food to which there is a sensitivity. Also, after a prolonged period (a few months) of avoidance, you may see the response when you try to reestablish the allergen on a rotation basis.

These methods may be used instead of deliberate efforts to evoke a response in the first few weeks of the diet, but regardless of the methods used, be aware of responses and keep a record of them to avoid confusion if the child is sensitive to a number of foods.

Mixed-Up Food

When a child has multiple food sensitivities, those containing a wide mixture of ingredients can complicate the pinpointing of which ingredient or combination of ingredients caused a reaction. A piece of cake made from scratch, for instance, may cause a reaction, but was it the flour, the eggs, the shortening, the baking powder, or the flavoring (vanilla, cinnamon, honey or the like)? So it is a good idea to avoid as many food mixtures as possible during the first few weeks of diet modification. If a food with a variety of ingredients is introduced later and causes an adverse reaction, then each ingredient should be tested separately to determine what is causing the problem. If this yields no answers, then it is possible that

1) Combining of the ingredients is causing the difficulty.
2) Perhaps you have overlooked something unobtrusive, such as pesticide residues or an ingredient within an ingredient[1] not listed on the product's label; or if you make the food at home, cinnamon or baking powder may have been overlooked.

Food mixtures also present the problem of containing derivatives of allergenic foods. When reading labels, you may be looking for "milk" or "cheese" but pass over such ingredients as "lactose" or "casein," not realizing that these are milk derivatives. The following are some of the common derivatives:

Milk—butter, whey, casein, caseinate, calcium caseinate, sodium caseinate, dried milk powder or solids, evaporated milk, condensed milk, lactose, cream, buttermilk, margarine, yogurt, lactate, lactalbumin, cheese

Wheat—bran, wheat germ, bread crumbs, seminola, flour, enriched flour, durum flour, wheat flour, whole-wheat flour, gluten, gluten flour, graham flour, malt

Corn—corn syrup, starch, cornstarch, corn sugar, corn sweeteners, hominy grits, dextrose, malt, dextrin, fructose,[2] maize, shortening, vegetable oil, glucose, sorbitol, cerelose

Eggs—albumin, whole eggs, egg yolks, egg whites, dried eggs, powdered eggs, ovomucin, ovomucoid, vitellin, ovovitellin, meringue, livetin

Often ingredients are listed in an evasive way, such as "starch," so that we are at a loss to know if it is cornstarch or another kind of starch. It is best to carefully avoid commercial foods wherever possible, as not only are the ingredients frequently questionable, but the derivatives of those ingredients may cause problems even though the whole natural food does not.

Food Families

It is not a steadfast rule, but multiple food sensitivities often follow a pattern in that foods to which the child is sensitive will tend to be within the same food family. Food families are groupings of foods which have similar characteristic structures.[3] A child who reacts to cashews, for example, may also be predisposed to react to pistachios and mangoes, since they are all within the same family.

The following are classifications of food families:

BIRDS

Duck Family—duck (eggs), goose (eggs)
Grouse Family—grouse, partridge
Guinea Family—guinea fowl (egg)
Pheasant Family—chicken (eggs), Cornish hen, pheasant, quail
Turkey Family—turkey (eggs)

FISH

Anchovy Family—anchovy
Bass (freshwater) Family—white perch, yellow bass
Bluefish Family—bluefish
Butterfish Family—butterfish, harvestfish
Catfish Family—catfish species
Codfish Family—cod, haddock, hake, pollack
Croaker Family—freshwater drum, sea trout, silver perch, whiting
Dolphin Family—mahimahi
Flounder Family—dab, flounder, halibut, plaice, sole, turbot
Herring Family—menhaden, sardine, sea herring, shad (roe)
Jack Family—amberjack, jack mackerel, pompano
Mackerel Family—albacore, bonito, mackerel, tuna
Marlin Family—marlin, sailfish
Perch Family—darters, sauger, walleye, yellow perch
Pike Family—muskellunge, pickerel, pike
Porgy Family—porgy
Salmon Family—salmon species, trout species
Scorpionfish Family—ocean perch, rockfish
Sea Bass Family—sea bass
Sea Catfish Family—ocean catfish
Shark Family—shark
Smelt Family—smelt
Snapper Family—red snapper
Sturgeon Family—sturgeon (caviar)
Sunfish Family—black bass species, crappie, sunfish species
Swordfish Family—swordfish
Tilefish Family—tilefish
Whitefish Family—whitefish

MAMMALS

Bovine Family—beef (gelatin, rennet, suet), buffalo, goat (cheese, milk), lamb, milk
    products (butter, cheese, dried milk, ice cream, lactose, yogurt), veal
Deer Family—caribou, elk, moose, venison
Hare Family—rabbit
Pronghorn Family—antelope
Swine Family—pork (bacon, gelatin, ham, lard, pork sausage)

SHELLFISH

Crustaceans—crab, crayfish, lobster, prawn, shrimp
Mollusks—abalone, clam, cockle, mussel, oyster, scallop, snail, squid

PLANTS

Algae Family—agar-agar, carageen, dulse, kelp
Amaranth Family—amaranth (leaf, seed)
Arrowroot Family—arrowroot
Banana Family—banana, plantain
Beech Family—chestnut
Birch Family—filbert (hazelnut), oil of wintergreen
Buckwheat Family—buckwheat, rhubarb, sorrel
Cactus Family—prickly pear
Carpetweed Family—New Zealand spinach
Carrot Family—angelica, anise, caraway, carrot, celeriac (celery root), celery, chervil, coriander, cumin, dill, fennel, lovage, parsley, parsnip, sweet cicely
Cashew Family—cashew, mango, pistachio
Citrus (Rue) Family—citron, grapefruit, kumquat, lemon, lime, mandarin, murcot, orange, pummelo, tangelo, tangerine
Comfrey Family—borage, comfrey
Conifer Family—pine nut
Daisy/Composite Family—artichoke (globe and Jerusalem; flour), burdock, chamomile, chicory, dandelion, endive, escarole, lettuce (head and leaf), safflower oil, salsify, sunflower seed (oil, sprouts), tansy, tarragon, yarrow
Dillenia Family—kiwi
Ebony Family—persimmon
Elm Family—hackberry, slippery elm
Flaxseed Family—flaxseed
Fungi Family—baker's yeast, nutritional yeast (brewer's, torula, primary), mushroom, mold (in some cheeses)
Ginger Family—cardamom, ginger turmeric
Goosefoot Family—beet (beet sugar), chard, lamb's-quarters, spinach
Gourd Family—cucumber, muskmelons (cantaloupe, casaba, Crenshaw, honeydew, Persian, watermelon), pumpkin (seed and meal), squash (acorn, butternut, crookneck, Hubbard, spaghetti, straightneck)
Grape Family—grapes (cream of tartar, currant, raisin, wine vinegar)
Grass Family—barley (malt, maltose), bamboo shoots, corn (cornmeal, cerulose, corn oil, corn sugar, cornstarch, corn syrup, dextrose, hominy grits, popcorn), millet, oats (oatmeal), rice, rye, sorghum grain (syrup), sugar cane (cane sugar, molasses), triticale (a crossbreed between rye and wheat), wheat (bran, bulgur, flour such as graham, gluten, and whole-wheat, wheat germ), wild rice
Heath Family—bearberry, blueberry, cranberry, huckleberry
Honeysuckle Family—elderberry
Horsetail Family—shavegrass
Laurel Family—avocado, bay leaf, cinnamon, sassafras
Legume Family—alfalfa (sprouts), beans (azuki, fava, kidney, lima, mung, navy, string), black-eyed pea, carob, chick-pea (garbanzo), fenugreek, gum acacia, gum tragacanth, jicama, kudzu, lentil, licorice, peanut (oil), peas, red clover, senna, soybean (lecithin, soy flour, soy grits, soy milk, soy oil, tofu)

Lily Family—aloe vera, asparagus, chives, garlic, leek, onion

Mallow Family—cottonseed (flour, oil), hibiscus, okra

Malpighia Family—acerola cherries

Maple Family—maple sugar, maple syrup

Mint Family—apple mint, basil, catnip, chia seed, dittany, horehound, hyssop, lemon balm, marjoram, oregano, peppermint, rosemary, sage, spearmint, savory, thyme

Morning Glory Family—sweet potato

Mulberry Family—breadfruit, fig, mulberry

Mustard Family—broccoli, brussels sprouts, cabbage, cauliflower, Chinese cabbage (bokchoy), colza, collards, horseradish, kale, kohlrabi, mustard greens, mustard seed, radish, rutabaga, watercress

Myrtle Family—allspice, clove, eucalyptus, guava

Nutmeg Family—mace, nutmeg

Olive Family—olive, black or green (olive oil)

Orchid Family—vanilla

Palm Family—coconut (coconut meal, coconut oil), date (date sugar), sagopalm

Papaya Family—papaya

Pedalium Family—sesame seed (oil, tahini)

Pepper Family—black and white pepper

Pineapple Family—pineapple

Pomegranate Family—pomegranate

Poppyseed Family—poppyseed

Potato Family—eggplant, green pepper, ground cherry, red pepper (cayenne, chili, paprika, pimiento), tomato, white potato, sweet red pepper

Protea Family—macadamia nut

Rose Family—A) pomes (seed): apple (cider, pectin, vinegar), crab apple, loquat, pear, quince, rose hips

B) stone fruits (pit): almond, apricot, cherry, peach (nectarine), plum (prune)

C) berries: blackberry, boysenberry, dewberry, loganberry, raspberry, strawberry, wineberry, youngberry

Sapucaya Family—Brazil nut

Saxifrage Family—currant, gooseberry

Sedge Family—chufa, water chestnut

Soapberry Family—litchi (lychee) fruit

Spurge Family—cassava meal, castor bean (castor oil), tapioca, yucca

Sterculia Family—chocolate (cocoa)

Walnut Family—black walnut, butternut, English walnut, heartnut, hickory nut, pecan

Yam Family—yam

The Rotation Diet

A rotation diet enables the body to clear itself of each food before a reexposure (four or more days later) to that specific food. A rotation diet:

1) unmasks food addiction by separating exposure to foods, thus indicating foods which are inappropriate to control the allergic condition.

2) helps to prevent new allergies from forming.

3) increases tolerance to particular foods when food is spaced out gradually.

A rotation diet is unique for each person, according to individual food allergies and taste preferences. The ingestion of simple, diversified foods may appear at first to be a phenomenal task, but truly it is an invaluable tool in strengthening the immune system.

Because sensitivities tend to run in a food-family pattern, it is a good idea to space foods from the same family just as you rotate individual foods. The best way to do this is:

1) to remove highly reactive foods from the diet for at least three months. Some foods may require a longer period of avoidance—six months to one year. Other foods (usually only one to three) may be fixed (permanently reactive) and cannot be reinstated in the diet.

2) rotate all other foods in such a way that no food is eaten more frequently than one day in four. Thus, if the child eats apples on Monday they cannot be eaten again until Friday. Some previously sensitive foods may require five, seven, ten, twelve, fourteen or more days' separation.

3) eat foods within the same family on the same day. For rotation of the potato family (cayenne, chili pepper, eggplant, green pepper, red pepper, tomato, white potato), for example, the child may eat one or more members of the family on Monday and wait until Friday to eat any of the members again.

Using the grass family (bamboo shoots, barley, corn, millet, oats, rice, rye, wheat, wild rice) as an example, the following chart demonstrates how to separate foods with respect to families:

Day 1—wheat
Day 2—no grain
Day 3—no grain
Day 4—no grain
Day 5—wheat
Day 6—no grain   four-day rotation of any individual food
Day 7—no grain
Day 8—no grain
Day 9—wheat
Day 10—no grain

or

Day 1—wheat
Day 2—no grain
Day 3—no grain
Day 4—no grain
Day 5—rice   four-day spacing of foods within the same
Day 6—no grain   food family
Day 7—no grain
Day 8—no grain
Day 9—rye
Day 10—no grain

or

Day 1—wheat, rye
Day 2—no grain
Day 3—no grain
Day 4—no grain
Day 5—millet
Day 6—no grain
Day 7—no grain
Day 8—no grain
Day 9—rice, corn
Day 10—no grain

More than one food-family member may be eaten on a 4-day-separation rotation. It is best for foods to be spaced as widely as possible; it would thus be optimal for wheat to be eaten every ten days or more.

Setting up this rotation diet may initially appear to be a difficult task. The very first thing most people respond with is "What's left to eat?" There are lots of things to eat, but a person who is addicted to or dependent upon processed foods often feels this way. Not everyone requires a strict rotation diet, but it is a good idea to become familiar with strict rotation so that you will be better able to vary food choices. Most children can manage without rotation provided they have a wide variety of foods, with consideration of food families, in their diet. Some children require a much more structured rotation diet, depending on the recommendation of their doctor and their ability to handle food. A complete "how to rotate" section is contained in "The Finish Line" chapter of this book. But to get you started, here is an example of a strict-rotation meal plan:

BREAKFAST	LUNCHEON	DINNER
1st Day		
millet cereal, sesame seeds, sesame milk (vanilla)	fruit salad: strawberries, papaya, pumpkin seeds, currants	turkey, brown rice, zucchini, yellow squash
2nd Day		
cinnamon almond (with arrowroot) pancakes, maple syrup, butter, almond milk	avocado stuffed with tuna, olives, olive oil, grapes	lamb, sweet potato, broccoli
3rd Day		
scrambled eggs, blueberry smoothie (unsweetened fresh or frozen blueberries, ice)	lentil soup (cooked lentils), celery with cashew butter	roast duck, asparagus, carrots, amaranth
4th Day		
sautéed banana slices (in safflower oil), bacon (chemical-free)	shrimp/pineapple kabob, sunflower seeds, pineapple juice	salmon, white potato, artichoke, spinach/red pepper/sunflower-sprout salad

New food choices not always consumed in the average diet, such as macadamia nuts, kiwi, jicama, mango, venison, avocado, and rutabaga, should always be encouraged. In this way the child's body is not overly subjected to common foods and more potentially allergenic (or preallergenic) foods. *Any* food that is overconsumed, however, may be pushed into the allergenic cycle. A rotation diet can be a creative, enjoyable diet that guides your child to optimal health.

A Matter of Beginning

Each child possesses a unique individual gauge or set of gauges which indicate foods, inhalants, or chemicals that on previous exposure have disrupted his or her body chemistry. These gauges serve as guides to feeding children properly. Determining these gauges is not difficult, as most of them are the predominant symptoms that led us to improve the child's diet in the first place.

Jeremy, at four, prominently displayed the "obnoxious" syndrome with constant whining, crying, mood swings, and irritability. Testing revealed sensitivites to about ten foods, wheat being a major allergen. With the elimination of wheat from his diet, his behavior improved substantially (an obvious sign of allergy) but also his appetite increased for protein foods, and a persistent bad breath, which his mother had not related to allergy, disappeared. Ingestion of wheat turns on this individual bad-breath gauge (putrefacation in the intestine of allergenic foods the body cannot break down), along with other gauges in the form of hyperactivity and extreme irritability and lack of control which usually climax in a screaming fit. Avoiding (and then rotating) wheat turns these symptoms off and keeps them off.

Eliminate! Rotate! Concentrate!

Children whose problems revolve around the ingestion of refined, empty foods require two steps—elimination of refined foods and concentration of nutritious substances—to alleviate their difficulties. Children with allergic manifestations require these two steps plus variation or rotation of foods to resolve their problems.

Step One: Eliminate

Processed foods are discontinued and replaced with fresh, whole foods. When allergens are isolated and eliminated (along with refined foods) from the diet, this period of avoidance lasts until the sensitivity cools down.

Jeremy's diet was fairly good, as his mother was careful to limit his refined-sugar intake. But it was necessary also to eliminate from his diet the white flour, white rice, hydrogenated fats, artificial ingredients, and all processed foods. A long list of foods to which he proved sensitive were eliminated as well.

Step Two: Rotate

Reinstatement of foods that previously caused flare-ups must be done carefully on a rotation basis so that the child does not redevelop sensitivities to them. Foods to be added back should first be tested with a trial ingestion of the food on an empty stomach in the morning, and if this proves the sensitivity has dissolved to some extent, then the foods may be added back one at a time (reintroduced at weekly intervals) on a rotation of every four days. Sometimes a wider spacing is needed and a five-, six-, or seven-day rotation may be required, so watch for the individual gauges (symptoms) to pop up. The length of time necessary for this is individual for each food to which the child is sensitive. Unfixed allergens may require a few weeks to many months before they can be returned to the diet; fixed allergens require a much longer time (six months to a year or more) or possibly can never be returned to the diet without evoking a profound response.

Initially Jeremy was sensitive to wheat, barley, citrus, most legumes, peanut, coconut, tomato, rye, oat, and potato. After avoidance of these foods for two months, peanut and potato were safely returned to his diet on a rotation basis, and within a few more weeks tomato, coconut, and oat were reinstated. Eleven months after the beginning of avoidance, legumes, wheat, and citrus continued to cause problems even when ingested in tiny amounts, such as an occasional whole-wheat cracker. Finally, after eighteen months these foods were successfully tolerated on a rotation basis of once per week with the digestive support of pancreatic enzymes. If food is not digested properly, these undigested materials—polypeptide molecules—can be absorbed into the bloodstream, evoking allergic responses.

Step Three: Concentration

Food is eaten to fulfill the body's needs; thus the more concentrated the nutrients in the foods within the diet, the more probability exists that these needs will be met. It is essential, however, that the foods we offer taste and look appealing as well as containing maximum nutrient content. To help speed improvement in the child's health, supplements may be administered by a physician, but the diet remains a child's main source for nutrients.

Jeremy's mother learned to concentrate foods in her child's diet. A milkshake became a vehicle for nutritious additions like nutritional yeast, lecithin, protein powder. Meat loaf might have any number of additions, such as a small amount of ground liver, shredded vegetables, lecithin. Jeremy slowly learned to like new snacks such as raw vegetables like jicama, carrots, zucchini, celery with a yogurt/green onion dip as well as enjoying cookies made with alternative ingeredients (no wheat).

Don't Forget the Water

One factor parents tend to overlook in nourishing children is the water they drink. Contaminants such as pesticides, industrial wastes, chlorides, molds, bacteria, heavy metals, herbicides, detergents, and so on that may be in the water supply need to be avoided. Pure spring water should be used to bypass unnecessary exposure to unknown or questionable contaminents.

Finding Replacements

Do remember that a child who is allergic to food doesn't adequately utilize the nutrients in it anyway. Nutritious foods that need to be removed from the diet because of sensitivity must be replaced with other foods or supplements that supply comparable nutrients. Milk is a good example, since it supplies most of a child's calcium requirements. If the child is sensitive to milk and must avoid it, then calcium will be inadequately supplied. Sesame seeds contain a large amount of calcium, but getting enough of them into a child to meet calcium requirements is difficult, besides increasing the possibility of the child's developing a sensitivity to sesame seeds, since they would be eaten in overabundance. Goat's milk or broccoli or canned salmon also could be used, but a sensitivity to these might occur if they were ingested on a daily basis in the quantity necessary to supply sufficient calcium. A multimineral supplement (chewable or one that can be crushed and added to food), a prebalanced mineral-nutritional yeast, or a combination of all these calcium sources (as well as the calcium content of other foods) could be used to ensure that enough calcium is obtained.

The discontinuance of other foods also may require alternative sources of nutrients. Elimination of citrus would drastically reduce the ingested quantity of Vitamin C and its complex. During spring and summer months, the availability of fruits and vegetables may fulfill Vitamin C needs, but during winter a supplement is usually necessary.

The nutrients in wheat, corn, and oats (as well as other grains) will not be especially missed as long as the diet contains concentrated whole foods. Eggs, however, supply many essential nutrients (iron, B vitamins, high-quality protein), so a sensitivity to eggs will remove some of these nutrients from the diet and will need to be made up elsewhere (liver, nutritional yeast, seeds, perhaps).

Sensitivities to nutritional yeast (children with *Candida albicans* infection are not allowed to eat any form of yeast) are possible, and other foods would need to be used (liver, wheat germ, eggs, seeds) to make up for the loss of this powerhouse of vitamins and minerals.

The elimination of most other foods to which a child is sensitive will not present much of a problem but keep in mind that the foods taken out of a diet may also have contained essential nutrients, and another source of those nutrients must be supplied.

Quieting the Storm

Children, as well as adults, often go through periods denying that particular foods affect them in an adverse way. This resistance may occur before, during, and/or after the successful removal of refined foods/allergens from the diet. Children below age six usually are more willing to go along with a change in diet—they do not yet have the wide freedom to obtain unacceptable foods that older children do. Children six and older are more capable of understanding the change, but often need convincing that their diet influences their mental (emotional, behavioral, perceptual, thinking, mood) and physical difficulties.

One doctor who works with children has found that the best way to establish the ironclad proof some children seem to need is to use the "You don't know how bad you feel until you feel good" approach. He asks the child to adhere to the new food diet for a week, and on the seventh day the child is permitted to gorge on sugary candy, cake, cookies, and the like. This method should be used only in extremely stubborn cases and under the care of a physician; responses following ingestion of so much refined and chemicalized "food" may be very intense.

Possibly just allowing the child to eat sugary foods on an empty stomach will provide enough evidence; or, if sneak eating of sugary foods occurs, gently pointing out why difficulties have flared may be enough.

An internal tug-of-war goes on within us all when we eat foods to which we know we are sensitive. We rationalize that this time the sugary food or fixed allergen won't affect us. Then when the negative reaction occurs, anger and frustration follow and often we set out again to prove we don't react, entrapping ourselves in a vicious circle.

Even when the new food diet is in full swing, resistance may be set up since the child is feeling so good and has forgotten previously feeling bad. Although physical craving for sugar goodies dies down, emotional cravings usually linger far longer. A child may give in to an emotionally irresistible food even though it tastes sickeningly sweet and initiates a response of nausea, hyperactivity, unprovoked anger, depression, drowsiness, headache, or whatever.

One child logically explained "the way it is" when he told his mother he had eaten candy at school, adding that it had tasted awful (because it was to sugary) but he had eaten it anyway. When his mother asked why he ate it if he didn't like it, he replied indignantly, "Because it was candy!"

If the child repeatedly forces down refined foods/fixed allergens after they have been successfully removed from the diet, the cycle will be reestablished, and the more the child eats the more is wanted. This is why "a little bit once in a while" of refined foods or fixed allergens simply does not work.

Our understanding of the physical and emotional struggles children experience is crucial to helping them overcome addictive bonds to foods that are detrimental to their health. We need to tell them what must be done, but also that we understand how difficult it is, and we need to tell about an experience we have had (or are having) in trying to avoid harmful foods. Supplying lots of nutritious fun foods will help the child over the stressful period, and talking about what you both are feeling can successfully quiet the storm and guide the child to a diet that is just right.

The *Rest* of the Family

The pace at which other family members revise their diets probably will be much slower than that of a child who is experiencing severe difficulties with food. Usually, though, if one member of the family has food sensitivities, then other members do also, although they may not be as noticeable. For instance, Daddy may be experiencing irritability and exhaustion which he attributes to overwork; Mother may have frequent headaches and attacks of dizziness which she attributes to the hustle-bustle of raising children. Sister may be withdrawn and lethargic, which is accepted as "normal" because she is the quiet one and causes no trouble; and baby brother may have colic, diaper rash, and congestion, and be fussy most of the time, but then "he's just a baby; he'll outgrow it."

So it is a good idea to take a close look at the rest of the family to see if anyone else is experiencing subtle difficulties. The improvement in the child whose problems caused you to improve your family's diet in the first place will give other family members a push in the right direction because they will see the improvement too. Patience will be needed to ride out the threats of "Yuk!" "I won't give up sugar!" "Grossning!" "I won't eat that!" But these outbursts will die down as we gear whole natural foods to our family's tastes.

Putting It All in Motion

With the thorough understanding of the dramatic influence food has upon your child's well-being, you are ready to:

1) Examine the diet for food allergy and isolate those foods to which the child is sensitive. This may require a physician's help, including a complete evaluation of your child's health and allergy testing.

2) Prepare your child (and the rest of the family as well) for modifications in diet, as the child *must* be knowledgeable as to exactly which foods cause reactions or are undesirable.

3) Summarize the diet briefly for teachers, friends, relatives, sitters who will be offering food to your child (give them a list of sensitivities if necessary).

4) Preplan meals and decide which recipes and foods will appeal to your child (and to the entire family).

5) Shop for foods you will need and organize your kitchen (it is best to sort out

foods that are not appropriate so you won't be tempted to use them up after the diet has started).

6) *Begin!*

Sound like a lot to do? This reconstructing and coordinating of food may seem difficult at first, but it is something that needs to happen only once. After you begin, it becomes something you do automatically, just a part of shopping and preparing meals. Minor alterations of the diet will continue as you gather more information on which foods are best suited for your family's needs, but these modifications occur slowly.

One Child's Beginning

Jasmine is three years old and most often a friendly, contented child. She has difficulties, however, with bed-wetting, dark circles under her eyes, congestion (a "cold that doesn't go away"), and ear infections and on awakening from sleep is extremely irritable, doesn't seem refreshed, and often begs for cookies and ice cream.

On occasion she has bouts of hyperactivity, unprovoked anger, hysteria. In other words, she has complete loss of control over emotions and behavior, which her mother already has connected with ingestion of sugar, a substance she eats infrequently (thanks to her mother's care in planning her diet). When she does eat sugar, these bouts seem to explode one hour afterward like clockwork.

Jasmine's diet is basically a good one, as her mother predominantly uses natural foods. Jasmine actively craves sugar (which she will gorge on when it is available), and milk, wheat, orange, broccoli, honey, yeast, and cheese were being consumed most frequently in her diet. Allergy testing of basic foods showed that Jasmine had unfixed sensitivities to milk, cheese, and yeast with an extreme (fixed) sensitivity to sugar.

Jasmine's mother wisely put off beginning an elimination diet until after an expected weeklong visit from Grandma was over. The preparations for Jasmine's diet went smoothly as her mother carefully planned alternative food choices; she already used whole foods in preparing meals.

After the absence from her diet (for several weeks to a few months) of milk, cheese, and yeast, and the complete avoidance of sugar and other refined foods, Jasmine probably will be able to ingest milk and yeast-containing foods on a rotation basis, since these sensitivities appear to be unfixed. Her sensitivities (milk, cheese, and yeast) will take planning to avoid at the same time, but should require a shorter period of avoidance than fixed allergies.

Every child's sensitivities are unique, just as responses to those sensitivities are unique. And as you attempt to fulfill your child's individual nutritional needs, you will also find your individual approach to fulfilling his or her "how to follow it through" needs.

The Emerging Child

The child who emerges from the mask of responses that once distorted true capabilities and personality is the child you had only short glimpses of before, but knew was there struggling to escape the confines of the hungry body and hungry mind. The relief of helping a child break free from this struggle is one of the most uplifting feelings you will ever encounter. It is a child you now can reason with, a child who is in control.

Of course, your child will not suddenly obey your every command. There will be further outbursts of anger, irritability, and crying, but these emotions will have a reason and purpose instead of being psychochemical responses. No longer will your child stumble uncontrolled down a jagged, unbalanced path.

FIFTEEN

The Ecologic Clues

One sensitivity often overlooked is that of chemical and natural inhalant allergens, which may occur in combination with food sensitivities. They can disrupt physical and mental health just as severely as food can, and may even become addictive.

The child who loves the odor, of say felt-tip markers or natural gas is often sensitive (and addicted) to that substance and will be able to detect it much sooner and more intensely than persons who are unaffected by the odor. I have such a sensitivity to perfume which is a petrochemical derivative. The odor of many perfumes, some more than others, bothers me so intensely I feel I must bolt from the room in order to breathe, yet others are oblivious to the odor.

The body does try to adapt to inhalant allergens (chemical or natural) by a phenomenon termed olfactory fatigue. The best example of this is the way in which the body becomes used to even an overpowering odor such as that of rotten eggs or ammonia. Continued exposure causes one to temporarily lose the capacity to smell the odor so that it becomes hardly noticeable. Although this fatigue may bring on a diminishing ability to smell strong odors, responses in sensitive persons may occur regardless of whether the odor can be detected. And this diminished capacity to detect allergens may be the prelude to "loving the odor"—and addiction.

Inhalant and contact allergens of a chemical origin include fluorocarbons, polyurethanes, epoxies, silicones, polyvinyls, polyethylenes, and polyesters.[1] However, some sensitivities may be due to natural substances such as tree, grass, and weed pollens or molds, dust, and danders. These may initiate the allergic response when the body's defense systems are not functioning efficiently, since they are potential allergens because of their prevalence in the environment. But chemical exposure (pesticides, exhaust) presents the most difficult problems, being unnatural to our environment and cast upon us without restraint.

The Onslaught Link

In our world of artificial everything (well, just about!), we ingest, inhale, and come in contact with an explosion of chemicals that are strewn in our food, water, soil, and air. The problem is adapting to this deluge of unnatural substances from twentieth-century technology which the body is unequipped to handle and should not be exposed to in the first place.

If these chemicals had been introduced *slowly,* one at a time, into the environment (requiring generations) perhaps they would not have become such a devasting threat to our existence. But we have become helpless in adapting to these substances because of the proliferation we are exposed to and with little or no investigation of the effects. This proliferation has vastly increased the incidence of stress to the immune system (most specifically to suppressor-T-cell dysregulation).

Volatile petrochemicals (hydrocarbons derived from petroleum) are a frequent source of childhood disturbances. Repeated exposure is unavoidable, as kids encounter such common things as perfume, felt-tip markers, insecticides, mothballs, auto exhaust, dry-cleaning fumes on clothing, plastics, printer's ink, waxes, polish, gas fumes, and paint, and even through the ingestion of sugar, which is exposed to hydrocarbons during the refining process!

Another major concern with unnatural substances is their unbelievable toxicity in incredibly minute amounts. Insecticides, for example, are close in structure to deadly nerve gases developed for wartime use that were designed to destroy the body's enzyme systems.[2] They also may block the oxidation processes by which the body receives its energy, prevent the normal functioning of various organs (especially the liver), and initiate in certain cells the slow and irreversible change that leads to malignancy[3] as well as immune dysregulation.[4]

This destruction occurs in minute amounts measurable in parts per million, per billion, and, in some cases, per trillion. These chemicals concentrate in the fat deposits within the body, and the cumulative effect is alarming. This centralizing of foreign chemicals is the body's attempt to prevent immediate poisoning, but as the body utilizes these fat deposits it is slowly poisoned over an extended period of time. Thus the delayed effect presents a far greater problem than immediate poisoning, since it is easily overlooked as the cause of the disturbance.

Nor do we do a good job of disposing of petrochemicals (and other chemicals). Tremendous quantities are dumped—many illegally—in unsafe sites. We watched as the horror of Love Canal unfolded, but now we are being told that that story is only the beginning. The Environmental Protection Agency (EPA) has determined[5] that there are millions of Americans taking involuntary health risks every day, simply because of where they live.[6] Concerned scientists describe the scope of the problem as staggering. No one even knows where all the dump sites are or what chemicals have been dumped. Nor does anyone seem to know the magnitude of the health risk, according to Dr. David P. Rall, director of the National Institute of Environmental Health and Human Resources in 1980.

Manipulating the environment with a deluge of untested chemicals to meet growing "needs" seems to have overshadowed what is basic to our survival—*our health*.

Inhalants That Alter the Mind

Natural inhalants to which a person is sensitive can affect the nervous system directly by triggering or inhibiting the transmission of nerve impulses or by initiating spasm or dilation of the blood vessels within the brain[7] in much the same way as the ingestion of allergenic foods. Thus exposure to inhalant allergens may cause the same frightening dysperceptions and other intense responses that ingesting of allergens produces, since they may interfere with cellular enzymes of the body and of the brain. In some children with learning difficulties, hyperactivity, schizophrenia, deviant behavior, autism, and related disorders, the problems may be complicated or even caused[8] by natural (pollen, mold) and/or chemical (formaldehyde, cleaning solutions) inhalants to which they are unknowingly subjected. Initial overexposure to a toxic compound (such as exposure to urea formaldehyde) may start an allergic manifestation by the stress induced upon the immune system.

On Contact

The skin absorbs substances with which we come into contact and they are passed into the body, often causing havoc. Lotions, oils, soaps, salves, deodorants that we lavish on our skin may cause difficulties, along with such items as synthetic fibers, detergents, fabric softeners in clothing, antiseptics, plants, dyes, and metals, to name just a few of a great many contactants which are potential allergens. The more obvious signs of exposure to contactants are severe itching, bumps, and blisters on the skin surface, but other responses may occur that interfere far more severely with the child's well-being.

At times it is difficult to ascertain whether something is absorbed or inhaled. If there is a reaction to soap, was it the odor of the soap or was it the contents of the soap rubbed into the skin? Often both inhalation and contact occur with exposure to the allergen. But regardless of what entry an allergen takes—ingestion, contact, or inhalation—it can produce profound difficulties in children.

Internal Potions

Our homes hold many potential allergens for the sensitive child—some natural, others synthetic. Although we cannot always remove from the environment substances to which a child is sensitive, we can be aware of them and avoid or substitute wherever possible. Here are some possiblities:

Beds-Carpets-Clothes—Some children are sensitive to the materials that make up or are on these items. In bedding, the problem may be in the pillow (filling of foam rubber, feathers, polyurethane, Dacron, Dynel, polyester, Acrilan); the mattress (chemically treated materials); or the sheets, pillow cases, and blankets (synthetic fibers, dyes, sizing, retardants). If problems arise with the bedding, it may need to be replaced with 100-percent-untreated cotton materials. Carpets are usually made of synthetics which cause trouble for some children and may need to be removed. Clothing may contain synthetic fibers, retardants, dyes, plastic finishes (permanent-press and the like) and may be washed with detergents and fabric softeners that are also potential allergens. Untreated natural clothing (cotton, linen, silk, wool) that is washed in pure soap may be needed in extreme cases of sensitivity.

Flying Fur—Pets are sometimes a problem because of flying fur. But before you zero in on your pet as an allergen, consider the flea collar that may be around its neck. Such collars contain extremely poisonous chemicals which should be avoided by everyone.

The Potted Plant—Plants may cause difficulties, but usually it's the mold that potted plants house rather than the foliage. Mold causes a great problem for some children, and areas where mold concentrates (such as the basement and bathroom) must be cleared of it, as well as any potted plants removed.

Cleaning with a Catch—Zeal in keeping homes spotless may cause us to expose children and ourselves to oven cleaner, polish, wax, air fresheners, mothballs, bleach (Clorox), scouring powder, disinfectants, ammonia, rug cleaners, and so on, any of which can produce sensitivities and must be eliminated.

Bath Moods—Sensitivities to perfume, nail polish and remover, hair spray, deodorants, toothpaste, colored and scented toilet and facial tissues, soap, alcohol, lotions, ointments, salves, oils, and sprays occur frequently and must be completely avoided in some cases (nail polish and remover, hair spray) and replaced in others with unscented, uncolored natural soaps, toothpaste, lotions, and the like.

The Garage Exposures—Auto exhaust often causes sensitivities when it seeps into the house through the attached garage. Items in the garage such as insect sprays, turpentine, gasoline, motor oil, paint, and so on are also potential allergens to which children may be exposed when these items are in use.

Cook-Heat-Cool—Cooking presents many difficulties such as gas fumes, and cooking odors,[9] and plastic cooking utensils, Teflon (and other) coatings, and aluminum cookware may need to be replaced or discarded. Gas fumes frequently produce negative responses, and not only might a gas oven need to be eliminated but gas heat as well. Cooling off has its problems too, with chlorine in the swimming pool and fumes from air conditioners.

Wrapping It Up—Plastics are trouble makers for many, and as a rule the softer and more odorous the plastic the more trouble it causes. Exposure to plastics is practically unavoidable, as they are all around us, but we *can* cut down on the use of plastics—especially heat-sealed packages. Foods such as meat contained in these packages are contaminated with plastic molecules when the plastic is heated. Application of heat to all plastics should be strictly avoided (such as using plastic utensils to cook with, heating a baby's milk in plastic disposable liners, or the heating of the electric blanket, which also heats up the plastic coating on the wires). Aluminum wrapping also presents difficulties for some, so the wrapping we choose may have to be pure cellophane rolls and bags.[10]

The Telephone Handset—Tucked into the earpiece of the telephone handset is a wad of cotton treated with fungicide that can be a source of irritation.

The Hard Stuff—The construction of the home (particleboard, insulation, paint, and so on) as well as furniture in the home causes problems for the sensitive. New homes are especially disturbing to many people because the insulation contains large concentrations of urea formaldehyde which migrates into the house during temperature and humidity changes. Urea formaldehyde is an unbelievably toxic insult to the immune system and must be avoided. Although the EPA has moved to stop the use of urea formaldehyde in construction of new homes, it is prevalent in houses previously built. Formaldehyde is also prevalent in carpeting and padding, waxes, adhesive, clothing dye, flame/water/shrink-resistant fabrics, and automobile exhaust (to name a few of many sources).

Blowing Out the Smoke—The air inside our homes is flooded with particles made up of dust, molds, synthetic fibers, and so on which are virtually impossible to remove. But one of the worst allergenic offenders that fly through the air is cigarette smoke, and this can be eliminated. Migrating particles inside the home are best dealt with by removal of the source of irritation, but in many cases this is not possible. The use of an ion machine[11] is helpful in settling these floating particles by spewing forth negative ions.

External Potions

The child encounters a multitude of potential sensitizing agents outside the home just as he does within it. Pollution is a primary factor, and this includes a very wide spectrum, the major sources being auto and diesel exhaust, industrial waste and fumes, insecticides, herbicides, radioactive materials, and so on. Natural substances [12] such as tree, grass, and weed pollens, molds, dusts, and danders also bother some children, causing many varied responses.

If the child responds severely to the environment, manipulating surroundings outside the home is quite difficult. The only alternative in some instances is to move to another locality or to obtain help for the child through ecologic and nutritional treatment.

Each of us is affected by the pollution in our environment, although some respond more than others. Testing has now revealed that the absorption of chemicals from the environment into the body varies in different people to a wide degree. Smog may make one person irritable and exhausted; perhaps someone else will experience tightness in the chest. These symptoms are tolerable, even though the person doesn't feel *well;* yet there are many people who respond to these chemicals in a devasting way. As we are exposed more and more to substances our bodies are not equipped to handle, the immune system weakens, our health weakens, and our reactions to chemicals are more crippling.

The School Dilemma

School is another allergenic area, presenting for some children quite a variety of potential inhalant and contact allergens:

The Academic Classroom—Chalk dust and freshly machine-copied papers bother many children, as do cosmetics and perfume worn by students and teachers. The furnishings of the room—draperies, desks, and fluorescent lighting—also may cause problems.

The Chemistry Classroom—Chemical experiments may involve inhalants or contactants to which the child is sensitive. The Bunsen burner (gas) also is suspect.

The Homemaking Classroom and the Lunchroom—Both may emit gas fumes from ovens and, of course, food odors to which a child may be sensitive.

The Rest Room—Older students may be exposed to cigarette smoke (it billowed out of rest rooms where I attended junior high and high school), and perfume, cosmetics, hair spray, and nail polish can be quite irritating in such an enclosed space. Sensitivities to soaps, disinfectants, and other cleaning chemicals also may occur.

Inside, Outside, Upside Down—Maintenance of the school, which includes the use of floor wax, polishes, cleaning solutions, germicides, detergents, deodorizers, and paint on the inside, as well as pesticides, asphalt, tar, and paint, used on the outside, may present problems.

The Ride Home—Sensitivities to plastic, rubber, upholstery, gasoline, and exhaust fumes may make riding home on the bus quite uncomfortable for the sensitive child.

Narrowing the Possibilities

Determining contact and inhalant allergens is not simple and usually requires the help of a clinical ecologist. But you may be able to isolate odorous allergens to which your children are exposed in the home by being aware of odors they seem to enjoy inhaling (machine-copied papers, marking pens, or whatever), ordors they complain about, or odors that seem to bring about a change in behavior. We can do a great deal to solve this puzzle ourselves.

Often, children already know that some odors bother them, yet these feelings may be evasive, since the child is unable to understand and verbalize. One helpful method in tracking down odorous allergens is to get the child out into the fresh air for a few hours and on returning to the house ask if any odors seem to stand out. Unnecessarily exposing any child to odorous chemical fumes should be avoided whether we notice responses or not.

The Proliferation Solution

The severe stress imposed on the immune system by environmental chemicals has led Stephen A. Levine, Ph.D.,[13] author of the book *Antioxidant Adaptation: Its Role in Free Radical Pathology* (Biocurrents, 1985), to conclude that

> individuals exposed to these chemicals are susceptible to oxidant stresses which can overwhelm the body's protective antioxidant mechanisms (supported by antioxidant nutrients) leading to neuropsychiatric effects, liver and lung pathology, and immune disorders. The protective antioxidant mechanisms maintain cellular oxidation–reduction potentials required for normal metabolism and to prevent free radical attack (destruction) of amino acids, proteins, and the lipid membranes necessary for functional and structural integrity of cells and tissues.

In simple language, chemicals can damage cell membranes, but if antioxidant nutrients are supplemented in the diet, the "oxidant stress" in the form of a chemical exposure can potentially be counteracted. Antioxidant nutrients (zinc, selenium, glutathione, beta carotene, Vitamin C, Vitamin E, pyridoxine, pantothenic acid) protect cell membranes by preventing lipid peroxidation (the combining of essential fatty acids in the cell membrane with oxygen) and the resulting free-radical damage that may lead to degenerative disease.

Obviously, total avoidance of all inhalant and contact allergens and environmental chemicals is beyond our capability. But building up the immune system with an optimal diet, avoiding environmental chemicals as much as possible in our homes, and identifying and treating food and inhalant allergies in conjunction with nutrient therapy (emphasis on the antioxidant nutrients) may serve as a successful antidote in withstanding the stresses of our brave new world.

SIXTEEN

Mom, Do I Have To?

As a rule, children do not joyously accept changes in diet, especially removal of foods they feel they must have (primarily of the sugar variety). Resistance may take such forms as hunger strikes, tantrums, gobbling goodies when no one is looking, threats, all-out refusals, and tears.

Guess who receives the brunt of it? You may already be grasping for a way to rationalize giving up; it's hard enough raising children without deliberately rocking the boat. But as you now know, children's nutritional problems are directly connected with their physical and mental difficulties and will remain intact until you move to resolve them.

I have observed that children (as well as adults) may at first resist diet changes, but as they begin to feel healthier and lose the addictive hold sugar has on them, their physical craving for fabricated foods recedes. At that point you must look for the emotional hold sugar goodies have. Examining your own emotional food cravings will offer insight that can help your children work through their cravings in their own way. Forcing a child to conform accomplishes little. Children must understand, accept, and be allowed to experience things themselves in order to believe what you teach them and to strive toward putting it into practice.

Won't, Can't, Why?

Various states of denial appear during the adjustment period of a new food diet. The main stages through which most children pass are the following:

"I won't do it!"—The first attempt at helping children make food choices is usually met with firm opposition, since it may be construed as a denial or punishment of some sort. (Remember all the times you said, "If you eat your dinner you get dessert"?) To emphasize their suspicions, children tend to use two basic ploys:

1) The sneaky-eating approach—hiding sugar goodies for later, gobbling or gorging on them at every opportunity.

2) The grouchy-bear approach—a buildup of negativism that is vocalized with "yuck!" "gross!" or gagging sounds.

Demonstrating to your children how sugar and other allergens affect them is necessary in helping them through the beginning of a new food diet, but talking with them about how they feel about the changes is just as important.

"I can't do it!"—With an understanding of the food/body mind effect, the child may conclude: "Yes, I do feel bad when I eat sugar, but it tastes so-o-o good!" To resist seems beyond their ability, and at this time (while physical cravings are in full swing) it may very well be. Reassurance that the "need" for sugar will pass and that natural fun foods will replace sugar goodies is helpful.

"Why me?"—After accepting sensitivity to food, chemicals, or inhalants the child may go through a period of trying to prove a cessation of reactions. Thus the stage of "Why me and no one else?" or "I can't eat anything!" has begun. Parents go through similar feelings of "Why can't my child be like other children?" The fact is that there are plenty of children and adults in this country who should be getting nutritional help.

Because deficiencies and imbalances come about slowly, connecting cause and effect is difficult. The "Why me?" stage is a normal part of learning to accept change and understand oneself. Encourage your children to express their feelings by communicating to them what you feel will speed their progress in accepting modifications in diet.

Standing Alone

Even though a great many children have nutrition-related problems, your child may be one of the select few whose parents are trying to get at the source of the problem. And that too can cause problems for the child. What a child eats is not obvious until meal or snack time, and other children often zero in on what your child eats and label him "different," especially if your child is insecure about it. Being different among peers is not exactly an "in" thing. The child who feels unsure about changes in diet will not easily handle teasing; the child who is secure about eating an optimal diet can disregard the teasing.

Developing a "comfortable feeling" about or acceptance of wholesome foods may include natural-food parties at school or at home; providing enough of a snack so it can be shared; inviting a few friends over on a Saturday to bake; giving a talk to your child's class about natural fun foods (with samples), or encouraging the teacher (if an interest is expressed) to teach nutrition and to demonstrate natural food.

Always keep food in its proper perspective, however. Optimal food choices should occur automatically, just as the child brushes his teeth or gets dressed without help; it is not something to carry on about—it is just done. Food is important, but it should never be emphasized to the point of being talked about incessantly.

The Parent's Responsibility

Your responsibility to your children's health is to guide them toward their own intelligent decisions about a diet that fulfills their nutritional needs. There will be high and low points as adjustments of their diets are made. The high points reflect successes in helping them overcome their problems, and the low points reflect frustrating times when the answers and the way to reach them are blocked.

One area of concern frequently encountered during a low-point episode is that emotional acceptance of the situation may not go along with intellectual acceptance. This difficulty hit me head-on several times on a personal level when my son was small; even though I knew why my son responded with hyperactivity, unprovoked anger, and general uncontrolled obnoxiousness after ingesting an allergen, and I knew he had no control over these responses, I still got angry and punished him for his behavior. After experiencing much guilt over my responses, I concluded that parents' emotional responses occur for three major reasons:

1) Deep down, many of us believe that a good swat is what the child really needs. This philosophy has been ingrained in us through our own parents. Spanking is used to teach a child what shouldn't be done, but if it is used when the child has no control over his reacting brain, it is unjust and cruel. Would you punish an epileptic child so that he would stop a seizure?

2) When children have behavioral problems, parents learn to live with them more or less because they have no choice. This increased tolerance to abnormal behavior, however, tends to decrease when parents discover that behavior improves with an optimal diet. The child who emerges is capable of behaving normally. If the child slips back into the old behavior (after ingesting an allergen or sugar, for instance), parental reaction may be "No! That's not you! I won't accept that behavior anymore!" No wonder parents react with anger. At all costs they want to avoid the nightmare that went on before.

3) The third reason is an obvious one that I knew but didn't think about much until my son, at four, figured it out for himself. Citrus was a major allergen for him. After he had eaten oranges for the third time at preschool and had come home with his third full-blown response (which I knew from experience would continue through the rest of the afternoon and evening), I reacted by shouting one of those delightful phrases parents use when we're at the end of our rope: "Sit down and shut up!" Not exactly what the child-care books tell you to say, but it can come out of your mouth automatically when you are angry. Shouting did not settle him down, so I tried screaming. And then spanking. It all resulted in a grand-mal tantrum. The next day when we were both calm after a nutritious allergy-free breakfast, we talked

about what had happened and why. I was explaining in my calmest voice how sorry I was for getting so angry when my four-year-old interrupted me: "Mommy, I know why you get grouchy and spank me! It's because you ate something you're allergic to!" An excellent point—but the little monkey also concluded that if I would get my act together and be in super-duper health, he could eat all the oranges he wanted. Then he could "act wild" (his definition of what happened after he ate oranges or wheat) uninterruptedly, since it would no longer bother me. That put our conversation back on square one.

Your own nutritional status is directly involved with how you react in stressful situations, and you need to remember that feeding yourself an optimal diet is just as important as feeding one to your child(ren). An optimal diet certainly won't guarantee that you will hold on to your temper, but it does give you a better chance to nourish your brain properly, which can help to keep you calmer and more relaxed.

Since I have crossed out shouting, screaming, and spanking, you may be wondering what you can do when your child has a low-point episode. Believe me, I know how hard it is to remain calm when the child knocks over lamps, jumps off the table, screams Indian war whoops and Tarzan calls interchangeably, practically strangles a pet or sibling, and so on, and so on. Since you, your house, and other family members might not survive this kind of onslaught, the child needs to be redirected.

The measures you use may take many forms. Whether you choose to handle the situation with a roughhousing or a run outdoors or restriction to a room will depend on what works best for you and your child. Keep in mind that these low-point responses will wear off. To buffer or possibly counteract them, your child's doctor may recommend allergy-neutralization drops, free-form amino acids, digestive supports (pancreatic enzymes, trisalts), pyridoxal-5-phosphate, Vitamin B_6, Vitamin C or other supplements to modify or stop biochemical or allergic reactions.

The easiest way to handle behavioral flare-ups is to prevent them from occurring in the first place by preventing the gobbling of detrimental foods. This often occurs because of a drop in the child's blood-sugar level, so it is a good idea to offer high quality mini-meals or supplement foods between meals in addition to basic high-quality breakfast/lunch/dinner meals. And allowing your children and yourself to express frustrations (instead of letting them smolder inside) will keep problems out in the open so they can be dealt with.

Inventiveness in keeping food enjoyable is important in making sure children willingly cooperate with modifications in their diet. Experimenting with recipes, varying diets as much as possible, keeping food especially attractive, creating recipes with the children or allowing them to create their own, including friends and relatives in testing creative food efforts, and making nutritious snacks and party food available where needed are ways to help children accept natural food as normal food. Take enough natural food on outings for everyone to have a taste, not just enough for your own child. Nutritious food should be shared and experienced by everyone.

On Their Own

Letting children figure out for themselves what brought on a response offers them the freedom they need to become responsible for their own diets. Demanding "What did you eat?" is not conductive to such understanding. Gentle nudging may be necessary at first ("You seem upset. Did something go wrong at school today?"), but as long as you are receptive and understanding of their resistance problems concerning food, they will volunteer the information needed to help resolve them.

Helping your children connect "I ate candy today" with the hyperactive (or other) response that followed also is important and can be accomplished by talking over what they feel inside and what you see on the outside during a response. Since cerebral responses usually strike within an hour or two after the ingestion of the allergen, you may not be able to hold a reasonable conversation immediately. The time to talk it over is the next day when the response has toned down.

Children are capable, even at an early age, of choosing nutritious food when confronted with both acceptable and unacceptable choices. This came as a surprsie to me at a school pot-luck when my son was four. I had been talking with Shawn's teacher while Shawn was looking over the food. He picked out what he wanted, then tugged at me to announce that the food would be all gone if I did not hurry. I turned to him and then saw the pride spread across his face. He had chosen the acceptable foods all by himself and knew just how great an accomplishment that really was.

Reality Strikes

Chances are that you will make mistakes and learn from those mistakes. Discovering how to reach your children in any matter, including their diet, can be turbulent at times. Although successes don't always come easily, they are rewarding—and what greater gift can we offer our children than a healthy body and a healthy mind?

PART IV

Specifics

Whether the psychosis is gene-dictated, or the price of intolerable strain, or the direct result of a derangement of the exquisitely concatenated chemistries of the brain and nervous system, in the end the mental sickness is a molecular disease, or it is not a disease at all.

DR. CARLTON FREDERICKS

The Finish Line

Your quest to obtain additional information bearing on children's health problems may make it necessary for you to seek out professional as well as practical help. Contained in this section you will find lists of:

Organizations offering information, seminars, newsletters, and physician referrals

Meal suggestions for home and travel

Snack suggestions that offer significant nutrient value

Buying suggestions for pure, alternative foods, including lists of companies supplying difficult-to-obtain foods

Rotation ideas and diet samples, including a program to form individual rotation diets

Supplement companies offering supplements free of allergy-provoking ingredients

Suggested reading for more information in particular areas of interest

These suggestions are a guide which you (possibly with the help of an orthomolecular physician) will mold to the child or children with whom you are working. Individual (biochemical, cultural, taste-preference, emotional) needs must be respected—encourage the child's involvement in planning the program. Changes may not occur overnight, but with the child's input there is a much better chance that the transition will be a smooth one.

The Meal Plan

Changing the diet toward pure alternative food choices does not have to be overwhelming if approached slowly. Discovering new foods can be a pleasant experience if approached slowly and as a challenge rather than a chore. You may want to begin by eating at restaurants where unusual foods are served (such as Chinese, Indian, Japanese, and so on). The next food-shopping trip could include some extra time for investigation of available fresh foods. Choose as many fresh foods as possible in their natural, unaltered state, including fresh fruits, vegetables, fish, poultry, meat, nuts, seeds, whole grains, legumes. Next consider frozen unaltered foods such as frozen vegetables (no sauces), unsweetened fruit, fish, and so on. Try new shopping experiences in Oriental food shops, fruit/vegetable markets, health-food stores, gourmet shops, and a farmers' market. Begin substituting alternatives for "the basics." Use rice pasta instead of wheat, cold-pressed safflower oil instead of processed corn oil, toasted-almond butter instead of peanut butter, romaine lettuce instead of iceberg, jicama sticks instead of carrot sticks, and guava or pineapple juice instead of orange, and coat chicken with ground seasoned sesame seeds instead of flour.

Trying new ingredients in favorite recipes may be the next step. Oat flour instead of wheat in a cookie recipe (start with half oat and half wheat), rice crepes instead of wheat, ground-nut piecrust instead of wheat, corn noodles instead of wheat in a casserole, ground almonds instead of bread crumbs. Continue by attempting new recipes and more new food choices—natural cold-pressed-oil mayonnaise, sugar-free ketchup, natural candy bars, ice cream with real flavor instead of artificial, pure maple syrup instead of corn syrup with maple flavoring. Be daring! There may be shouts of "Eeoo, gross!" "Barf me out," or the old faithful childhood comment "yuk"; but do not succumb to begging, yelling, bribing, or the old faithful parental command "Eat it—it's good for you!" Accept the child's physical and emotional need for a time to change.

In Search of . . . Food

The availability of particular foods varies somewhat in different parts of the country; thus you may wish to order some specialty foods from distributors in other areas (see product source list in this chapter). However, as long as you utilize your local resources (Oriental, health, gourmet, farmers' markets) you should be able to acquire plenty of alternative foods. Products not carried in stores can be ordered if you speak with the manager. Health-food stores usually have access to different distributors and can fill most special orders within a few days.

Although the American diet forces us into ingesting the same foods over and over again (wheat, corn, milk, sugar, orange, potato, beef, carrot, and so on) alternative food choices are widely available, just not utilized. The following food-replacement ideas may help you get started on alternative food choices.

To replace:	Use:
MILK	Nut or seed milk (½ cup raw seeds or nuts blended with one cup spring water; strain and add natural flavoring if desired), pure juice, Lakewood coconut milk (this also contains grape juice), Ah Soy nondairy milk (soy milk in plain, vanilla, carob) or Heath Valley soy moo (plain, carob)

CHEESE	Tofu, goat's-milk cheese
BUTTER	Soya lecithin spread (Canadian Soya), cold-pressed oils (safflower, sesame, or the like)
PEANUT BUTTER	Roasted almond butter, cashew butter, sesame butter, sunflower butter
JAMS, JELLY	Westbrae and Sorrel Ridge unsweetened jam, DeSousa jelly (Some jams are sweetened with honey and barley malt or other grain syrup—read labels carefully.)
SUGAR	Desert Gold honey (some honey has refined sugar added even though it is not stated on the label!) Tupelo honey, unsulfured blackstrap molasses, real maple syrup, date sugar, maple sugar, fruit-juice concentrate
CORNSTARCH	Arrowroot powder, tapioca, or potato flour
EGGS	Jolly Joan egg replacer, gelatin (1 tbsp. or 1 pkg. of Knox gelatin equals one egg when dissolved in hot liquid), or 1 tsp. additional baking powder added to recipes in place of each egg needed; Dr. Tima Soyannaise (egg-free) will replace mayonnaise (egg-free)
FOOD COLORING	Earth Grown natural food color (green, red, yellow, orange), or use fruits and vegetables (beet, carrot, blueberry, grape juices)
SOFT DRINKS	Calistoga or A Sante water (plain, lemon, lime, cherry, mint oil added for flavor), Pierre with or without fruit juice added, Dr. Tima (kola, root beer, black cherry, lemon/lime) or R. W. Knudsen natural soft drinks
PASTA	DeBoles pure corn pasta (noodles, shells, macaroni, spaghetti) and Food for Health rice pasta (macaroni, and so on), which can be found in health-food stores; rice noodles, potato or rice sticks (for spaghetti), bean threads (mung bean starch or green bean starch—may use like spaghetti), rice flake (wide noodles), and fresh mung bean sprouts or cooked spaghetti squash (use like noodles or spaghetti), Westbrae Japanese potato pasta (use as spaghetti)
LEAVENING	Baking powder may contain grain products (corn) and aluminum; it is best to purchase Cellu grain-free baking powder or make your own (see recipes)
BREAD	Food for Life sprouted-grain (no flour) breads, Essene sprouted breads (rye, multigrain, cinnamon-date, wheat) Guisto breads (millet/soy, rice, lima potato, rye), Ener-G breads (brown rice bread, hamburger buns, cinnamon rolls, hot dog buns, doughnuts, and pizza shells); if allergies are a problem it's a good idea to make your own breads, using ingredients you can best tolerate (see recipes)

CONDIMENTS   Westbrae soy sauce (wheat-free), relish, mayonnaise, pickles, ketchup; Health Valley salad dressing, mustard, ketchup; Hain mayonnaise, barbecue sauce, spahgetti sauce, salad dressing, brown-gravy mix, taco and chili seasoning mix, teriyaki marinade, various mixes for chip dip. Robbie's sweet-and-sour, Worcestershire, and barbecue sauces, and so on. Some of these products are far too complex for most rotation diets but are acceptable in varied diets.

COLD CUTS   Health Valley or Health Is Wealth hot dogs (in turkey, beef, or chicken), cold cuts (beef or chicken), liverwurst (pork), bacon (beef or pork); Blossom Distributors pure beef jerky, Garden of Eaten Soy Jerky, Bob's turkey jerky (regular and hot/spicy)

SAUSAGE   Health Valley pork or beef sausage, Rich's turkey sausage

BRAN   Instead of wheat bran try oat, rice, or corn bran

BEAN DIP   Hain natural bean dip (onion, hot pepper, and taco flavors) made with soybeans

CRACKERS/CHIPS   Rice cakes and crackers, Health Valley carrot, potato, and parsnip chips, corn chips, cheese puffs, Barbara's sweet potato chips, rye crackers (various brands), Khalsa Kettle potato chips (red chili, salted, unsalted)

FLOUR   Many flours can be used that are free of wheat and other allergens; grain flours to use as substitutes equivalent to 1 cup of wheat flour include 1⅓ cups oat flour, ⅞ cup rice flour, 1 cup soy or millet flour with 2-cup addition of starch such as arrowroot, 1 cup corn flour. It is often necessary to use a starch such as arrowroot, tapioca, taro, or potato flour in conjunction with variety flours; other additions might include ground seeds and nuts, protein powder (Richlife Glo Pro or Dynamite protein, Superprogest, or Crystal Springs Amino), nutritional yeast, seaweed, noninstant milk powder, lecithin, eggs, wheat, or corn germ; Jolly Joan and Ener-G Foods make various boxed mixes of variety flours for breads, cookies, cakes, and the like

BREADING   Any ground seed or nut flour can be used as a breading (grind dry in blender); dry acceptable breads (rice, soy, and so on) or variety flours may be used.

CEREALS   Hot cereals such as brown or wild rice, millet, oat, bran, amaranth, and so on are acceptable if tolerated; cold cereals must be simple; thus if you make granola you need to make your own from carefully controlled ingredients; available for purchase are El Molino puffed millet brown rice or corn and New Morning crispy brown rice or Oatios

CHOCOLATE	Carob (make sure the carob you buy does not contain sugar; pure carob powder is available; most bars contain milk and soy; Burry makes a milk-free carob bar), Chacopa (a new chocolate substitute from the dahlia plant)
GELATIN DESSERTS	Knox gelatin (1 T per 2 cups of liquid) with pure fruit juice or Hain gel mix (contains no gelatin but agar-agar) in wild cherry, lemon, orange, mixed fruit
PUDDING	Hain pudding mix in banana, carob, vanilla, and butterscotch, and tapioca pudding in various flavors
DRIED FRUIT	Sonoma dried fruit (organically grown); unusual fruits available, such as star fruit; GoodBody freeze-dried fruit snacks
ICE CREAM	Soy ice bean (vanilla, carob, toasted almond, strawberry, pineapple-orange, ice bean sandwiches), Rice Dream (made in various flavors from rice), and for those who can tolerate regular cow's-milk products, Haägen Dazs honey vanilla and carob, Alta Dena, Natural Nectar, and others; see recipes for homemade ice cream
ICES ON A STICK	Just Juice bars are available in strawberry, orange, grape, pineapple, and apple cider; also see recipes to make your own ices and ice bars
CANDIES	Good Life yogi bars, Cougar Crunch bars, Absolutely Nuttin bars, Dynamite protein bars, Robinson bars, Shady maple popcorn, Burry carob bars, Natural Nectar bars, Glenny's brown rice treats, Protein Aide sesame chew, Sunfield granola bars and fruit leather, and the list goes on . . .
WHITE POTATO	Yam, sweet potato, cauliflower (steam and mash to use in place of mashed potatoes)
VINEGAR	Lemon juice, ascorbic acid (Vitamin C)
SALADS	In place of lettuce/tomato salad, try new salad combinations. Sprouts can and should be used liberally in them to offer a vibrant source of nutrients. You may try: 1) spinach, jicama, alfalfa sprouts 2) shredded cabbage, watercress, radish 3) shredded zucchini, yellow squash, cucumber 4) shredded carrot, celery, pineapple, coconut 5) avocado, sunflower sprouts, red pepper

Incorporating alternative foods into meals will require usual as well as unusual meal plans:

Breakfast without toast, cereal, and orange juice?

Breakfast may still include pancakes, waffles, bread, doughnuts, cereal, breakfast cake, and so forth with alternative flours. Turkey sausage and beef bacon may be used even if pork must be avoided. Duck (or other) eggs may replace chicken eggs if they cause problems.

The freshly squeezed juices of pineapple, carrot, cherry, apple, and other fruits are delicious substitutes for orange juice. If you don't own a juicer, blend fresh fruit and ice to make a smoothie. Fresh slices of unusual fruits are a colorful treat.

Hot carob milk (with cow's milk if tolerated or soy, seed, or nut milk if not) is great for cold mornings. Just stir milk, carob powder (1 tablespoon) and honey (1 teaspoon) and heat gently—a dollop of fresh whipped cream and cinnamon optional.

Breakfast on the go may include milkshakes or smoothies laced with supplement foods (see recipes) and power-packed muffins, breads, and the like that may be removed from the freezer and warmed in the toaster oven. Fruit, seeds, and nuts are also great gobble-and-go foods when you're running late. Breakfast can be any nutritious food that your child enjoys such as a hamburger, shrimp, hot dogs, homemade soup, potato skins, nachos, or pizza as long as they are prepared from wholesome, alternative ingredients.

Lunch without a sandwich?

Lunch may or may not include bread for a sandwich. Commercial breads are available that do not contain wheat, but they do tend to be very dense. Toast these types of bread (brown rice, millet, soy, rye, potato are available for purchase) to make them more appealing. If wheat is tolerated or allowed occasionally, try different breads such as whole-wheat buns or pita (pocket) bread or sprouted-wheat bread. Sandwich fillings may include roasted-almond butter and unsweetened raspberry jam instead of peanut butter and sugary jelly, or chemical-free chicken bologna instead of nitrate/ beef bologna. Tuna, chicken, duck, cheese, and turkey also make good sandwich fillings if tolerated.

Homemade soup, chili, stew, and spaghetti (alternative pasta) are great for wintry days. Leftovers such as chicken legs, deviled eggs, meat loaf, turkey sausage, or shrimp may also be enjoyed. String cheese and turkey or beef jerky are fun foods to eat at lunch or on the run at recess.

Salads should be encouraged, but add a little imagination to them such as potato salad with lots of egg, tofu, and cheese, taco salad (ground turkey with taco seasoning, corn chips, avocado, sprouts, tomato), hot dog salad (sliced natural hot dogs, mayo, lettuce, sprouts, cheese, chopped vegetables), or walking apple salad (core apple, fill with chopped celery, walnuts, raisins, nut butter, sunflower or sesame seeds, and so on, and fit top back on apple).

Crunchy foods include nut/seed/dried-fruit mix, popcorn, carrot chips, cheese puffs, fresh fruits, vegetables cut in appealing shapes and possibly served with a yogurt or avocado or bean dip.

Such tidbits may be offered as natural-dried-fruit rolls or a fruit kabob (cubes of fruit on a stick).

Good goodies may be included such as homemade cookies, brownies, gingerbread, cupcakes, or occasionally a natural candy bar from the health-food store or health section of the supermarket.

Beverages may include natural-fruit smoothies, milkshakes, fresh juice, sparkling mineral water, or carob milk.

Snack without sugar cookies and milk?

Natural snacks are widely available. There are alternatives to cookies and milk. Try popcorn, seeds, nuts, dried fruit, jerky, raw fruits or vegetables with dip, soup . . .

Dinner without meat and potatoes? No dessert?

Eating beef and potato for dinner (in different forms) day after day isn't a good idea for anyone's health. Introducing more fish and poultry is good for the entire family. Try stir-frying vegetables; try different salad combinations for a change of pace. Shred a variety of vegetables into casseroles; chop them very fine and sauté them; or add them to soups. Homemade muffins or breads with alternative flours may be accepted if flavored with appealing ingredients (blueberries, cinnamon, vanilla, and so on). Whole grains as a side dish may take longer to be accepted, such as millet, brown rice, or amaranth (try mixing with a little of more accepted foods first, such as half white rice, half brown rice or tiny chopped vegetables). Dessert may include natural pie, cake, cookies, custard, brownies, ice cream, and so forth made with natural ingredients or fruit, seeds, and nuts.

Eating in a restaurant is easiest if simple foods are chosen—steak, roast beef, broiled or poached fish, lamb chops, roast duck or chicken, steamed vegetables, rice, baked potato, salad bar, fresh fruit, and shrimp, and strawberries with real whipped cream, custard, or a baked apple for dessert. Avoid casseroles, soup, sauces, and salad dressing (order lemon and olive oil).

Rotation Information

Using a variety of foods in the diet offers the body a wider spectrum of nutrients and reduces the exposure to particular foods that may be inappropriate. Rotating foods within the diet helps control the allergic state by diminishing the exposure to allergenic and potentially allergenic foods. The transit time for food to leave the body is 3.5 days; thus individual foods should be consumed no more often than every four days. The same is true for foods in the same food families. You probably now associate citrus fruits (orange, lemon, lime, grapefruit, tangerine) together and would assume they are in the same food family. But some food families are more unusual—the daisy family, for example, with artichoke, lettuce, safflower oil, sunflower seeds.

A rotation diet is unique to each person according to his or her food allergies, taste preferences, cultural background, and lifestyle. There are several variations of the rotation diet that can fulfill your needs and lifestyle. But the severity of the rotation diet is dependent upon the degree to which you are allergic.

The first response most people make when told they cannot eat wheat, sugar, milk, eggs (or any abused, addictive food) on a daily basis is "There's nothing left to eat!" This is because we so often stuff food into our mouths not to nourish or taste but to merely feed our addictions. With rotation, we begin to enjoy the taste of foods that may not have seemed interesting before. No longer is eating a means of feeding addictions to particular foods; it becomes a discovery of flavors not riveted in the taste of sugar and salt. Breaking a food addiction often requires a period of total abstinence from the food until it can be consumed in rotation without provoking symptoms. Symptoms that may be experienced after a particular food is ingested may occur anywhere in the body and may begin within seconds or take days to surface. If a symptom should occur when a food is eaten, make a note of it so that the information is avilable to the doctor or for reference later on.

The Diet Diary

This is where the diet diary can be an invaluable tool for uncovering problems because you can refer back to food intake/reactions and use the information to more easily isolate allergy-provoking foods.

The diary should include:

1) all foods eaten;
2) approximate quantity and time of day eaten;
3) symptoms observed.

The simpler the meals (two to three foods per meal is a simple meal), the easier it is to identify the troublemakers. All ingredients in food mixtures must be counted. For example, a spaghetti dinner may contain as many as twenty ingredients, and any one of the ingredients may cause a problem. If beef, asparagus, and sweet potato are consumed for dinner it narrows down the allergen considerably. These would have to be served simply, however —as steak, asparagus, baked sweet potato. If the steak is served with horse-radish, the asparagus with hollandaise sauce, and the sweet potato with butter there may be an additional five foods in this meal that must be considered.

Because meals will be simpler (avoiding complex sauces, salad dressing, soups, seasonings), containing only a few foods, it may be necessary to offer larger portions. Larger quantities of fewer foods per meal is the very best strategy until the allergens are identified and under control.

Coordinate foods whenever possible with respect to their derivatives. For example, if you make fish with a coating of ground almonds, use almond oil to dip and/or cook the fish in. If you choose pineapple as a fruit for a snack and want to serve a juice with it, use pineapple juice. Or if lettuce is used in a salad, try to use safflower oil in the dressing for the salad, as lettuce and safflower oil are in the same food family.

Encourage the unusual! Foods rarely or never eaten have a lesser chance of causing problems. Some unusual food choices might be

Protein—duck, lamb, rabbit, Cornish hen, venison, shark, swordfish
Vegetables—jicama, water chestnuts, sweet potato, parsnip, yam
Fruit—mango, guava, blueberry, raspberry, pomegranate, kiwi
Seeds/nuts—filbert, pine nut, macadamia nut, chia seeds

Some new food choices may be intensely disliked, and if so, skip them and move on to something else. But once the addictive cycle is broken (be it wheat, corn, milk, citrus, or whatever) the acceptance of new foods escalates. This is true of children of any age, including adults!

Move into food rotation slowly. First and foremost, remove processed, refined foods from the diet. In the second step, add new foods that have a good chance of being accepted, such as unusual fruits. The third step is to use more variety in the diet. Instead of eating beef, wheat, milk, citrus every day, substitute other proteins, starches, beverages, and fruits. Once you've made these changes you can try preparing your favorite recipes and the recipes in this book with a variety of flours and nutrient-rich ingredients. Be careful not to overuse any one ingredient when converting or choosing recipes. Cookies, for example, can be eaten daily if made of oat flour one day, potato flour another, tapioca flour another, and ground nuts or seeds on still another.

Another consideration in achieving variety in the diet is coordination of the ingredients used in recipes with the simpler foods in the diet. For example, if oatmeal and millet are consumed as cereals, it is best to use flours other than oat or millet when making muffins, cookies, breads, or any other recipes. It is also important not to eat foods from the same family throughout the day. Try to group them into the same meal or the same four-hour period. For example, a sandwich on soy bread at lunch could be accompanied by soy cookies. If you do this, you shouldn't be eating any soy foods at breakfast or dinner.

If you go out to eat in a restaurant, you'll find that it's hard to control the foods. You will probably be eating common, abundant foods. For example, if you have pasta, the noodles will be made from wheat. That is why it is best to try to eat "unusual" foods at home. You can serve pasta at home the next day if you choose noodles made from rice or corn flour; it would be foolish to use wheat-flour noodles at home when that is what you'll probably have to eat if you dine out.

Implementing the Rotation Diet

The structured rotation diet requires advance meal planning so that parent and child know well in advance what is available to eat on particular days. Organizing the kitchen can make this type of rotation more fun than restrictive:

1) Post the rotation diet on the refrigerator so that it is always at hand to refer to at home.
2) Work out some acceptable food combinations with your child and change these every two weeks so that the diet does not become boring.
3) Remove temptation—the sugar goodies have to go.
4) Organize the refrigerator and pantry into four sections (or more; some rotation diets may be five, six, seven, eight days instead of four) with acceptable foods for each of the corresponding four (or more) days of rotation.
5) Always consider snack foods for each day, as hunger often pushes children into grabbing the wrong food.
6) Create new recipes with your child from simple ingredients.
7) Freeze and label cookies, breads, cakes, crepes, and so on, for appropriate rotation days.
8) Plan meals with the whole family in mind. While chicken, baked potato, and carrots may be too simple for other members of the family, you can "spice up" their chicken with dumplings, their potatoes with gravy, and their carrots with a honey glaze—yet the allergic child can enjoy the same foods in a simpler form (add the sauces, gravy, seasonings after you remove the allergic child's portion).

The length of time a strict rotation diet must be adhered to depends on the severity of the allergic condition. Support with nutrient therapy (vitamins, minerals, digestive enzymes) is essential and shortens the severity of rotation considerably. Even after the strict rotation diet is no longer necessary the allergic individual should always vary his/her diet, with special attention to previously allergenic foods.

Zeroing In on the Allergic Offenders

You may be better able to isolate suspected allergenic offenders by examining your child's diet in detail. Begin by writing down all the foods the child eats. List those foods most frequently consumed in all meals, snacks (which may occur at any time), and beverages. Next, uncover the contents and quantity of specific foods eaten such as what kind of sandwich, casserole, beverage, cereal; store-bought or homemade; and so on. Consider ingredients within an ingredient. Does your child consume many complex foods (bread, cookies, cake, crackers) that are related to a common food denominator (wheat)? If your child has milk on cereal for breakfast, yogurt for a snack, cheese at lunch, milk with cookies for a snack, milk and cheese within the meal at dinner, ice cream for dessert, and a glass of milk at bedtime, that is a large daily consumption of milk. You may not realize how much milk is being consumed because it is in different forms and mixed into so many different foods. Consider carefully those foods to which your child is frequently exposed as you fill out the Diet in Detail dietary assessment.

The Diet in Detail

Fill in all the foods your child usually eats throughout the day. If you list a food mixture, like tuna casserole or cake, write down what is in the casserole besides tuna and what kind of cake it is. Think about how many times a day your child eats the same food like milk, orange juice, wheat, and so forth. When this portion of the diet diary is completed, list each food in the diet in the appropriate column in Table 2.

TABLE I. FOOD LIST BY MEAL

BREAKFAST:_____

_____

_____

SNACKS:_____

_____

LUNCH:_____

_____

_____

_____

SNACKS:_____

_____

DINNER:_____

_____

_____

_____

Snacks:_____

_____

List Medications_____

List Supplements Taken_____

List Average Daily Water Consumption and Source_____

List Favorite Foods_____

List Craved Foods_____

List Those Foods Child Will "Sneak to Eat"_____

TABLE 2. FOOD LIST BY FREQUENCY

Complete the isolation of potentially allergenic foods by listing foods appearing
on the next page in the appropriate columns below:

A	B	C	D	E	F	G	H	I	J
Eats more than once per day	Eats daily or almost daily	Eats large amounts when served	Eats 2–3 times a week	Eats about once per week	Eats about 2–3 times per month	Eats but is a suspected allergenic food	Will not eat/hates	Cannot eat —allergic to	Previous allergy to

List these foods in the appropriate columns in Table 2:

alfalfa sprouts
allspice
almond
amaranth
apple
apricot
arrowroot
artichoke
asparagus
avocado
banana
bamboo shoots
barley
basil
bay leaf
beans:
  fava
  garbanzo
  green
  kidney
  lentil
  lima
  pinto
beef
beet
bell & red
  peppers
blackberry
blueberry
black-eyed pea
boysenberry
bran
brazil nut
buckwheat
broccoli
brussels sprouts
cabbage
cauliflower
caraway
carob
carrot
cashew
celery
cheese (list type)
cherry
chia seed
chicken

chicory
chili pepper
chocolate
cinnamon
clam
cloves
coconut (oil)
coffee
cola
collards
cottonseed
corn
crab
currant
curry
date
dill
duck
egg
eggplant
endive
escarole
fennel
flaxseed
fig
fish:
  bass
  catfish
  cod
  haddock
  halibut
  herring
  lobster
  mackerel
  red snapper
  salmon
  sardine
  scallop
  shrimp
  sole
  sturgeon
    (caviar)
  trout
  tuna
garlic
ginger
goose

grape (raisin)
grapefruit
guava
hazelnut
honey
hops
horseradish
jicama
kale
kiwi
kumquat
lamb
leek
lemon
lettuce
licorice
lime
litchi fruit
macadamia nut
mace
malt
mango
maple syrup
melon
milk—cow's
milk—goat's
millet
molasses
mushroom
mustard
mustard greens
NutraSweet
nutmeg
nectarine
oats
okra
olive (oil)
onion
orange
oregano
oyster
papaya
paprika
parsley
parsnip
pea
peach

peanut (oil)
pear
pecan
black and white pepper
pimento
pineapple
pine nut
pistachio
plum, prune
pomegranate
poppyseed
pork
potato—white
pumpkin (seeds)
rabbit
radish
raspberry
rhubarb
rice
rutabaga
rye
saccharin
safflower
sage
sesame (oil)
soy (oil)
spinach
squash
strawberry
sugar (table)
sunflower (oil
sweet potato
tangerine
tapioca
tea (regular)
thyme
tomato
turkey
turnip
vanilla
vinegar
walnut
wheat (whole &
white)
yam
any other food
  consumed

Consider ingredients within ingredients in complex foods. Some examples:

Cereal	What grains is it made from? Is the grain refined (white flour) or in its natural state (whole wheat)? Is sugar or other sweetener added? Are preservatives or other additives contained in the cereal? Is the cereal consumed with milk or fruit or added sweetener?
Tuna casserole	Is the tuna packed in oil, and if so what kind of oil? What seasoning is contained in the can of tuna? Are eggs, milk, cheese, and wheat noodles added to the casserole?

All ingredients count.

Consider the nonfood contents of food. Examples:

Nitrates/nitrites/cereal fillers/sugar found in luncheon meats

Hydrogenated vegetable oils found in margarine, peanut butter, salad dressing, mayonnaise, shortening, cake, cookies, candy, and just about any processed food you can think of

Monosodium glutamate found in soups, salad dressing, seasoned mixes, TV dinners, canned spaghetti, sausage

Artificial colors and flavors in cereals, cookies, cakes, TV dinners, candy, "juice" drinks, breads, ice cream, maraschino cherries

Preservatives like BHA and BHT in crackers, candy, cereal, salad dressing, instant potatoes.

Be sure to list "filler" foods such as potato chips, candy, soft drinks, chewing gum, mints, refined sugar.

At the bottom of the chart note any odd cravings for butter, salt, and any other particular foods or for inedible substances.

Here is how Corey's mom filled out his food lists by meal and frequency:

BREAKFAST:

Cheerios (oat) or corn flakes with sugar and milk
Toast with margarine (refined wheat, hydrogenated fat)
Scrambled eggs, bacon (pork, nitrates, nitrites)
Pancakes (refined wheat, egg, milk) with syrup (corn syrup)
Orange juice, milk, tea

SNACKS:

Chocolate-chip cookies (refined wheat, hydrogenated fat, vanilla, sugar)
Apple, peanuts, cheese (cheddar) and crackers (refined wheat), orange juice

LUNCH:

Bologna (beef, cereal solids, onion, garlic, additives) or peanut butter (sugar, hydrogenated fat) sandwich on white bread (refined wheat).
Potato or corn chips (hydrogenated fat)
Orange, apple, or banana; carrot and celery sticks; pickles
Chocolate granola bar (oat, sugar, vanilla, additives)
Milk

SNACKS:

Crackers (refined wheat) and cheese (cheddar), bread (refined wheat, yeast) with peanut butter (sugar, hydrogenated fat), Cheerios (oat) with sugar and milk, chocolate granola bar (oat, sugar, additives) orange juice, cola

DINNER

Hamburger, steak (beef), chicken, hot dogs (beef, additives) and beans (pinto), pork chops, meat loaf (beef, pork, refined-wheat bread crumbs, egg, onion), pizza (refined wheat, tomato, cheese, oregano, garlic, onion, basil, thyme, olive oil, additives)
Peas, carrots, corn, potatoes (baked or as french fries—hydrogenated fat)
Pasta, noodles (refined wheat, margarine), white rice, mushrooms
Salad (lettuce, tomato, cucumber, olive oil–and–vinegar dressing)
Milk, orange juice, cola
Chocolate ice cream (milk, chocolate, vanilla, additives), cake or pie occasionally (refined flour, hydrogenated fat, sugar)

SNACKS:

Popcorn, cheese (cheddar) and crackers (refined wheat), Cheerios with sugar and milk, chocolate granola bars (oat, vanilla, sugar, additives), orange juice, cola, chocolate candy (sugar, vanilla, milk, additives)

LIST MEDICATIONS:

Ritalin for hyperactivity

LIST SUPPLEMENTS TAKEN:

Flintstones chewable

LIST AVERAGE DAILY WATER CONSUMPTION AND SOURCE: 3 cups, tap water
LIST FAVORITE FOODS:

Chocolate, pizza, orange juice, french fries

LIST CRAVED FOODS:

Chocolate, cola, salt, sugar, Cheerios (oat)

LIST THOSE FOODS CHILD WILL "SNEAK TO EAT":

Chocolate, ice cream, candy

Evaluation of Corey's Diet

On the basis of this list, what can we say about this child's diet?

1) Overall, Corey eats a lot of processed, empty-calorie foods. Foods with refined flours, sugar, additives, and hydrogenated fat predominate in his diet, and those foods need to be withdrawn.
2) He eats wheat, oat, orange, cheese, milk, sugar, corn, and chocolate all day long. These may be allergenic troublemakers for Corey.
3) Corey had a previous allergy to milk. Most likely he still has it. He drinks a lot of milk, eats a lot of cheese, and loves ice cream.

COREY'S DIET

A	B	C	D	E	F	G	H	I	J
Eats more than once per day	Eats daily or almost daily	Eats large amounts when served	Eats 2–3 times a week	Eats about once per week	Eats about 2–3 times per month	Eats but is a suspected allergenic food	Will not eat/hates	Cannot eat —allergic to	Previous allergy to
wheat	lettuce	dessert!	peas	chicken	sole	strawberry	fish	cashew	milk
milk	egg	pizza	carrot	rice	honey		mint		
oat	apple	popcorn	celery	pinto bean	rye		spinach		
hydrog. fat	vinegar	corn chips	pork	lemon	turkey				
orange	tomato	french-fries	banana	oregano	walnut				
chocolate	cole slaw	chocolate	mushroom	basil					
cheese	bl. pepper		tea	thyme					
peanut	vanilla		olive						
sugar	onion		cinnamon						
yeast	garlic								
potato	cucumber								
salt	beef								
corn	pickles								

4) He refuses most vegetables, whole grains, and fish. Is he getting all the nutrients he needs?

5) He craves sugar, chocolate, salt, and cola. He is using "stress" foods to obtain a temporary lift of his blood-sugar level.

6) He eats a lot of sugary and yeast/mold-type foods—pickles, cheese, bread with yeast, vinegar, mushrooms. He may have a yeast/mold sensitivity or a *Candida albicans* infection.

7) He gorges on desserts (chocolate, sugar), corn chips, popcorn, pizza, and french-fries (potato) when offered. These are other possible allergy-provoking foods.

Corey is hyperactive, destructive, and irritable much of the time. Corey's mother eliminated all refined foods from his diet. Testing revealed that Corey was in fact allergic to all the foods he craved and many of those he overconsumed. He also had hypoglycemia, a *Candida albicans* infection, and deficiencies of many nutrients. Now Corey is a calm, happy child.

Easing into Rotation

If a structured rotation diet seems out of the question, the adult or child who hears about the idea and shouts, "No way!" can be eased into rotation gradually. Don't give up before you even start! A little more variety in the diet is better than doing nothing, and is really the first step toward rotation. As time goes on you may try some new foods, experiment with a few recipes once in a while, eat out at restaurants offering unusual foods occasionally, and slowly decrease processed-food consumption. Putting these suggestions into practice can offer quite a lot of benefit for a minimal amount of effort. Let's consider the following in which a sample meal plan is altered slowly toward more pure, varied foods:

The Old American Standby Diet

Breakfast: Mr. T, Count Chocula, or Pac-Man cereal, sugar, milk
White toast, margarine, strawberry (sugar) jam
Tang or orange juice, milk
Pancakes (sugar syrup), bacon, eggs on weekends

Lunch: White-bread sandwich with bologna and mustard or peanut butter (hydrogenated fat, sugar) and jelly or processed cheese/lettuce/mayo.
Hamburger/hot dog on a white bun, canned spaghetti
Chips or fries, carrot sticks, fruit cocktail (sugar)
Cookies, candy, ice cream, Popsicles, Twinkies
Soda, chocolate or reg. milk, artificial punch, juice

Snacks: Cheese and crackers, peanuts, apple, orange, sugar cookies or small cakes, milk, artificial punch

Dinner: Beef (in meat loaf, steak, spaghetti, hamburger, hot dogs, casseroles), pizza, fried chicken, pork chops
Corn, green beans, carrots, applesauce
Pasta, rolls or bread (white flour), margarine
White potato (mashed, fried, baked)
Salad—iceberg lettuce, tomato, bottled dressing
Dessert (spells sugar)—ice cream, Jell-O, cookies, cake, pie

Lights!

Breakfast: Shredded Wheat, milk, honey
Whole-wheat toast/butter/honey-sweetened jam
Orange, grape, or apple juice (unsweetened)
Eggs, bacon, sausage (2–3 × week)
Yogurt (plain) with fresh fruit and honey
French toast or pancakes (whole-wheat) with real maple syrup (1× week)

Lunch: Whole wheat sandwich with—fresh peanut butter/honey
                                        —chicken salad/celery/mayo
                                        —jack cheese/lettuce/mustard
                                        —tuna salad/cucumber/tomato
Hamburger or natural beef or chicken hot dog (1–2× week)
Yogurt with honey-sweetened fruit
Corn or potato chips (natural), carrot or celery sticks, orange, apple, banana
Granola bar (no sugar), natural cookies or candy, raisins
Milk, fruit juice

Snacks: Popcorn, peanuts, almonds, celery with peanut butter, natural cookies, whole wheat crackers and cheese

Dinner: Beef (3–4× week), chicken, Chinese food, sautéed sole
Potato, whole-grain pasta and rolls, rice, butter
Carrots, zucchini, broccoli, peas, green beans, corn, vegetable casserole or soup
Salad—iceberg lettuce, cucumber, carrots, sprouts (a tiny bit), tomato, natural dressing
Dessert—natural ice cream, cookies, gelatin, or fresh-fruit salad with fresh whipped cream, nuts

Camera!

Breakfast: Granola or crispy brown rice or puffed-millet cereal with honey and soy milk
7-grain English muffin or bread with butter and unsweetened jam
Grape, pineapple, guava or apple juice; or a smoothie made of fresh fruit and ice blended

Yogurt with fresh fruit (banana, strawberry, and so on) and chopped almonds

Scrambled eggs, pork sausage or bacon (chemical-free)

Pancakes (mixed-grain or buckwheat) with butter and real maple syrup (1× week)

Hot carob milk, milk

Lunch: Homemade soup, stew, chili, leftover spaghetti (whole wheat)

String cheese, natural beef jerky, natural chicken or turkey hot dogs

Sandwich on multigrain, rye or sprouted-wheat bread
    with—almond or peanut butter/honey
        —chicken or tuna salad/water chestnuts/sesame
        —colby cheese/avocado/sprouts /tomato
        —turkey/lettuce/cream cheese

Carrot, sweet potato, or parsnip chips (like potato chips)

Jicama, carrot, cucumber, or celery sticks (fresh), potato salad, fruit salad

Trail mix, cashews, dried apricots, homemade cookies or gingerbread (made with alternative ingredients)

Snack: Homemade cookies (alternative ingredients), trail mix, fresh fruit, raw vegetable sticks with dip, brown-rice cakes or crackers with cream cheese, sunflower seeds

Dinner: Beef, chicken, turkey, lamb, fish, ethnic food

Stir-fried vegetables (use all different kinds of veggies—zucchini, carrots, broccoli, snow peas, green beans, bok choy, bamboo shoots, cauliflower, spinach, yellow squash, and so on and maybe even a little seaweed!)

Brown rice, white or sweet potato, whole-grain pasta—mixed-grain, corn, w/w, or rice

Salad with romaine lettuce, sprouts, avocado, jicama, carrot, tomato, cucumber, bok choy, spinach, and so on with homemade or natural bottled dressing with cold-pressed oils; or confetti salad of finely chopped vegetables

Dessert of fresh-fruit salad, homemade cookies, cake, or pie with alternative ingredients, custard, baked apple with pecans and honey, natural ice cream

Action!

Breakfast: Oat, millet, brown rice, or amaranth hot cereal or puffed-corn, millet, or brown-rice cold cereal with cinnamon, honey, or date sugar, fruit, ground seeds or other supplement foods mixed in, and soy, coconut, goat's or cow's milk.

Brown rice, soy, millet, or other toast or homemade muffin with alternative ingredients

Yogurt with sunflower or sesame seeds, fresh fruit

Kiwi, papaya, strawberries, pineapple, guava—any fresh fruit

Eggs, turkey/pork sausage, beef/pork bacon (chemical-free)

Leftover protein from dinner (lamb chop, chicken leg, and so on)

Pancakes or waffles made from alternative ingredients with butter and real maple syrup

Smoothie with fresh fruit and ice or milkshake laced with supplement ingredients (protein powder and the like)

Carob milk, fresh-squeezed juice

Lunch: Turkey, chicken leg, salad (chicken, tuna, salmon, shrimp with lettuce, sprouts, seeds, various chopped vegetables)

Celery with almond or cashew butter, beef or turkey jerky, string cheese; sandwich on alternative bread or rice, bran, or rye crackers

Homemade soup with varied ingredients, chili

Any nuts or seeds mixed with chopped dried fruit

Raw vegetables—jicama, cucmber, broccoli, carrot, etc. with dip (bean, avocado, yogurt, and so on)

Varied fresh fruit or frozen, unsweetened fruit

Homemade cookies and small cakes with alternative ingredients

Sparkling mineral water (may purchase with oil of lemon, orange, cherry added or mix with pure fruit juice), fresh-squeezed juice, smoothie, milk (or alternative)

Snack: Homemade soup, nuts, seeds, fruit, vegetables, egg, tuna, chicken or salmon salad, homemade cookies made with alternative ingredients

Dinner: Salmon, trout, flounder, scallops, duck, halibut, Cornish hen, turkey, chicken, lamb, beef

Artichoke, broccoli, spaghetti squash (use as pasta), acorn squash, zucchini, cabbage, spinach, eggplant, rutabaga, cauliflower, asparagus, carrots, and so on

Salads with many varied ingredients including sprouts and homemade dressing

Yam, sweet potato, white potato, brown or wild rice, amaranth, millet, pasta (corn, rice, mung bean, potato, noodles or spaghetti squash)

Dessert of melon, berries, baked apple with pecans, seeds, homemade cake, cookies, pie, custard, gelatin

Beverages of herbal tea, sparkling mineral water, or milkshake or smoothie laced with supplement ingredients

Rotation Creation

Creating an individualized rotation diet is easier with a diet-plan guide. The rotation guides in this book were developed after many, many trial programs in helping patients structure a rotation diet to fit their own needs. Working with a dynamic woman, Ms. Jessica Denning, who suffered from a severe allergic condition herself, I was able to find a program that was interesting and fun to work with. If you are interested in a personalized rotation diet, rotation games, or a prefabricated worksheet, you may write to Jessica Denning, 4160 Friendly Lane, Lincoln, CA 94648, for further information.

We know that foods sharing characteristic structures are called food families. The following food-plan guide separates food families by boxing them off. For example:

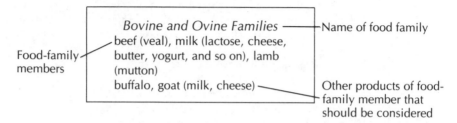

Foods within the same family should be eaten on the same day of the rotation diet. You may extend the rotation of one food family to more than four days (to eight-day rotation) if you eat, for example, beef and cheese on the first day of rotation and when you start the rotation over again on day five you eat lamb and/or goat's milk (or any other family member). This is sometimes necessary when the individual's allergic condition warrants a longer separation of foods. If a food (or foods) within a food family proves to provoke intense symptoms when your child is tested or when you challenge your child with that food, cross it out in pencil, as it should not be used in the rotation diet until it can be tolerated; it should be avoided for at least three months.

A rotation diet may be four, five, six, seven, or eight days in length. Some particular foods may be easily tolerated every four days, but you may find that some foods require a two-week-or-more separation to be well tolerated. This knowledge of individual tolerance will come with time and is something that you and your child can work with and discover together.

Every day the rotation menu will include these food groups: meat/poultry, fish, vegetables/complex starches, seasonings, fruit, oils/nuts/seeds, so that a balanced diet can be maintained. You may wish to color-code these groups of foods to make them easier to work with. For example:

Meat/Poultry	—RED
Fish	—ORANGE
Vegetables/ Starches	—GREEN
Seasonings	—YELLOW
Fruit	—BLUE
Oils/Nuts/Seeds	—WHITE

A few food families span more than one food group. The cashew family, for example, consists of cashew, mango,* and pistachio and is mainly in the nut/seed/oil group. Mango,* however, belongs in the Fruit group and is marked with an asterisk to indicate that it belongs in a different food grouping.

To plan your child's individual rotation diet, you will use the charts on pages 198–203.

Food-family Chart

This lists the names of all the food families and the foods that are within those families. After coloring the chart, cut the families apart along the lines. Place the food families in small piles according to color on the table you are working on. The red pile will then contain meat/poultry, the orange pile fish, the green, vegetables/starches, the yellow, seasonings, the blue pile fruit, and the white, oils/nuts/seeds. Each rotation day will contain at least one food from each food group (color) to keep the diet balanced. But since you are working with 4 rotation days and 96 food families, you will be able to choose from more than one food family in each group per day. Some foods to which an individual child is allergic will need to be crossed out because the child will not be including these in his or her diet.

Diet Planner

This helps you choose the food families by food group (meat, poultry, fish, and so on) for each of the four days of the diet. Using the example on the following pages you would divide a large rectangular piece of white cardboard into four vertical sections and label them across the top Day 1, Day 2, Day 3, and Day 4. Draw horizontal lines for the six food groups (meat/poultry, fish, vegetables/starches, seasoning, fruit, oils/nuts/seeds). The color-coded food families that you previously cut apart can now be arranged on the diet planner. Move the food families around on the diet planner so that foods your child enjoys eating together appear on the same day. Use a little cellophane tape or white paste to stick the food families onto the diet planner once you decide on which days to use each of the food families. It's a good idea to wait until you have completed *all* the charts before doing this. You may want to move families around a little as you begin planning meals.

Available Foods

This helps you to list all the foods you have to work with on each rotation day. Following the example on the next pages, divide a sheet of paper into four vertical columns, labeled across the top Day 1, Day 2, Day 3, and Day 4. Draw horizontal lines so that there are 10 sections that I

FOOD FAMILY CHART

RED

- **Bovine and Ovine Families:** beef (veal, gelatin), milk, lactose, cheese, butter, yogurt, lamb (mutton), buffalo, goat (milk, cheese)
- **Swine:** pork (bacon)
  - **Duck:** duck, goose, & their eggs
- **Pheasant:** chicken (egg), Cornish hen, pheasant & their eggs
- **Turkey:** turkey
  - **Hare:** rabbit
- **Deer:** venison—caribou, elk, moose
  - **Pronghorn:** antelope
- **Crustacean:** shrimp, prawn, lobster, crab
  - **Frog:** frog's legs
- **Mollusk:** abalone, clam, oyster, mussel, squid, snail, scallop

ORANGE

- **Salmon:** trout, salmon
  - **Shark:** shark
  - **Smelt:** smelt
- **Flounder:** flounder, dab, sole, halibut, turbot, plaice
  - **Anchovy:** anchovy
- **Cod:** cod, haddock, pollack, hake
  - **Croaker:** whiting, drum, croaker, sea trout, silver perch
- **Bass:** bass, sunfish, grouper, white perch
  - **Bluefish:** bluefish
  - **Porgy:** porgy
- **Mackerel:** mackerel, tuna, bonito, albacore
  - **Swordfish:** swordfish
  - **Sturgeon:** sturgeon-caviar
- **Pike:** pike, muskellunge, pickerel
  - **Butterfish:** butterfish, harvestfish
- **Scorpion:** ocean perch, rockfish
  - **Snapper:** snapper
  - **Herring:** sardine, shad, roe, herring
- **Dolphin:** mahimahi
- **Catfish:** catfish
- **Mullet:** mullet
- **Marlin:** sailfish

GREEN

- **Legume:** alfalfa (sprout), pea, carob, clover, jicama, kudzu, fenugreek, peanut (oil), lentil, beans: azuki, fava, mung, garbanzo, navy, soy (oil, milk, flour), string, kidney
  - **Arrowroot:** arrowroot
- **Carrot:** carrot, celery, dill, parsley, caraway, parsnip, anise, coriander, fennel
  - **Sedge:** water chestnut
  - **Amaranth:** amaranth (leaf, seed)
- **Mustard:** broccoli, cabbage, brussels sprouts, bok choy, cress, cauliflower, kale, mustard, radish, rutabaga, turnip, horseradish
  - **Buckwheat:** buckwheat, sorrel, rhubarb
- **Grass:** bamboo shoots, corn (oil, starch), barley, millet, rice, triticale, rye, oat, wheat (oil), wild rice, sugar cane (molasses)
  - **Morning Glory:** sweet potato, yam
- **Daisy:** lettuce, endive, artichoke, chamomile, escarole, safflower (oil), sunflower* (seed, oil), dandelion, tarragon, chicory
  - **Goosefoot:** beet, chard, sugar beet, spinach
- **Potato:** eggplant, potato, tomato, pimento, chili, red & green pepper, paprika
- **Mallow:** okra, hibiscus, cottonseed (oil)
- **Spurge:** tapioca

YELLOW			
Lily asparagus*, garlic, onion, chives, leek, aloe vera, shallot, sarsaparilla	*Mint* basil, chia seeds*, rosemary, savory, sage, thyme, mint, marjoram, hyssop, oregano, lemon balm, horehound	*Myrtle* allspice, clove, eucalyptus, guava*	*Pepper* black/white pepper
Laurel avocado*, bayleaf, cinnamon, cassia, sassafras	*Comfrey* comfrey, borage	*Ginger* cardamom, ginger, turmeric	*Ginseng* ginseng
			Nutmeg nutmeg, mace
Citrus orange, lemon, tangelo, kumquat, grapefruit, lime, tangerine, citron, murcot, pummelo, mandarin		*Caper* capers	*Horsetail* shavegrass
		Orchid vanilla	*Iris* saffron
		Fungus mushroom, molds in cheese, yeast (baker's, brewer's, torula)	*Elm* hackberry*, slippery elm
		Algae agar-agar, carrageen, seaweed	
		Honey	
		Maple Syrup	

BLUE			
Heath blueberry, cranberry, huckleberry	*Soapberry* litchi	*Rose—berry* black/rasp/dew straw/boysen/logan berries	*Rose-pit* almond* (oil), peach, apricot (oil), cherry, plum (prune)
Papaya papaya	*Starfruit* starfruit	*Rose—seed* apple, pear	*Palm* coconut (oil, milk), date (sugar), sago palm
Banana banana, plaintain	*Grape* grape (raisin)	*Mulberry* fig, mulberry	
Dilleni kiwi	*Saxifrage* currant		
Cactus prickly pear			
Pineapple pineapple			
Pomegranate pomegranate			
Ebony persimmon			

WHITE		
Cashew cashew, mango*, pistachio	*Walnut* walnut—English & black (oil), pecan, hickory, butternut	*Sapucaya* Brazil nut
Beech chestnut	*Palm* coconut (oil, milk), date* (date sugar), sago palm*	*Conifer* pine nut
Flax flaxseed	*Birch* filbert, oil of wintergreen	*Olive* olive (oil)
Pedalium sesame seed (oil, tahini)	*Poppy* poppyseed	*Protea* macadamia
Psyllium Psyllium seed		

DIET PLANNER

	DAY ONE	DAY TWO	DAY THREE	DAY FOUR
MEAT/ POULTRY (red)				
FISH (orange)				
VEGETABLES/ STARCHES (green)				

				SEASONING (yellow)
				FRUIT (blue)
				NUTS/ SEEDS (white)

AVAILABLE FOODS

	DAY ONE	DAY TWO	DAY THREE	DAY FOUR
PROTEIN				
VEGETABLES				
FRUIT				
COMPLEX CARBOHY-DRATES				

NUTS/ SEEDS			
FATS			
SEASONING			
SWEETENERS			
BEVERAGES			
SNACKS			

suggest be labeled: Protein, Vegetables, Fruit, Complex Carbohydrates, Nuts/Seeds, Fats, Seasoning, Sweeteners, Beverages, Snacks. After placing the food families on the desired days on the diet planner, list the individual foods within each family that you will have to work with on the Available Foods guide. The Available Foods guide enables you to see at a glance exactly what foods are available to work with on each day.

Meal Planner

The meal planner on pages 206–7 will help you combine foods that make up individual meals on each of the four rotation days. Using the list of Available Foods, you can plan meals day by day.

Combining foods is challenging but can be fun. If you and your child make some mistakes, try again; mistakes have to be made for one to learn from the experience. If you go on a vacation for a few weeks, loosen the diet but don't abandon it completely. Use lots and lots of variety wherever possible. You and your child will grow tired of the same menus after a month, so change the rotation around and experiment with new food combinations. Changes in the rotation will occur as you develop more ideas and more experience in food combining. Even when strict food rotation can be left behind as the child's allergies improve, variety should be a major goal of an optimal diet.

Sample Rotation Diet One

Scott, age eight, has severe allergic problems that provoke hyperactivity, learning difficulties, and mood swings. His doctor has suggested that he adhere to a strict rotation diet and avoid those foods found through allergy testing to provoke allergic responses.

Provocative foods to be avoided: Wheat, oat, barley, rye; pork; sugar; chocolate; peas, white potato; banana, apple, orange; peanut

Scott's mother read over the rotation material in detail. She considered factors that were important to her and to her child. Scott, like most eight-year-olds, liked foods such as pizza, spaghetti, ice cream, hot dogs, hamburgers, cakes, cookies, and milkshakes. Scott's mother, on the other hand, had to consider the time element she had to work with for different meals —lunches that had to be packed for Scott to take to school, snacks that Scott asked for throughout the day, dinner menus that would be agreeable to the rest of the family, and desserts (in Scott's opinion the reason for eating a meal).

Scott and his mother picked a Sunday afternoon to sit down and plan the rotation diet. Scott's mother drew up the Diet Planner, Available Foods, and Meal Planner ahead of time. On Sunday morning she gathered all the things they needed—paper, regular and colored pencils, erasers, scissors, tape—and began work on the dining-room table, where they would have plenty of room.

They began by listing some of the foods that Scott liked to eat. Next they discussed how foods belonged in different families and how each day should contain protein, vegetables, fruit, and so forth. They colored in the Food Family Chart with colored pencils and cut apart the food families. Scot placed the food families in piles according to color.

Scott's mother then pulled out the cardboard Diet Planner and explained that the food families would be placed on this chart according to what day the foods would be eaten. Scott shouted out that he wanted spaghetti, so his mother asked him if he knew what ingredients went into a spaghetti dinner. "Meat?" Scott asked. What kind of meat? his mother asked. "Beef," Scott answered after thinking about it. His mother then asked what food family beef belonged in, and they found it under the name of Bovine. The Bovine Family contained more than just beef, though. It also had milk, cheese, yogurt, veal, lamb, gelatin, butter, and cream. The cheese could be used on top of the spaghetti, but what about the other foods? The other foods could be used throughout Day 1—yogurt at breakfast, gelatin for a snack (mixed with a fruit juice), ice cream for dessert. Scott's mother placed the Bovine family on the Diet Planner under Day 1 and beside the Meat/Poultry group.

"What else goes into a spaghetti dinner?" asked Scott's mother. Together Scott and his mother found that tomato was in the Potato Family, which also contains eggplant, potato, red and green peppers, chili powder, paprika, and pimento. Scott's mother wrote Potato Family under Day 1 beside Vegetables/Starches. But she crossed out potato because this was a food that provoked symptoms and Scott's doctor had directed that this food be avoided. They found oregano in the Mint Family and placed that under Day 1 beside Seasoning. The Mint Family also contained basil, chia seeds, rosemary, savory, sage, thyme, mint, and marjoram, and any of these could also be used on Day 1. Onion and garlic are needed for a spaghetti dinner, and they belong in the Lily Family along with asparagus, chives, leek, aloe vera, and shallot. The Lily Family was listed on the Diet Planner under Day 1 beside Seasoning. Olive oil would be used in spaghetti, and this belongs in the Olive Family, right along with olives, as one would expect.

"Now, what about the most important part, the pasta?" asked Scott. Because Scott could not eat wheat and some other grains, only corn or rice pasta could be used. These belonged in the Grass Family, which also contains bamboo shoots, millet, triticale, rye, oat, wheat, wild rice, barley, and sugar cane. They listed the Grass Family under Day 1, beside Vegetables/ Starches, but crossed out wheat, oat, barley, triticale (this is a wheat/rye grain), and rye because these foods provoked symptoms and were to be avoided. (They could also have used spaghetti squash for pasta, or mung bean sprouts, or noodles; Scott was allergic to potato, so they could not have used potato pasta.)

MEAL PLANNER

DAY ONE	DAY TWO	DAY THREE	DAY FOUR
BREAKFAST:			
LUNCH:			

DAY ONE	DAY TWO	DAY THREE	DAY FOUR
SNACK:			
DINNER:			

SAMPLE DIET PLANNER FOR SCOTT

	DAY ONE	DAY TWO	DAY THREE	DAY FOUR
MEAT/ POULTRY (red)	Bovine and Ovine Families	Duck Family Shellfish Family	Turkey Family	Pheasant Family Mollusk Family
FISH (orange)	Swordfish Family Cod Family	Dolphin Family	Salmon Family Mackerel Family	Flounder Family
VEGETABLES/ STARCHES (green)	Grass Family Potato Family	Legume Family Gourd Family Goosefoot Family	Carrot Family Daisy Family Morning Glory Family Spurge Family Buckwheat Family	Sedge Family Mustard Family Amaranth Family Arrowroot Family

SEASONING (yellow)	Lily Family Fungus Family Laurel Family Myrtle Family Orchid Family Nutmeg Family Mint Family	Honey	Ginger Family Maple Family
FRUIT (blue)	Grape Family Heath Family Mulberry Family Starfruit Family	Rose (seed) Family Papaya Family Saxifrage Family	Pineapple Family Dillenia Family Citrus Family	Rose(berry) Family Rose(pit) Family Soapberry Family
NUTS/ SEEDS (white)	Olive Family Flax Family Birch Family	Protea Family Walnut Family	Cashew Family Palm Family Beech Family	Pedalium Family

SAMPLE AVAILABLE FOODS FOR SCOTT

	DAY ONE	DAY TWO	DAY THREE	DAY FOUR
PROTEIN	milk, cheese, yogurt, lamb, beef, gelatin, swordfish, cod	duck, eggs, tofu, mahi-mahi, lobster, crab, prawn, shrimp	turkey, mackerel, salmon, trout, whitefish, tuna, albacore	chicken, eggs, Cornish hen, scallops, clams, oysters, flounder, sole, agar-agar
VEGETABLES	asparagus, olives, bamboo shoots, avocado, mushroom, tomato, green/red peppers, eggplant, fresh corn	alfalfa sprouts, jicama, mung sprouts, spinach, cucumber, beets, chard, squash, string beans, pumpkin	celery, parsley, parsnip, carrot, lettuce, endive, artichoke, sunflower sprouts	cabbage, broccoli, radish, brussels sprouts, turnip, cauliflower, rutabaga, watercress, water chestnut, bok choy, kale
FRUIT	grape (raisin), blueberry, cranberry, fig, starfruit, guava	pear, rose hips, papaya, currants, melon	mango, pineapple, kiwi, coconut, dates, rhubarb, lemon, grapefruit, lime	apricot, peach, plum, cherry, nectarine, prune, strawberry, boysenberry, blackberry, raspberry, litchi fruit
COMPLEX CARBOHYDRATES	corn, millet, brown rice, wild rice	lentils, soy, navy, lima, pinto, mung, kidney, garbanzo, azuki beans	sweet potato, yam, tapioca, buckwheat, sago starch	arrowroot, amaranth

NUTS/SEEDS	flaxseed, filberts, chia seeds	macadamia nuts, pecans, walnuts, pumpkin seeds	cashew, pistachio, chestnuts, sunflower seeds	almond, sesame seeds
FATS	butter, cream, linseed oil, corn oil, olive oil, avocado oil	soy oil, lecithin, walnut oil	coconut oil, sunflower oil, safflower oil	sesame oil, almond oil, apricot oil
SEASONING	onion, garlic, allspice, vanilla, cloves, yeast, cinnamon, basil, nutmeg, pepper, oregano	carob, licorice, soy sauce (wheat-free) fenugreek	dill, fennel, anise, caraway, lemon, lime, coconut	ginger, mustard, horseradish
SWEETENERS	rice syrup, grape-juice concentrate	honey, bee pollen, pear concentrate	date sugar	maple syrup, maple sugar
BEVERAGES	milk, grape juice, cranberry juice	papaya or pear juice, soy milk	coconut/pineapple juice, sunfl. milk, lemonade	apricot/prune juice, almond/sesame milk
SNACKS	raisins/filberts, beef jerky	milk-free carob candy, carob cookies, melon	cashews, pistachios, sunflower seeds, dates	dried apricots/almonds, sesame-maple cookies

SAMPLE MEAL PLANNER FOR SCOTT

	DAY ONE	DAY TWO	DAY THREE	DAY FOUR
BREAKFAST:		rose-hip tea	buckwheat cereal, date sugar,	sesame/arrowroot/egg pancakes
	millet puffs and milk	pecan muffins (ground pecans,	sunflower milk and seeds	with maple syrup
	beef patty, lamp chop	soy oil, honey soy flour)	grilled turkey slices	amaranth cereal with almond or
	yogurt/flaxseed/raisins	pumpkinseeds and fresh papaya	yam with date sugar and chest-	sesame milk
	brown rice toast/butter	acorn squash baked with honey	nuts	amaranth bread with strawberry
	rice crepes/blueberries	and walnuts	kiwi and pineapple	jam
	starfruit	hot carob soy milk	fresh pineapple juice	scrambled eggs
	milk/protein shake			apricot juice
	cranberry/grape juice			
LUNCH:		shrimp salad (spinach, soy oil,	tuna salad (lettuce, parsley,	crunchy chicken (baked with
	natural beef hot dogs or ham-	Vitamin C, sprouts, jicama)	sunflower seeds/sprouts/oil)	ground sesame seeds)
	burger patty, ketchup	bean soup, papaya smoothie	celery with roasted-cashew	prunes, apricots, litchi, berries
	cheese corn puffs	walnut crackers, soy nuts	butter	(frozen, unsweet)
	cheese/br. rice crackers	cucumber/jicama slices	carrot/celery sticks	sesame/maple cookies
	grapes, starfruit, guava	pear, currants/pecans	toasted coconut chips	roasted-almond or tahini butter/
	cinnamon rice cookies	walnuts dipped in honey/carob	pineapple/mango/kiwi	sesame crackers
	olives, peppers, filberts		cold rhubarb/date sugar	strawberry smoothie

SNACK: raisins/filberts, beef jerky green/red peppers brown rice crackers	currants/pecans, melon carob cookies and candy jicama slices pumpkinseeds	pineapple/pistachios sunflower crackers sunflower seeds/date pieces, coconut/cashews	almonds/dried apricots strawberries sesame-maple cookies Brazil nuts
DINNER: nachos or tacos (beef, salsa, cheese, tomato, avocado, olive, sour cream) pizza (rice crust), spaghetti (corn pasta), corn tortilla steak, lamb chop, swordfish asparagus, eggplant coated in ground filbert/sauté wild rice, millet, fresh corn salad—avocado/bamboo shoots/ sweet red pepper grape gelatin/whipped cream blueberries, ice cream	crispy duck, lentil soup sautéed tofu/soy sauce mahimahi topped with macadamia nuts string bean, spaghetti squash spinach/jicama/beet/sprout salad/soy oil/Vit. C salad sautéed zucchini/yellow squash carob cookies melon soy ice cream	roast turkey/chestnuts grilled salmon steak trout with dill/lemon sweet potato, artichoke shredded carrot, pineapple, coconut, sunflower seeds carrot/parsnip/caraway salad—lettuce, endive, sunflower sprouts, carrot with sunflower oil/lemon pineapple tapioca pudding pineapple/cashew/coconut bars or cookies	chicken, broccoli, water chestnuts, apricot stir-fry Cornish hen with Bing cherry topping sautéed scallops, clams flounder (almond topping) rutabaga, cauliflower salad—shredded cabbage, Vit. C, sesame oil/seeds agar-agar mold with Bing cherries berry pie (almond crust) raspberry ice

Scott commented that they had worked awfully hard on that one spaghetti dinner; but his mother explained that he had chosen a very complex food with lots of ingredients. However, there would be other food combinations that used similar ingredients. Pizza, tacos, and nachos might be used instead of spaghetti when the rotation began again. For example, if Scott had spaghetti for dinner on Monday, when the rotation started over again on Friday he had the same individual foods to choose from but he might have pizza or nachos instead of spaghetti.

Now they started adding more food families to Day 1 on the Diet Planner. They added the Swordfish and Cod families beside the fish section. The Laurel (avocado, bay leaf, cinnamon), Fungus (mushroom, brewer's yeast, the mold found in cheese), Myrtle (allspice, clove, guava), Orchid (vanilla), and Nutmeg (nutmeg, mace) families were listed beside the Seasoning section. The Fruit section of the Diet Planner was empty, so they added the Grape (grape, raisin), Heath (blueberry, cranberry, huckleberry), and Mulberry (fig, mulberry) families. The Flax (flaxseed) and Birch (filbert) families were added to the Nut/Seed section. They had finished Day 1 and moved on to Day 2, then to Day 3, and finally to Day 4. A few food families were not used, such as Frog, Elm, Swine, and Smelt because Scott refused to eat them; these food families were placed in an envelope in case they were needed at a later time.

When the Diet Planner was completed, Scott's mother pulled out the Available Foods chart and they began listing all the available Protein foods. On Day 1 the Bovine Family provided quite a few protein foods; swordfish and cod were also listed. Next they listed all the Vegetables they had to choose from. Asparagus, mushroom, and avocado were hiding in the Seasoning food families, whereas the other vegetables were easier to find in the Grass and Potato families that were colored green in the Vegetable/Starch section. The Grass Family supplied the Complex Carbohydrates. The flaxseed and filberts were already in the Nuts/Seeds section and were easy to find, but the chia seeds, in the Mint Family, also had to be added to the Nuts/Seeds area under Day 1. The Fats were found in several different food families and listed. The seasonings were listed in the Seasoning area. Sweeteners for Day 1 were rice syrup and grape-juice concentrate. Beverages to have on hand were milk, grape juice, and cranberry/grape juice, or a fruit smoothie could be made with frozen, unsweetened blueberries, grape juice, and ice. Snacks might be beef jerky or a raisin/filbert mix. Scott and his mother continued with Day 2, then Day 3, and finally Day 4.

Now they were ready for the Meal Planner and discussed what Scott was willing to eat and what Scott's mother was willing to prepare for meals and snacks on each day. Breakfast was often a busy time, so they listed quick-meal ideas like brown rice toast with butter, protein shake, millet puffs and milk, and yogurt with flaxseed and raisins, as well as rice crepes with blueberries and yogurt/whipped cream on special days when they had more time for breakfast. Scott took his lunch to school, so they planned foods that he enjoyed like hot dogs with ketchup, corn puffs, cheese and brown rice crackers, grapes, raw green pepper slices, filberts, and cinnamon-rice cookies. Snacks might be raisins/filberts, homemade beef jerky, brown rice crackers, fruit gelatin. Dinner might be the spaghetti Scott liked to have or pizza, nachos, steak, hamburger, meat loaf, lamb chops, veal, cod, or swordfish. The vegetable might be asparagus, corn on the cob, eggplant, or a stir-fry of available vegetables (bamboo shoot, mushroom, tomato, eggplant, red peppers). A side dish of brown or wild rice or millet might be used with some meals. A salad could be made with avocado, bamboo shoots, and sweet red pepper. Dessert might be something baked like a cake (filbert flour, millet flour, butter, rice syrup, cornstarch, vanilla, raisins), cinnamon cookies (cinnamon-filbert), pie (blueberry with a filbert crust), or something easier to prepare like vanilla ice cream, grape gelatin with whipped cream, or blueberries and yogurt. Meal planning continued for Day 2, Day 3, and Day 4.

Scott's mother taped magnets on the backs of the Diet Planner, Available Foods chart and Meal Planner and placed them on the refrigerator so that they could refer to them. Now they were ready to begin the food-rotation experience!

Sample Rotation Diet Two

Lauren, age fifteen, has been directed by her physician to adhere to a strict rotation diet with avoidance of yeast/mold foods (due to her *Candida albicans* infection) and those foods which provoked reactions during testing. A lower-than-average carbohydrate intake is also suggested because of her hypoglycemic and *Candida albicans* complications.

Provocative foods to be avoided:

cheese, beef	apple, banana
wheat, corn	sugar
sole, shrimp	pork
chicken, eggs	carrot, tomato
orange, grapefuit	garlic, onion

Candida-stimulating foods:

all cheese	all melon
malt	peanuts
yeast	gluten grains—wheat, oat,
refined sugar	buckwheat, rye, barley
natural sweeteners (honey, maple	smoked, dried, or processed meats
syrup, and the like)	or fish
mushrooms	vinegar and foods containing
refined flour	vinegar—pickles, salad dressing,
dried fruit	mayonnaise, relish, mustard,
soy sauce	ketchup

SAMPLE DIET PLANNER FOR LAUREN

	DAY ONE	DAY TWO	DAY THREE	DAY FOUR
MEAT/ POULTRY (red)	Deer Family Turkey Family	Hare Family Pheasant Family Crustacean Family	Bovine Family Mollusk Family	Duck Family
FISH (orange)	Swordfish Family Flounder Family	Croaker Family Herring Family Salmon Family	Mackerel Family Sturgeon Family	Butterfish Family Snapper Family Scorpion Family Cod Family
VEGETABLES/ STARCHES (green)	Legume Family	Carrot Family Grass Family Buckwheat Family Goosefoot Family Arrowroot Family	Potato Family Gourd Family	Mustard Family Daisy Family Morning Glory Family Amaranth Family Spurge Family

SEASONING (yellow)	Lily Family Myrtle Family Pepper Family	Algae Family Laurel Family Honey	Mint Family Orchid Family	Nutmeg Family Ginger Family
FRUIT (blue)	Papaya Family Heath Family Maple Family	Rose (pit) Family Dillenia Family	Rose (seed) Family Pomegranate Family Rose(berry) Family	Citrus Family Pineapple Family Grape Family
NUTS/ **SEEDS** (white)	Olive Family Birch Family Protea Family	Pedalium Family Conifer Family	Flax Family Walnut Family	Cashew Family Palm Family Beech Family

SAMPLE AVAILABLE FOODS FOR LAUREN

	DAY ONE	DAY TWO	DAY THREE	DAY FOUR
PROTEIN	venison, turkey (eggs), swordfish, halibut, flounder, tofu, soy milk	rabbit, sardines, trout, salmon, whiting, crab, Cornish hen, agar-agar	lamb, milk (cow/goat), yogurt, shark, caviar, tuna, oyster, scallop	duck (and eggs), red snapper, ocean perch, butterfish, cod, haddock
VEGETABLES	jicama, chives, string beans, olives, mung bean/alfalfa sprouts, asparagus	celery, parsnip, parsley, avocado, bamboo shoots, spinach, chard, beets, seaweed	eggplant, squash (all varieties), cucumber, bell and sweet red pepper	broccoli, cabbage, turnip, cauliflower, bok choy, rutabaga, radish, kale, lettuce, brussels sprouts, artichoke, endive, chicory, sunflower-seed sprouts
FRUIT	papaya blueberry cranberry gauva	apricot, cherry peach, plum rhubarb kiwi	pear, pomegranate strawberry blackberry raspberry, rose hips	lemon, lime mango pineapple, grape coconut
COMPLEX CARBOHYDRATES	peas, soy, navy, pinto, azuki, kidney, garbanzo, soy and garbanzo flour	arrowroot, wild rice, br. rice—flour/noodles, millet (flour)	white potato—flour and noodles water chestnuts	yam, sweet potato amaranth (flour/) tapioca, Jerusalem artichoke flour

NUTS/SEEDS	filbert macadamia	almond sesame seeds pine nut	flaxseed, chia seeds pumpkin seeds pecan, walnut	cashew, pistachios chestnut, coconut sunflower seeds
FATS	soy oil lecithin olive oil	almond oil apricot oil sesame oil	butter, cream linseed oil walnut oil	safflower oil sunflower oil coconut oil
SEASONING	carob, allspice, clove, black/white pepper	dill, fennel, caraway cinnamon, bayleaf coriander, parsley	chili, paprika oregano, basil, rosemary vanilla, mint	nutmeg, ginger horseradish, mustard cardamom
SWEETENERS	maple sugar/syrup papaya concentrate	honey	pear concentrate	date sugar grape-juice concentrate
BEVERAGES	carob/soy milk blueberry smoothie	sesame/almond milk cherry smoothie	peppermint tea yogurt/berry shake	lemonade, cashew milk pineapple smoothie
SNACKS	roasted soy nuts, jicama, carob brownie	almond cookies, kiwi rice cakes/almond butter	pumpkin seeds, yogurt, pecans, berries, walnuts	cashews, sunflower seeds, pineapple

SAMPLE MEAL PLANNER FOR LAUREN

	DAY ONE	DAY TWO	DAY THREE	DAY FOUR
BREAKFAST:	filbert/soy-flour pancakes with blueberry (unsweet.) jam soy/cranberry muffins sautéed tofu and turkey filberts and guava baked halibut papaya/soy protein drink carob/maple soy milk	millet-cinnamon cereal with chopped almonds and almond milk almond or sesame pancakes with unsweet. peach jam roast Cornish hen (cook the night before—warm up) sesame/arrowroot muffin cinnamon tea	lamb patty or chop potato-walnut pancakes frozen unsweet. raspberries sautéed eggplant pumpkin seeds/pear baked potato with yogurt and caviar yogurt-raspberry shake peppermint tea	amaranth cereal with date sugar & sunflower milk/seed scrambled (duck) eggs baked sweet potato and chestnuts sunflower seeds and pineapple pineapple smoothie cashew milk
LUNCH:	bean soup turkey, jicama, sprouts, garbanzo bean salad with dressing of soy oil/Vit. C macadamia nuts/guava roasted soy nuts jicama with bean dip	sardines/rice crackers roasted almond butter on celery or rice crackers spinach, crab, avocado, sesame salad with sesame oil/Vit. C dressing kiwi, Bing cherries pine nuts	yogurt with blackberries and flaxseeds pecan crackers bell/sweet pepper strips tuna salad with cucumber, tuna, walnut oil oyster stew pear, walnuts	lettuce, sunflower sprouts roast cold duck salad baked red snapper/lemon pineapple-coconut-cashew pistachios/mango sunflower crackers with cashew butter lemonade

SNACK: jicama sticks roasted soy nuts carob brownie	almond cookies rice crackers/tahini celery/almond butter	blackberries, pear yogurt, pumpkin seeds pecans, walnuts	sunflower seeds, cashews pineapple coconut amaranth cookies
DINNER: venison stew (peas, string beans, jicama, peppercorns) baked flounder topped with chopped macadamia nuts bean/pea or sprout/jicama salad asparagus carob crepes/blueberry filling	trout almondine stuffed with wild rice and dill rabbit, spinach, rice noodle soup parsnip, parsley, caraway steamed spinach spinach/beet/celery salad fresh kiwi rhubarb pie (almond crust)	roast leg of lamb with spearmint baked scallops in cream sauce, paprika spaghetti squash/oregano zucchini/potato muffins baked potato/butter sauteed eggplant/chili strawberries/fresh whipped cream with vanilla	baked perch with cashew coating lemon-ginger codfish mashed rutabaga or cauliflower stir-fried cabbage, cashew broccoli, bok choy steamed artichoke, lemon baked yam/pineapple/coconut lemon tapioca pudding

A rotation diet low in carbohydrates that also avoids yeast/mold foods is quite restrictive. But Lauren understood that to overcome her severe allergic condition it was necessary to follow a strict dietary regimen. Lauren and her mother discussed the new diet, but the actual planning was completed by Lauren herself.

Using the color-coded Food Families, Diet Planner, Available Foods chart, and Meal Planner, Lauren arranged her diet around her needs and lifestyle. She enjoyed experimenting with recipes and different food combinations and found that the following examples worked best for her:

Rare Food Elimination Diet

This elimination diet is one in which the most common allergic foods are strictly avoided and low reactive foods are exclusively consumed. If any of the foods appearing on this list are commonly consumed foods, favorite foods, or intensely disliked foods then they should also be avoided:

Salmon	Millet	Jicama	Papaya	Sunflower seeds/oil,
Scallops	Amaranth	Kale	Kiwi	butter, sprouts
Trout	Brown rice	Parsnip	Blueberry	Sesame seeds/oil,
Shark	Arrowroot	Parsley	Mango	tahini
Flounder	Taro	Rutabaga	Guava	Macadamia nuts
Rabbit	Yam	Eggplant	Rhubarb	Filberts/hazelnut
Duck	Tapioca	Asparagus	Avocado	Poppyseed
Venison		Artichoke		Flaxseed
Lamb		Bamboo shoots		Chia seed
		Alfalfa sprouts		
		Water chestnuts		

After the allergic condition is stabilized (this usually takes approximately one week) a new food may be introduced each day until the offending foods are isolated. The menu would be very basic with meals prepared simply but attractively. This type of diet would be used when an individual has a very complex allergic manifestation and would need to be under the care of a qualified clinical ecologist or orthomolecular physician.

Sample meals might be as follows:

Breakfast: Hazelnut pancakes (one cup ground hazelnuts, 2 tablespoons arrow-root; add water; mix to pancake consistency and cook as regular pancakes in sunflower oil). Top with blended, frozen unsweetened blueberries

OR: Baked yam with roasted chestnuts

Lunch: Crispy duck, water chestnuts, mango

OR: Salmon salad (salmon, diced jicama, sesame oil), kiwi

Snack: Guava smoothie (guava juice and ice; blend), macadamia nuts

OR: Fresh papaya, sunflower seeds

Dinner: Lamb chops, eggplant (dip in sesame oil and ground sesame seeds; bake), salad with alfalfa sprouts and avocado, dressing made with sesame oil and Vitamin C

OR: Baked trout, asparagus, amaranth, salad of shredded parsnip and Jerusalem artichoke

Knife-Fork-
Spoon

Before any self-respecting child will even consider it's-good-for-you food, it must look good, smell good, and taste good. It matters little how nutritious food is if it is not eaten! Expanding the dimensions of children's eating patterns will occur automatically if you concentrate on creatively combining supplement foods with familiar foods and varying the diet. Certainly your children will not be thrilled with everything you make; personal preference, like nutritional needs, are unique. But through a few creative efforts of their own (and your helpful hints) they can discover what tastes good and guide you in the right direction.

As I began modifying familiar food into healthy new food, it became apparent that the best way to create recipes for children was to have them closely involved. So thanks to the efforts of my son and his friends (they distributed samples throughout the neighborhood) I acquired many small and medium-sized helpers to do taste testing. Quickly I caught on to which recipes were yum and which were yuk by my son Shawn's saying, "All right!" or "You blew it, Mom!" when they rated the recipe. Often, I had to prepare a second or third batch of a recipe to give the adults and myself a chance to taste-test. It got rough in the end because so many children decided to "help with tasting" that they constantly knocked on the door, peeked in the kitchen window, and finally lined up outside the door in anticipation of the next recipe to sample.

The recipes contained in this section can be a springboard for your own creativity. Food that satisfies your family's needs and tastes is, of course, unique to them. These preferences require modifying favority family recipes as well as trying new ones.

Choosing New Food

Finding alternatives to the staples—sugar, flour, eggs, milk—may appear to be quite a challenge. Whether and how you modify the use of these staple foods will depend primarily on your child's sensitivities and the rotation or variation of all nonreactive or low-reactive foods. Regardless of the child's health status, all refined sugar, hydrogenated fat, white flour, and artificial ingredients should be entirely eliminated. These are the hardest to avoid by reason of their massive infiltration into our food supply.

To Sweeten

The use of sweetening is unavoidable. If natural goodies are not made available on occasion, children soon will cheat on any new food diet. We can, however, use a minimum amount of sweetening, choose more nutritious sweetening agents over others, and balance sweeteners in recipes with high nutrient additions. The more favorable sweetener choices include:

Fruit (dried, frozen, or fresh) may be used as sweetening to flavor many recipes. Blending whole fruit and using juice both work well, but check labels carefully when using frozen or dried fruit to ensure purity.

Fruit concentrate (unsweetened, frozen or bottled) is appropriate in many recipes in place of honey or sugar. Pure grape, pear, orange, papaya, apple, pineapple, and others are available bottled and as a frozen, unsweetened concentrate.

Honey may be obtained in very deep colors (such as buckwheat) to light colors (such as wildflower). The deeper the color, the stronger the taste, so lighter honey may be preferred for baking. Choose raw, unfiltered honey, with its unaltered nutritional content, over commercial heated honey. Tupelo honey appears to be better handled by many people with blood-sugar problems because of its higher content of levulose. Honey is sweeter than refined sugar, and usually one-half as much is needed when honey is substituted for sugar in recipes.

Date sugar made from crystallized dates may be substituted for refined sweeteners in recipes. Date sugar is not as sweet as refined sugar, and more will thus be needed to achieve the deisred taste of sweetness. Date sugar does have a heavy, grainy texture.

Coconut sugar, which you prepare by grinding unsweetened shredded coconut, may be used as a substitute for powdered sugar.

Pure maple syrup and sugar may be used in conversion of recipes in the same manner as honey; it is not quite as sweet as honey but has its own distinctive, delicious flavor. Maple syrup may be purchased in different grades. Generally Grade B or Grade C contains a slightly higher percentage of minerals than Grade A.

Blackstrap molasses is the syrup left after the final extraction of sugar from cane or beets. Because of this derivation, it may cause an allergic reaction in children who have a strong sugar sensitivity, although some can handle it without problems. It does have a higher content of vitamins and minerals than most sweeteners, but its strong taste limits its use.

Grain and malt syrups are derived from rice, wheat, barley, and sorghum. If no sensitivity to grain is evident these are acceptable sweeteners.

To Replace Dairy Products

Sensitivities to dairy products may require substitutions for eggs, butter, milk, and cheese.

Liquid milk may be replaced with:

Coconut milk which you prepare by mixing one-half cup shredded unsweetened coconut with one cup of pure water in your blender until smooth. A dab of sweetening may be added if desired.

Goat's milk, if tolerated; this is delicious if obtained truly fresh. Goat's milk may be used exactly like cow's milk, provided there is no reaction to it.

Nut or seed milk, which you prepare by mixing in your blender one-half cup of raw seeds or nuts with one cup of pure water until smooth.

Soy milk which may be used like cow's milk and is available from Health Valley as Soy Moo, sweetened with honey, and Ah Soy, sweetened with barley malt.

Juice, pure and unsweetened, may be substituted for milk in recipes.

Butter (pure and uncolored) is often tolerated by milk-sensitive individuals, but if not it may be replaced with:

Lecithin spread, a butter substitute available in health-food stores from Soya Canadian Industries. It contains no hydrogenated fats and has an excellent taste, but is rather expensive. Pure liquid soya lecithin may be used to grease pans to keep foods from sticking.

Pure oils, which must be cold-pressed—safflower, soy, sesame, walnut, linseed, wheat germ, olive, and sunflower. Erewhon and Westbrae make excellent high-quality unrefined oils.

Cheese may be replaced with:

Goat's-milk cheese, which is available through health-food stores and gourmet shops.

Tofu, a soy-milk cheese that is soft and bland. It may be used in other foods (potato salad, scrambled eggs) but is not very appealing to children when eaten alone.

Eggs may be replaced in recipes (this works for no more than 2–3 eggs) with:

Baking powder, by addition of one teaspoon of baking powder for each egg in addition to whatever baking powder the recipe calls for.

Gelatin at the ratio of one tablespoon or one package of pure gelatin (Knox brand) for each egg. Be sure to dissolve gelatin in hot liquid before using in a recipe.

Jolly Joan egg replacer, which contains arrowroot; it may be used as directed to replace eggs.

Duck (or other fowl) eggs, in place of chicken eggs. One duck egg is equivalent to two chicken eggs. Duck or other eggs may be frozen for use when fresh eggs are unavailable.

To Replace Flour

Wheat flour (white or whole-wheat) is the most difficult ingredient to replace in conversion of recipes to allergy-free food. Wheat is the basis of most recipes! And yet wheat is one of the most common allergenic offenders, so a replacement for wheat flour is a must.

Sensitivity to wheat usually extends to other grains as well. Barley and rye are the most common, and therefore recipes in this book do not contain wheat (except for wheat germ, which is a high-nutrient food and may be used in rotation if tolerated), rye, or barley. Rice, oats, corn, and millet are used in the recipes, but sensitivites may exist to any of these. If so, you will have to switch flours to avoid those grains to which your child is sensitive. Oat and corn may accompany wheat sensitivity, but with lesser frequency than barley and rye. Rice and millet are least likely to cause problems. But keep in mind that grains to which a child is not sensitive must be rotated to prevent sensitivities from developing to any foods eaten in overabundance.

Flour does not need to be made from grains, but can also be made from nuts, seeds, potato, beans, protein powder, and milk powder. Grainless flours may also act as superior nutritive additions and should always be used in conjunction with grain flours where possible.

The alternative grain flours to wheat, rye, and barley include:

Corn flour, which may be of coarse or fine texture. It is difficult to use alone in baking because it yields a rather grainy product, so another flour (milk powder, arrowroot, or the like) should be used along with it. One cup of fine corn flour is equal to one cup of wheat flour. Corn germ is available from Fearn Products and may be used in place of wheat germ.

Millet flour, which is made from a grain that is infrequently used in this country. It has a slightly heavy texture, and can be used in place of soy flour. One cup millet flour plus one-fourth cup starch (arrowroot or other) will replace one cup of wheat flour.

Oat flour; this is light in texture and easy to work with and yields light breadstuffs. One and one-third cups of oat flour is needed to replace one cup of wheat flour.

Rice flour/rice polish; this is a bit gritty in texture, and thus recipes made with it need to be chosen carefully. Seven-eighths cup of brown rice flour equals one cup of wheat flour in the conversion of a recipe. But to make it more nutritious, substitute rice polish for some portion (up to half) of the rice flour. When baking with rice flour you may need to add a portion of starch (about one-fourth cup) to give it more substance.

Nongrain flours include:

Amaranth flour; this comes from a nutritious plant and can be used as a cereal or flour in recipes containing a starch such as arrowroot. This flour is well tolerated by acutely allergic people.

Desiccated liver; this is an extremely potent addition, and it will probably be possible only to add it by the teaspoon to strongly flavored foods.

Milk powder, of the noninstant, nonfat, low-heat variety (found in health-food stores or health sections in supermarkets), which is preferable for baking. Its addition yields a delicious product, but it mandates a lower baking temperature (by 25 degrees), as it browns more quickly. Usually one-fourth to one-half cup of milk powder can be used in conjunction with heavier flours like seed flour or soy flour. Milk powder will, of course, be unsuitable for those with milk sensitivity, in which case arrowroot (or other starch) or protein powder may be substituted in most recipes.

Potato flour; this may be used to replace wheat flour in many recipes. Light in texture, it does not affect the flavor of baked goods. Use three-eighths cup potato flour to replace one cup of wheat flour.

Nut flour, which you make by grinding fresh, raw nuts dry in the blender or small electric coffee grinder until powdery. Almonds, Brazil nuts, filberts, cashews, walnuts, pecans work well. Nut flour usually has to be used with another flour, grain, starch, or milk powder. For convenience, grind up nut flour ahead of time and store in the refrigerator or freezer. All nut and seed flour must be refrigerated.

Seed flour; this is essentially the same as nut flour—ground-up raw seeds. And because seeds tend to have a higher nutritional value than nuts, seed flour should be used liberally in recipes. Sunflower, sesame, and pumpkin all make fine flours. Grind and store in the refrigerator or freezer.

Nutritional yeast—a superior source of nutrients. This is an exceptional supplement food (and flour) as long as your child shows no sensitivity and has no *Candida albicans* infection. Because of its strong taste it must be used sparingly, yet even in small amounts it is a nutrient-rich addition. The taste of yeast is hidden well in baked goods (like cookies, cakes, breads, crackers) and strongly seasoned foods. There are many different nutritional yeasts available, but try to obtain one with balanced minerals. The following recipes contain Dr. Donsbach's Yeast 500. Using a large amount of nutritional yeast (2–3 tablespoons) can cause a niacin flush reaction in some people (red flush on face, ears, neck) but it is nothing to be concerned about.

Protein powder; this may be of many different derivations, such as egg, milk, soy, beef, yeast, so be sure to check labels for a protein powder free of those ingredients to which your child may be sensitive. Protein powder should be unsweetened and without artificial ingredients. Plain soy protein powder, egg protein, milk protein, and predigested protein derived from gelatin (such as Super Progest or Crystal Springs Crystal Amino powder) may be used in recipes. Protein powder used in the following recipes was Dr. Donsbach's Glo-Pro, but because it contains milk, soy, and beef derivatives it is not appropriate for everyone. When using protein powder in baking, one-fourth to one-half cup may be used with other flours.

Soy flour, which is made from soybeans, offers a much higher nutritional value than wheat flour. It does have one major drawback, however: it has a strong, raw taste before it is heated. Licking a bowl of cake batter (or whatever) is out of the question when soy flour is used. Too much soy flour in a recipe also will overpower the food you are preparing. Use one cup soy flour and one-fourth cup starch to replace one cup wheat flour. Other legume flours such as garbanzo flour can also be used.

Wheat germ, which may be used as is or ground to a finer texture. Be very careful to obtain fresh wheat germ, or buy it packaged in the health-food store by Fearn, in which the inside of the package is flushed with nitrogen to keep it from becoming rancid. Wheat germ adds bulk to baked goods, but can be used only in one-fourth- to one-half-cup quantities along with other flours. Always refrigerate or freeze wheat germ. Individuals allergic to wheat must avoid wheat germ—replace with corn germ or seed flour in recipes.

To Leaven

Baking powder may contain grain products, usually corn derivatives. To avoid this grain, a cereal-free baking powder may be purchased (Cellu brand), or a baking powder can be prepared at home from equal portions of baking soda, cream of tartar, and arrowroot starch. Use either as you would regular baking powder.

To Season

Pure herbs and spices may be used to season food as well as sea salt (use sparingly), apple-cider vinegar (if sensitivity to vinegar exists, use as-corbic acid instead, which yields a similar taste in salad dressing), wheat-free soy sauce, natural mayonaise, mustard, ketchup, bouillon, and the like.

Where to Buy

The ingredients for the recipes contained in this book may be obtained in the health-food sections of supermarkets, health-food stores, catalog sales (see list of food catalogs in "The Finish Line"), and farmers' markets.

Recipes

BREADS, BISCUITS, AND BUNS

Breads containing wheat flour rise with the action of baking yeast on the gluten content of the flour. Flours not containing gluten will not rise with yeast. Eggs, baking powder, arrowroot, and baking soda may be substituted as rising agents in place of yeast.

Different varieties of bread are required for the grain-sensitive child, which is why so many different kinds of flour are used in the following recipes. Freezing bread is a must, both for convenience and to successfully accomplish the rotation of the different grains. If a child shows no sensitivity to grains, whole-wheat bread may be used, but the following recipes offer an optimal variety of grain.

In purchasing bread for your family, do not be misled by confusing labels. That which is called soy bread usually contains wheat, rye bread nearly always contains wheat, and whole-wheat bread often contains a percentage of white flour. Read those labels carefully!

BREAKFAST CAKE

¼ cup butter
¼ cup honey or apple-juice concentrate
1 egg, beaten, or egg replacer
½ cup milk (or milk alternative)
¾ cup seed flour
½ cup soy flour or garbanzo flour
¾ cup milk powder (or alternative)

2 T nutritional yeast (optional)
2 tsp baking powder
1 tsp cinnamon
½ tsp vanilla
2 T melted butter, 2 T honey or apple juice concentrate, 1½ tsp. cinnamon plus ½ cup chopped pecans or walnuts for topping

1. Cream butter and honey
2. Beat in egg and milk with honey mixture
3. Mix dry ingredients
4. Combine dry and honey mixtures, vanilla
5. Spread dough in 8 × 8 oiled baking pan
6. Mix and swirl on topping, dot with butter
7. Bake at 325° for about 45 min.

SUPER SOY BREAD

1 cup soy flour
¼ cup soy protein powder
⅓ cup milk powder or nut flour
1 tsp baking soda
  pinch of sea salt
5 eggs, separated

1 tsp lemon rind, 1½ tsp lemon
  juice
1 T lecithin granules
¾ cup yogurt or milk alternative
3 T honey

1. Mix dry ingredients
2. Beat egg whites till stiff, set aside
3. Blend egg yolks, lemon juice/rind, lecithin, yogurt, honey
4. Combine yogurt mixture and dry ingredients
5. Fold in egg whites
6. Pour into oiled loaf pan $8 \times 5 \times 2$
7. Bake at 375° for 10 min. and 350° for 35 min.

SESAME CRUNCH BREAD

½ cup sesame flour
½ cup protein powder or milk
  powder
½ cup arrowroot or other starch
1½ tsp baking powder
1 tsp baking soda

2 T whole sesame seeds
  pinch of sea salt
⅓ cup yogurt or milk alternative
3 eggs, separated
2 T cold-pressed oil
3 T honey

1. Mix all dry ingredients except sesame seeds
2. Beat egg whites until stiff first reserving a small amount for step 6; set aside
3. Mix yogurt, egg yolks, oil, honey
4. Blend yogurt and dry mixtures
5. Place in $8 \times 5 \times 2$ oiled loaf pan
6. Brush top of bread with egg white and sesame
7. Bake at 375° for 15 min., 350° for 30 min.

CHEESE BISCUITS *(yield: 8 biscuits)*

6 T butter
½ cup soy flour or ⅔ cup oat
  flour or ½ cup rice flour
2 T nutritional yeast (optional)
¼ cup arrowroot or other starch

1 T baking powder
¾ cup milk or milk alternative
¾ cup shredded cheese, or use
  another flavor if milk allergy is
  a problem

1. Mix dry ingredients
2. Cut butter into dry ingredients with two knives or fingertips

3. Make a well in dry ingredients and add milk; mix
4. Knead cheese into dough on a floured board (use appropriate flour)
5. Roll dough out to ½-inch thickness and cut with a 2-inch biscuit cutter
6. Bake at 375° on a greased cookie sheet for 15 to 20 min.

DATE NUT BREAD

2 T melted butter
¾ cup date sugar
1 egg or egg replacer
2 cups nut flour
½ cup milk powder or alternative
½ cup protein powder

⅓ cup arrowroot or other starch
½ tsp cinnamon
2 tsp baking powder
½ cup chopped nuts
½ cup chopped, soaked dates

1. Blend butter, date sugar, then egg
2. Mix dry ingredients
3. Combine dry and date sugar mixtures, adding milk and mixing well
4. Mix in chopped nuts and dates
5. Bake at 325° for about 1 hour

CINNAMON ROLLS *(yield: 18 rolls)*

½ cup butter
1 cup soy flour or flour alternative
½ cup seed flour
½ cup arrowroot or other starch
1 tsp cinnamon
⅓ cup protein powder

4 tsp baking powder
2 T nutritional yeast (optional)
1 egg or egg replacer
¼ cup honey
¼ cup chopped nuts, ¼ cup raisins, ½ tsp cinnamon, ¼ cup honey for filling

1. Mix dry ingredients
2. Cut butter into dry ingredients
3. Combine egg and honey
4. Blend honey mixture with dry ingredients
5. Knead dough one minute and turn onto floured (soy) board
6. Roll out dough, spread with 3 T melted butter, then filling
7. Roll up dough like a jelly roll and slice in 1-inch-thick slices; handle carefully
8. Place rolls in buttered muffin tins for small rolls or on a buttered cookie sheet for medium-sized rolls
9. Top rolls with butter, nuts, raisins, and cinnamon, and drizzle with honey
10. Bake at 325° for about 20 min.

MIX AND MATCH BREAD

2 tsp gelatin
⅔ cup milk or milk alternative
¼ cup protein powder
1 cup rice flour and 1 cup rice
polish
   or 2¼ cups oat flour
   or 2¾ cups millet flour
   or 2½ cups fine corn flour

2 tsp baking powder
1¼ cup fruit-juice concentrate
3 T cold-pressed oil
2 beaten eggs or egg-replacer
equivalent
optional flavoring

1. Soak gelatin in ⅓ cup milk and then dissolve gelatin by warming in a saucepan
2. Combine dry ingredients
3. Mix fruit-juice concentrate, oil, eggs (egg white may be beaten and folded in)
4. Blend all ingredients
5. Pour into oiled 8 × 5 × 2 loaf pan
6. Bake at 375° for 15 min., 350° for 35 min.

BIG BRAID, LITTLE BRAID

2 cups millet, soy or alternative
flour
3 T nutritional yeast (optional)
1 cup seed flour
1 cup arrowroot or other starch
⅔ cup protein powder
2 tsp cinnamon
2 T baking powder

1 cup butter
2 eggs
½ cup honey
2 T melted butter, 2 T honey, ½
tsp cinnamon, ¼ cup chopped
nuts or chopped dried fruit for
topping

1. Mix dry ingredients
2. Cut butter into dry ingredients
3. Blend eggs and honey
4. Mix dry ingredients with honey mixture
5. Knead dough one minute and place on a floured (appropriate) board
6. Remove small amount of dough so child can make own braid or make a small braid surprise
7. Divide dough into three sections and roll each section into a long strip
8. Braid strips carefully on an oiled cookie sheet. Place small braid on the same sheet
9. Top braids with optional topping
10. Bake at 325 for about 25 min.

There are many variations of Big Braid, Little Braid that you can create. Try separating the dough into two long braids by using six long strips of dough. Form two braids into a ring by pinching them together (use a bit of water for this). Also you may roll dough out onto a floured board, place filling on top, and roll up like a jelly roll. Form into a ring and cut gashes into the dough on a slight angle every 1½ inches. Bake these, and any other ideas, with the same directions as Big Braid, Little Braid.

DOUGHNUTS AND MUFFINS

Doughnuts and muffins are convenient for children because they can be eaten on the run. They also help erase breakfast blahs and may open closed mouths for the first meal of the day. Doughnuts require a doughnut machine. Muffin tins should be lined with white cupcake papers to avoid the dye used in colored ones.

CAROB DOUGHNUTS *(yield: 12 doughnuts)*

½ cup seed flour
1 T nutritional yeast (optional)
¼ cup soy flour or flour
    alternative
¼ cup carob powder
1 T baking powder

¼ cup honey
¼ cup cold-pressed oil
¼ cup milk or milk alternative
1 egg or egg-replacer equivalent
½ tsp vanilla

1. Combine dry ingredients
2. Blend honey, oil, milk, egg, and vanilla
3. Mix everything together
4. Bake in a doughnut machine for about 7 minutes (extra cold-pressed oil will be needed)
5. Doughnuts may be eaten plain or topped with melted unsweetened carob chips, natural icing, coconut, and so on

BLUEBERRY YOGURT MUFFINS *(yield: 12 muffins)*

1½ cups oat flour
1 cup nut flour
½ cup milk powder or protein
    powder
1 T baking powder
2 eggs or egg-replacer equivalent
1 tsp vanilla

½ cup yogurt
¼ cup melted butter or cold-
    pressed oil
½ cup honey
⅓ cup blueberries (fresh or
    frozen, unsweetened)

1. Mix dry ingredients
2. Blend eggs, vanilla, yogurt, butter, and honey

3. Combine both mixtures and stir in blueberries
4. Pour into muffin tins lined with paper and bake at 375° for 20 min.

APPLE SPICE DOUGHNUTS *(yield: 12 doughnuts)*

½ cup nut flour
¼ cup potato flour
½ cup milk powder or protein powder
2 T arrowroot
½ tsp nutmeg
½ tsp cloves

1 tsp cinnamon
1 T baking powder
½ cup apple-juice concentrate
¼ cup cold-pressed oil
¼ cup applesauce
1 egg or egg-replacer equivalent

1. Combine dry ingredients
2. Mix wet ingredients
3. Blend both mixtures
4. Bake for about 7 min. in a doughnut machine (extra cold-pressed oil will be needed)

MAPLE PECAN MUFFINS *(yield: 12 muffins)*

1½ cups pecan flour
½ cup protein powder
½ cup milk powder (or increase protein powder to 1 cup and cut out milk powder)
½ cup wheat germ or corn germ

1 T baking powder
3 T melted butter
3 eggs, slightly beaten
¾ cup maple syrup
½ cup milk or milk alternative
18 pecan halves

1. Mix dry ingredients
2. Blend butter, eggs, syrup, milk
3. Combine the two mixtures
4. Fill lined muffin tins and top each with a pecan half
5. Bake at 350° for 25–30 min.

JAM MUFFINS *(yield: 12 muffins)*

2½ cups sesame-seed flour
1 cup milk powder
2 T arrowroot or other starch
1 T baking powder
1 tsp cinnamon
½ cup honey

3 eggs, slightly beaten
2 T cold-pressed oil
1 tsp vanilla
unsweetened blackberry (or other) jam

1. Mix dry ingredients
2. Blend honey, eggs, oil, vanilla

3. Combine the two mixtures
4. Fill bottom of a paper-lined muffin tin with 1 T batter, add 1 tsp of jam, and cover completely with more batter
5. Bake at 350° for 25 min.

PUMPKIN SPICE MUFFINS *(yield: 12 muffins)*

⅔ cup soy, millet, or alternative flour
½ cup protein powder
2 T nutritional yeast (optional)
¼ cup seed flour
2 tsp baking powder
1 tsp cinnamon
¼ tsp cloves

½ tsp nutmeg
⅔ cup maple syrup
1 cup pumpkin puree
2 eggs or egg-replacer equivalent
¼ cup cold-pressed oil or melted butter
⅓ cup milk or juice

1. Mix dry ingredients
2. Blend syrup, pumpkin, eggs, milk
3. Combine the two mixtures
4. Pour batter into lined muffin tins and bake at 350° for 25–30 min.

CARROT-COCONUT MUFFINS *(yield: 12 muffins)*

1 cup seed flour
1 cup rice flour
½ cup rice polish
¼ cup arrowroot or other starch
2 tsp baking powder
1 tsp cinnamon
4 eggs
1 cup pear-juice concentrate

¼ cup melted butter or cold-pressed oil
1 tsp vanilla
½ cup coconut
½ cup shredded carrot
¼ cup crushed pineapple
handful of chopped nuts or raisins

1. Mix flours, baking powder, and cinnamon
2. Combine eggs, pear concentrate, oil, vanilla
3. Blend the two mixtures and stir in coconut, carrot, pineapple, nuts, raisins
4. Pour into lined muffin tins and bake at 350° for 25 min.

BREAKFAST MUFFINS

Soy Buns (see recipe) or other natural buns
slices of cheese

slices of cooked Rich's turkey sausage
eggs

1. Slice each bun into three horizontal portions
2. Warm ends of soy buns with cheese on top until it begins to melt

3. Cut a hole in the center portion of each middle piece of soy bun, butter both sides of bread, and place in a buttered frying pan. Break an egg in the well in the bread and cook until egg yolk is slightly firm.

4. Put breakfast muffin together in this order:
   a) bottom of bun
   b) middle of bun with cooked egg
   c) slice of cooked sausage
   d) top of bun with melted cheese

PANCAKES, WAFFLES, CREPES

Sunday breakfast just wouldn't be complete without pancakes, waffles, or crepes. Most families enjoy pancakes and waffles, but crepes might still remain an undiscovered treat. Crepes are a popular, versatile food that children enjoy as much as adults. Pancakes, waffles, and crepes no longer have to be nutritional nightmares of sugar and white flour topped off with sugary, artificially flavored syrup. They can offer high nutritional value and taste great at the same time.

A NEW KIND OF PANCAKE *(yield: 4 medium-sized pancakes)*

(It's good for you!)

3–4 eggs or Jolly Joan egg replacer
   splash of milk or milk
   alternative
1 cup any nut or seed flour
1 T arrowroot or other starch

1 T protein powder (optional)
½ tsp cinnamon, ½ tsp vanilla, ¼
   cup blueberries or any favorite
   flavoring or eat 'em straight

1. Simply beat eggs and milk (or milk alternative) with a fork and stir in nut or seed flour until a pancake-batter consistency is reached

2. Add any desired flavoring

3. Cook as you would traditional pancakes in butter or cold-pressed oil

Sesame-cinnamon and almond pancakes are a hit at our house!

BANANA NUT WAFFLES *(yield: 6 waffles)*

1⅓ cups oat flour
1 cup seed flour
½ tsp nutmeg
2 tsp baking powder
3 egg yolks
1 cup pineapple juice

1 cup mashed ripe banana
3 T melted butter or cold-pressed oil
¼ cup chopped nuts
3 egg whites, beaten stiff

1. Combine flours, nutmeg, baking powder
2. Mix egg yolk, juice, banana, butter
3. Combine two mixtures just to moisten, stir in nuts, fold in egg whites
4. Bake on a waffle iron 5–6 min.

CAROB CREAM WAFFLES *(yield: 6 waffles)*

1 cup soy, millet, or alternative flour
¼ cup arrowroot or other starch
2 tsp baking powder
2 T nutritional yeast (optional)
½ cup milk powder

3 egg yolks
1 T honey
3 T melted butter
1 cup milk
½ cup cream
3 egg whites, beaten stiff

1. Combine dry ingredients
2. Mix egg yolks, honey, butter, milk, cream
3. Stir the two mixtures together just to moisten
4. Beat egg whites and fold into batter
5. Bake on a waffle iron for 5–6 min.
6. Waffles freeze well; just pop in the toaster to warm

Dessert crepes can be filled with fruit, nuts, whipped cream, yogurt, or anything else you happen to think of. Instead of rolling up your crepes, try stacking them, with layers of filling in between. My family's favorite layering is carob soya crepes with whipped cream, slivered almonds, and unsweetened carob chips. The oat and rice crepes, found on the next page, may be easily changed to dessert crepes if your child is sensitive to milk or soya. Recipes for using lunch or dinner crepes will be found in the main-dish section. Tip: always double or triple crepe recipes so there will be some left to freeze—they disappear fast!

MAPLE-NUT DESSERT CREPES *(yield: 6 crepes)*

2 T almond flour
6 T soy, millet, or alternative
  flour
3 eggs
1 T melted butter or cold-pressed
  oil

½ cup cream
2 T maple syrup
½ tsp cinnamon
2–3 T milk

1. Blend all ingredients till smooth
2. Cook according to crepe-machine directions

RICE CREPES *(yield: 6 crepes)*

¾ cup rice flour
3 T rice polish
3 eggs

1 cup milk or milk alternative
1 T melted butter or oil

1. Blend all ingredients till smooth
2. Cook according to crepe-machine directions

CAROB SOYA DESSERT CREPES *(yield: 6 crepes)*

2 T carob powder
6 T soy, millet, or alternative
  flour
3 eggs
1 T melted butter or cold-pressed
  oil

½ cup cream
1 T honey
1 tsp cinnamon
1–2 T milk

1. Blend all ingredients till smooth
2. Cook according to crepe-machine directions

OAT CREPES *(yield: 6 crepes)*

⅔ cup oat flour
2 T protein powder
1 cup milk or milk alternative

4 eggs
3 T melted butter or cold-pressed
  oil

1. Blend all ingredients till smooth
2. Cook according to crepe-machine directions

AMARANTH APPLE CREPES *(yield: 6 crepes)*

¾ cup amaranth flour
¼ cup arrowroot
2 eggs

1 cup apple concentrate
1 T melted butter
½ tsp cinnamon

1. Blend all ingredients till smooth
2. Cook according to crepe-machine directions

CROUTONS, PASTA, CRACKERS

Nonwheat pasta, crackers, and chips may be (happily) purchased in both grocery and health-food stores. Croutons are not yet available without wheat but can be made from breads to which your child is not sensitive.

Pasta made at home without wheat is hard work (believe me, I *tried*)! But since rice, mung bean, potato, arrowroot, and corn pasta are now available, the struggle to make pasta can be avoided. Health-food stores, Oriental sections in supermarkets, and gourmet shops carry pasta in various shapes and kinds. Look carefully at labels, though, as a product may be labeled "spinach macaroni" or "sesame spaghetti" and contain wheat in the form of "semolina."

Crackers and chips made of corn, rice, rye, or potato are available at health-food stores and in health-food sections in supermarkets. Crackers, unlike pasta, are fairly easy to make, and your child may enjoy some of the following recipes more than crackers that you purchase.

BASIC CROUTONS

2 cups cubed (tolerated) bread
¼ cup melted butter
season with Parmesan cheese, garlic

powder, sea salt, or any Italian
herbs

1. Dry cubed bread in oven for about 10 min. at 350°
2. Remove from oven and sprinkle on desired seasoning and melted butter; mix well
3. Return to oven, stirring occasionally
4. Continue baking until bread cubes are crisp and lightly browned

CHEESY OAT CRACKERS *(yield: 2½ dozen)*

½ cup oat flour
¾ cup nut flour
¼ cup baking soda
½ tsp sea salt
1 T cold-pressed oil

1 cup finely shredded cheese
2 T sesame seeds
Earth Grown natural orange food coloring
2 T ice water (approx.)

1. Combine dry ingredients
2. Mix oil into dry ingredients
3. Add cheese and sesame seeds; mix
4. Gradually mix in water until a ball is formed; natural food coloring may be added if desired
5. Roll out dough thinly on an oat-floured board; cut dough into small squares or rounds

CINNAMON WHEAT GERM CRACKERS *(yield: 1½ dozen)*

1 cup ground wheat germ or corn germ
1 tsp cinnamon

2 T honey
1–2 T ice water (approx.)

1. Mix wheat germ and cinnamon
2. Stir in honey, then use fingertips to mix until mixture is crumbly
3. Add water slowly until a cohesive ball is formed
4. Place dough on a cookie sheet, cover with foil and roll out thinly, score dough
5. Remove foil and bake at 325° till browned

COCONUT SEED-NUT CRACKERS *(yield: 2 dozen)*

½ cup nut flour
½ cup seed flour

½ cup shredded coconut
3–4 T ice water (approx.)

1. Combine all dry ingredients
2. Mix in water by the tablespoon until a ball is formed
3. Roll out thinly on a lightly oiled baking sheet
4. Score dough into triangles or squares
5. Bake at 325° until lightly browned and crisp

PRETZELS

2¾ cups soy flour
   or 2 cups rice flour and ½ cup rice polish
3 beaten eggs

water to moisten
¼ cup sesame seeds
½ tsp sea salt

nbine dry ingredients

flour mixture with eggs, adding liquid as needed

l into ropes and curl into pretzel shapes. Form fat or thin, large or small pretzels as desired. Gently pinch dough where two overlap to seal, brush on a bit of egg white, and sprinkle with sesame seeds and sea salt

4. Bake at 350° for about 35 min. for soy pretzels and 15 min. for rice pretzels. Pretzels should be crisp and lightly browned

CEREALS

Cereals tend to be too starchy for many children and should be used with caution in the diet. If you choose to make cereals a part of your child's diet and the child seems able to handle them, it's a good idea to serve them in conjunction with high-nutrient foods. This may be accomplished by addition of supplement foods to the cereal (as listed below).

HOT STUFF

To prepare hot cereal, bring 2 cups of water to a rolling boil, add 1 cup of millet (cook 30 min.) or rolled oats (cook 5 min.) or amaranth (cook 30 min.) or buckwheat groats (cook 20 min.) or soy grits (cook 30 min.) or a combination cereal of bran, wheat germ, and 2 tsp flaxseed (cook 15 min.), reduce heat, and allow to boil gently. Add ground seeds, wheat germ, milk powder, protein powder, nutritional yeast, lecithin, bran, carob powder, chopped nuts, seeds, chopped dried or fresh fruit, cinnamon, or whatever your child enjoys. Top with milk or milk alternative.

COLD STUFF

Cold cereals may include natural puffed cereals such as puffed millet, puffed corn, and puffed rice available from El Molino Mills or New Morning Oatios (like Cheerios) or Crispy Brown Rice (like Rice Crispies). Homemade granola is preferable to store-bought (even if purchased without brown sugar in a health-food store) because you can control the ingredients (avoiding what your child is sensitive to) and maximize the nutrient content. Homemade granola is not difficult to make: Just combine 4 cups rolled oats; ½ to 1 cup wheat germ, wheat bran, corn germ, or soy grits; ½ cup or more of milk powder or protein powder (optional); 1 to 2 cups any seeds or chopped nuts; 1 or more cups chopped, dried fruit; 1–2 T nutritional yeast; and flavoring such as carob powder, cinnamon, spices. Blend ⅓ to ½ cup honey, fruit concentrate, or maple syrup, 1 tsp vanilla, and ⅓ to ½ cup melted butter or cold-pressed oil; then stir thoroughly into dry mixture. Bake at 325°, stirring occasionally, until desired crunchiness is obtained (approx. 2½ hours).

APPLE-CRUNCH GRANOLA

4 cups rolled oats
½ cup slivered almonds
½ cup wheat germ
¼ cup soy grits
¼ cup sesame seeds
½ cup sunflower seeds
2 tsp cinnamon

1 T nutritional yeast
1 cup chopped crunchy dried apples (redry chopped dried apples in oven till they are crisp)
⅓ cup apple concentrate, ⅓ cup melted butter, and 1 tsp vanilla

1. Follow directions given for "Cold Stuff," page 242.

CINNAMON-SEED CEREAL

1½ cups any seed flour
1 tsp cinnamon
½ cup milk powder or protein powder

½ cup chopped dried fruit or coconut
½ cup chopped nuts

1. Mix and refrigerate
2. Serve in ¼-cup portions cold or hot (cook in water) with milk or milk alternative

COOKIES, CAKES, BARS, SQUARES

The cookie is a time-honored snack that children thoroughly enjoy. Cookies, however, should be nutritious additions to a child's diet instead of a white-sugar/hydrogenated-fat/white-flour blend. The following recipes are traditional cookies that were snatched and gobbled up as if by magic by my "helpers." Be bold, be daring . . . convert some of your own favorite cookie recipes into wholesome ones.

DOUBLE CAROB NUT COOKIES I *(yield: 1½ dozen)*

½ cup butter
⅓ cup honey
2 eggs, slightly beaten
½ cup seed flour or almond flour
¼ cup carob powder
½ cup milk powder or protein powder

2 T nutritional yeast (optional)
½ cup chopped nuts
¼ cup unsweetened carob chips
½ tsp vanilla

1. Cream butter and honey
2. Add beaten eggs to honey mixture; blend well

3. Mix flour and powders
4. Combine the two mixtures and stir in vanilla, nuts, chips. Drop from tsp onto a buttered cookie sheet
5. Bake at 350° for about 12 min.

DOUBLE CAROB NUT COOKIES II (chewy)
(yield: 1½ dozen)

½ cup butter
2 T honey
¾ cup date sugar
2 eggs, slightly beaten
½ cup filbert or pecan flour
½ cup milk powder or protein
  powder

2 T nutritional yeast (optional)
¼ cup carob powder
½ tsp vanilla
½ cup chopped nuts
¼ cup unsweetened carob chips

1. Cream butter, honey, date sugar
2. Add beaten eggs to honey mixture, blend well
3. Mix flour and powders
4. Combine the two mixtures and stir in vanilla, nuts, chips. Drop from tsp onto a buttered sheet
5. Bake at 350° for about 12 min.

LEMON DROPS *(yield: 1 dozen)*

⅓ cup honey
2 T butter
1 egg, beaten or egg replacer
  equivalent
3 T lemon juice

1 T lemon rind
½ cup protein powder or milk
  powder
¼ cup arrowroot
1 tsp baking powder

1. Cream honey and butter; mix in egg and lemon juice and rind
2. Mix dry ingredients
3. Combine dry and lemon-honey mixtures
4. Drop from teaspoon onto an oiled cookie sheet and bake at 325° for about 20 min.

PEANUT BUTTER CRUNCH *(yield: 2 dozen)*

½ cup butter
⅔ cup honey
1 egg, beaten, or egg-replacer
  equivalent
¾ cup crunchy natural
  (unhydrogenated) peanut
  butter *or* substitute almond,
  cashew, or sesame butter

1 tsp vanilla
2 T nutritional yeast (optional)
½ cup protein powder
½ cup milk powder
¾ cup wheat germ or almond
  flour
1 cup seed flour
½ tsp baking soda

1. Cream butter and honey; add egg, then peanut butter and vanilla; mix well
2. Mix dry ingredients and combine with peanut butter mixture
3. Form into balls and flatten with the bottom of a glass (dip glass in ice water to prevent sticking); small, medium and large cookies all work well
4. Bake at 325° for 20–25 min.

MISTY MINT CHIP COOKIES (crisp) *(yield: 1½ dozen)*

½ cup butter
⅓ cup honey
2 eggs, beaten
¾ cup wheat germ or nut or seed flour

¾ cup milk powder
1 T nutritional yeast (optional)
½ tsp baking soda
½ tsp mint extract
¼ cup unsweetened carob chips

1. Cream butter and honey; mix in eggs
2. Mix dry ingredients, then combine with honey mixture
3. Add mint extract and stir in carob chips
4. Drop batter from tsp onto a buttered cookie sheet
5. Bake at 350° for 12 min.

PINWHEELS *(yield: 1½ dozen)*

½ cup butter
⅔ cup honey
1 egg, slightly beaten, or egg-replacer equivalent
2 tsp vanilla
1 cup soy flour and ¼ cup arrowroot
     or 1⅓ cups oat flour or alternative

¾ cup milk powder or protein powder
1 tsp baking powder
2 T carob powder (to add to half of dough)
2 T soy (or appropriate) flour (to add to other half of dough)

1. Cream butter and honey; add egg and vanilla
2. Mix dry ingredients (except for 2 T of flour and 2T of carob powder
3. Combine honey and dry mixtures
4. Halve dough and mix carob powder with one portion and flour with other portion
5. Chill both portions for a few hours
6. Roll out each portion separately between two sheets of foil, about ⅛ inch thick
7. Place one layer of dough on top of the other and roll up firmly; slice thinly with a sharp knife and bake at 350° for 12–15 min.

CAROB GINGERBREAD PEOPLE *(yield: 1 dozen)*

½ cup carob powder
1¼ cups seed flour
½ cup arrowroot powder
¾ cup soy flour or flour
  alternative
2 T nutritional yeast (optional)
1 tsp ginger

¼ tsp nutmeg
½ tsp cinnamon
1 egg, beaten, or egg alternative
½ cup cold-pressed oil
¼ cup blackstrap molasses
½ cup honey

1. Mix all dry ingredients
2. Blend egg, oil, molasses, honey
3. Blend the two mixtures
4. Roll out dough between two pieces of foil; cut into people shapes
5. Bake at 300° for 20–25 min.

THUMBPRINTS *(yield: 2½ dozen)*

½ cup butter
½ cup honey
1 egg, beaten
1 tsp vanilla
1¼ cups oat flour

¼ cup arrowroot
2 cups seed or nut flour
1 T nutritional yeast (optional)
honey-sweetened or unsweetened
jam for filling

1. Cream butter and honey; mix in egg and vanilla
2. Mix dry ingredients; combine with honey mixture
3. Roll dough into small balls and dip in slightly beaten egg white, then in nut flour
4. Place on buttered cookie sheet and depress center of each cookie with your thumb
5. Bake at 350° for about 20 min.; fill centers of cookies with natural jam

CINNAMON SMILES *(yield: 2 dozen)*

1 cup butter
½ cup honey
1½ tsp vanilla
1 cup soy, millet or alternative
  flour

1½ cups seed or nut flour
⅓ cup arrowroot or other starch
2 T nutritional yeast (optional)
1½ tsp cinnamon
¾ cup finely chopped nuts

1. Cream butter and honey; add vanilla
2. Mix dry ingredients; combine with honey mixture
3. Chill dough four hours or overnight

4. Roll out dough, sprinkle on cinnamon and chopped nuts, and dot with butter; roll up dough carefully and slice thin

5. Pinch into the shape of smiles and sprinkle with cinnamon

6. Bake at 300° for 35 min. or until nicely browned; allow to cool for a few min. before removing from baking sheet

OATMEAL CRISPS *(yield:1½ dozen)*

¾ cup butter
½ cup honey
1 egg, beaten, or egg-replacer
  equivalent
1 T nutritional yeast (optional)
½ cup milk powder or protein
  powder

2 T arrowroot powder
1 cup nut or seed flour
½ cup oat flour
1 tsp cinnamon
1 tsp vanilla
1½ cups rolled oats
½ cup raisins

1. Cream butter and honey; mix in egg
2. Mix dry ingredients and combine with honey mixture
3. Stir in vanilla, rolled oats, and raisins
4. Drop from a tsp onto a buttered baking sheet and bake at 350° for 15 min.
5. Allow cookies to cool about 15 min. on sheet before removing, as they are delicate when warm

MAPLE-WALNUT COOKIES *(yield: 1½ dozen)*

¼ cup butter
½ cup maple syrup
1 egg, beaten, or egg-replacer
  equivalent
1 tsp vanilla
1½ cups walnut flour

½ cup protein powder or milk
  powder
1 T nutritional yeast (optional)
2 T arrowroot or other starch
1 tsp baking powder
walnut pieces for tops of cookies

1. Cream butter and syrup; mix in egg and vanilla
2. Mix dry ingredients; combine with maple-syrup mixture
3. Drop onto buttered cookie sheet and top with walnut halves or pieces
4. Bake at 325° for 20–22 min.

HAYSTACKS *(yield: 1 dozen)*

2 stiffly beaten egg whites
½ tsp vanilla
2 T honey
¾ cup finely shredded
  unsweetened coconut

handful of finely chopped nuts
variation: add 2 T carob powder
and 1 more T honey

1. Beat egg whites till stiff; beat in vanilla and honey slowly
2. Mix coconut and chopped nuts, then fold into egg-white mixture
3. Drop onto greased cookie sheet and bake at 300° for about ½ hour

CAROB ALMOND MINT BARS *(yield: 1 dozen)*

½ cup butter
⅓ cup honey
2 eggs
½ tsp vanilla
1 tsp peppermint extract

¼ cup carob powder
1¼ cups almond flour
2 T arrowroot or other starch
½ cup chopped almonds

1. Cream butter and honey; beat in eggs, vanilla, peppermint
2. Mix dry ingredients; combine with peppermint mixture
3. Stir in nuts, then pour batter into a buttered 8 × 8 pan and bake for about 45 min. at 325°

LEMON COCONUT SQUARES *(yield: 1 dozen)*

½ cup butter
½ cup honey
1 egg, beaten, or egg-replacer
   equivalent
¾ cup rice flour
¼ cup rice polish

2 T arrowroot or other starch
1 tsp baking powder
3 T lemon juice
2 T lemon rind
1 cup finely shredded
   unsweetened coconut

1. Cream butter and honey, add egg, and mix
2. Mix dry ingredients; combine dry and honey mixtures
3. Stir in lemon juice and rind and coconut
4. Pour and spread into an 8 × 8 oiled pan
5. Bake at 325° for about 45 min.

TOPPING:
2 T butter
1 T honey
2 T lemon juice

1 T lemon rind
1 cup ground coconut

1. Mix all ingredients and spread on top of cooled squares

CAROB CHERRY NUT SQUARES *(yield: 1 dozen)*

1 cup millet flour
   or ½ cup potato flour
2 T carob flour
1 cup seed or nut flour

¼ cup arrowroot or other starch
1 T nutritional yeast (optional)
½ cup butter
¼ cup honey

1. Mix dry ingredients
2. Cut butter into flour mixture
3. Blend honey into mixture and press into a 9 × 13 buttered pan
4. Bake at 325° for about 20 min.

TOPPING:

1 cup water blended with ½ cup fresh or frozen unsweetened Bing cherries
2 T arrowroot

2 T sweetener of choice
½ cup halved Bing cherries
¼ cup chopped nuts
¼ cup unsweetened carob chips

1. Mix arrowroot in cold cherry juice; then heat mixture till thickened, adding sweetener and cherry halves
2. Cool mixture slightly, then pour over cake; sprinkle on nuts and carob chips

FUDGY NUT BROWNIES *(yield: 1 dozen)*

¼ cup melted butter
½ cup honey
½ cup carob powder
2 eggs, beaten
1 tsp vanilla
½ cup milk powder or protein powder

1 cup nut or seed flour
1 T nutritional yeast (optional)
1 tsp baking powder
½ cup chopped nuts

1. Mix melted butter with honey and carob powder; add eggs and vanilla
2. Combine dry ingredients; blend with honey mixture
3. Pour into an oiled 8 × 8 pan and bake at 350° for 35 min.

RASPBERRY-JAM SQUARES *(yield: 1 dozen)*

CRUST:

¾ cup soy or alternative flour
½ cup seed flour
¼ cup milk powder or protein powder
1 tsp baking powder

½ tsp cinnamon
½ cup butter
1 egg, beaten
3 T honey

1. Mix dry ingredients; cut butter into this mixture
2. Blend egg and honey with flour/butter mixture; press into an oiled 8 × 8 pan

FILLING:

¾ cup Westbrae unsweetened   raspberry (or other) jam

1. Spread filling over crust

TOPPING:

¼ cup melted butter   1 tsp vanilla
1 egg, beaten   1 cup soy or alternative flour
¼ cup honey   2 T arrowroot or other starch
                               ½ cup seed flour

1. Mix all topping ingredients and spread on top of jam filling in pan
2. Bake at 325° for 40–45 min.

CAKES

Developing a cake recipe without wheat flour was difficult, to say the least. The cakes *refused* to rise, and one cake after another looked like a large pancake. I became so frustrated with my failures (two failures I can handle without hysteria, but not ten!) that I stopped baking for two days just to sort out what I was doing wrong. Sheet cakes and angel-food cakes came out beautifully, so why not layer cakes?

After much thought, I decided to try expanding the recipes to three layers. Success! And thank goodness, for I had reached the end of my idea rope. Of the following cake recipes, the Maple Spice Cake was rated the favorite by adults (my best friend insists she cannot get through her birthday unless I make this token cake for her each year). My "helpers," on the other hand, said they like the Fruit Basket Cake "the bestest," but they practically inhaled every new flavor of cake offered.

The following recipes include cake icings that contain milk powder to boost nutritional value and give the proper texture. If your child is sensitive to milk, substitute a starch such as arrowroot or protein powder (some protein powders work better than others).

MAPLE SPICE CAKE

¾ cup maple syrup   2 tsp baking powder
¾ cup butter   ½ tsp baking soda
1 tsp vanilla   1½ tsp nutmeg
4 egg yolks, beaten   1½ tsp cinnamon
2¼ cups nut flour   ¾ tsp cloves
4 T arrowroot   ½ cup yogurt
½ cup milk powder   4 stiffly beaten egg whites
¼ cup protein powder

1. Cream maple syrup and butter and add vanilla
2. Mix dry ingredients and combine with syrup mixture; add cloves
3. Blend in yogurt and fold in egg whites
4. Pour into three 9-inch buttered, nut-floured cake pans and bake at 325° for about 45 min.

PECAN ICING

1 T butter
½ cup maple syrup
1¼ cups milk powder

4 T cream
1 tsp vanilla
½ cup chopped pecans

1. Cream butter and maple syrup
2. Beat in milk powder slowly along with cream and vanilla; add pecans
3. Icing will be thick and sticky; ice cooled cake and refrigerate to harden icing

GERMAN CAROB CAKE

¾ cup butter
¾ cup maple syrup
3 egg yolks, beaten
1½ tsp vanilla
6 T carob powder
1 cup soy or alternative flour

⅓ cup arrowroot or other starch
¾ cup seed or nut flour
2 T nutritional yeast (optional)
1 T baking powder
¾ cup soy milk or alternative
3 egg whites, beaten stiffly

1. Cream butter and syrup; blend in egg yolks and vanilla
2. Mix dry ingredients and combine with syrup mixture
3. Pour in soy milk slowly, mixing well; fold in egg whites
4. Pour into three buttered, round 9-inch cake pans and bake at 350° for 40–45 min.

COCONUTTY ICING

¾ cup butter
½ cup maple syrup
½ cup arrowroot or protein
  powder

½ cup chopped pecans
¾ cup coconut
1 tsp vanilla

1. Cream butter and sweetening; beat in milk powder slowly; add vanilla
2. Mix in nuts and coconut
3. Spread icing over cake layers

THE ELEGANT DESSERT

1 recipe Double Carob Nut
  Cookies I
1 pint real whipping cream

1 tsp vanilla
honey to taste, chopped nuts

1. Prepare cookies (see recipe, page 243); cool
2. Whip cream; add vanilla and honey
3. Coat both sides of each cookie with whipped cream, sticking them together in a row (use a long, narrow serving plate; cake cannot be moved to another plate later on)
4. Now cover entire roll with whipped cream so the cookies do not show through
5. Sprinkly with finely chopped nuts
6. Refrigerate 4–6 hours; serve

GINGERBREAD SHEET CAKE

½ cup honey
½ cup butter
½ cup blackstrap molasses
3 eggs, beaten, or egg replacer
¾ cup yogurt or milk alternative
½ cup soy or ⅔ cup oat flour
½ cup milk powder or protein
  powder
2 cups seed or nut flour

¼ cup arrowroot or other starch
2 T nutritional yeast (optional)
1 tsp baking soda
2 tsp cinnamon
1 tsp ginger
1 tsp allspice
½ cup chopped nuts
½ cup raisins

1. Beat honey and butter; mix in molasses, eggs, yogurt
2. Combine all dry ingredients
3. Blend dry and molasses mixtures; stir in nuts and raisins
4. Pour batter into oiled 9 × 13 pan and bake at 325° for about one hour

FRUIT BASKET CAKE

½ cup butter
¾ cup honey
2 eggs
1 tsp vanilla
1½ cups nut flour
1 cup milk powder or protein
  powder
⅓ cup arrowroot or other starch

1 tsp cinnamon
¼ cup wheat germ or seed flour
2 tsp baking soda
2 tsp baking powder
½ cup drained crushed pineapple
¾ cup grated carrot
¼ cup coconut (optional)

1. Cream butter and honey; add eggs and vanilla
2. Mix dry ingredients and combine with honey mixture
3. Stir in pineapple, grated carrot, and coconut
4. Pour into three 9-inch buttered pans and bake at 325° for 45 min.

FRUITY FROSTING

Whip 2 cups of cream, adding 1 tsp of vanilla and honey to taste. Smooth whipped cream on one layer of Fruit Basket Cake, top with sliced fresh fruit (strawberries banana, pineapple, etc. as you like), top with another layer of cake, and continue. Cover sides of cake with whipped cream and decorate top with fresh fruit; refrigerate.

LEMON MIST CAKE

¾ cup butter
¾ cup honey
4 egg yolks, beaten
¾ cup rice polish
1½ cups rice flour
1 cup nut or seed flour
4 T arrowroot or other starch

1 T baking powder
3 T lemon juice
2 T lemon rind
¾ cup liquid (water, soy milk, or other)
4 egg whites, beaten stiffly

1. Cream butter and honey, add egg yolks, and mix well
2. Mix dry ingredients, combine with honey mixture, and stir in lemon rind/juice
3. Gently mix in the beaten egg whites
4. Pour into three buttered, rice-floured 9-inch pans; bake at 350° for 35 min.

LEMON YELLOW ICING

½ cup very light-colored honey
¾ cup butter
1 egg yolk
½ cup milk powder or arrowroot

3 T lemon juice (or may use ½ tsp oil of lemon instead)
1 tsp lemon rind

1. Cream honey and butter; blend in egg yolk and milk powder (or arrowroot)
2. Mix in lemon juice and rind
3. Frost cooled lemon cake

PINK PEPPERMINT CAKE

¾ cup honey
½ cup butter
3 egg yolks, beaten
2 cups oat flour
1 T nutritional yeast (optional)
¾ cup nut or seed flour
¾ cup milk powder or protein
    powder

½ tsp baking soda
2 tsp baking powder
½ cup yogurt or milk alternative
¾ tsp peppermint extract
3 egg whites, beaten stiffly

1. Cream honey and butter; blend in egg yolks
2. Combine dry ingredients and blend with honey mixture
3. Add yogurt and peppermint extract; fold in beaten egg whites
4. Pour into three buttered, oat-floured pans and bake at 350° for about 35 min.

PEPPERMINT SWIRL ICING

¾ cup butter
½ cup honey
½ cup milk powder or arrowroot

drops of Earth Grown natural red
coloring (will appear pink in icing)
swirled at strategic points

COCONUT SNOWSTORM CAKE

8 eggs, separated
½ cup + 2 T honey
1 tsp vanilla

¼ cup milk powder
2 cups filbert flour
1 cup ground coconut

1. Beat egg yolks, honey, vanilla
2. Combine milk powder, nut flour, and coconut; mix with egg mixture; add vanilla
3. Beat egg whites till stiff and fold into batter
4. Pour into lightly oiled angel food cake pan and bake at 325° for about one hour

COCONUT FROSTING

Whip 1 cup of cream and beat in ½ tsp vanilla and 2 tsp honey. Frost coconut cake with whipped cream and sprinkle about ½ cup coconut on whipped cream.

CINNAMON-APPLE CAKE

½ cup butter
¾ cup apple-juice concentrate
3 egg yolks
1 tsp vanilla
½ cup applesauce
2 cups seed or nut flour
2 T nutritional yeast (optional)

½ cup milk powder or protein
   powder
⅓ cup arrowroot or other starch
2 tsp cinnamon
1 T baking powder
¾ cup chopped apple
¼ cup raisins

1. Cream butter and apple-juice concentrate; and blend in eggs, vanilla, applesauce
2. Combine dry ingredients and add to mixture
3. Stir in chopped apple and raisins
4. Pour into a buttered 9 × 13 pan and bake at 325° for 65–70 min.
5. Serve with a dollop of whipped cream and a sprinkle of cinnamon

SIMPLE SIMON'S FAVORITE PIES

For a change of pace, pies are fun to make. However, they do tend to contain more carbohydrates and less of nutritive additions than other desserts, so they should be prepared less often. However, adding wholesome ingredients boosts nutritional value.

Crusts may be made from natural graham cracker crumbs, natural granola, nut flour, seed flour, or other variety flours. Butter, cold-pressed oils, and honey work well to hold the crust together.

Fillings for pies can be prepared from scratch with natural ingredients or purchased in packaged form at health-food stores—various natural pudding and pie mixes are available.

CAROB SILK PIE

CRUST:
1½ cups almond flour
½ tsp cinnamon

3 T butter
1 T honey

1. Mix almond flour and cinnamon; cut in butter
2. Mix in honey, press into pie pan, brush with egg white, and bake at 350° for 15 min.

FILLING:

1¼ cups milk	3 egg yolks, beaten
4 T carob powder	1 T butter
3 T water	1 tsp vanilla
3 T arrowroot	1 cup fresh whipped cream
½ cup honey	

1. Mix 1 cup milk, carob powder, and water
2. Mix arrowroot and ¼ cup milk, then stir into carob mixture. Add honey and stir entire mixture over medium heat for about 15 min. or until thick and bubbly
3. Beat in egg yolks, 1 T butter, and vanilla; mix a dollop of hot carob mixture into eggs, then pour eggs into carob mixture. Mix constantly over heat for a few minutes
4. Remove carob mixture from heat, pour into a bowl, and chill till firm (3 to 4 hours)
5. Whip cream, blend with carob mixture, and pour into prebaked pie shell. Chill till firm enough to cut

FLUFFY LIME PIE

CRUST:

1 T honey	3 T butter or cold-pressed oil
1½ cups nut flour	

1. Cut butter into flour until a bowl of crumbs is formed; mix in honey
2. Press into a pie pan and brush on egg white; bake at 350° for 15 min.

FILLING:

⅔ cup water	2 tsp lime rind
⅓ cup lime juice	2 egg whites, beaten stiffly
⅓ cup light-colored honey	1 cup whipped cream
1 T unflavored gelatin	1 tsp Earth Grown natural green
2 egg yolks, beaten	food coloring

1. Combine water, lime juice, honey, and gelatin in a saucepan over medium heat; add egg yolks; cook till gelatin is dissolved
2. Remove mixture from heat, stir in lime rind, and chill until slightly thickened
3. Beat egg whites and add to gelatin mixture along with whipped cream and food coloring; chill again for 1 hour
4. Spoon lime mixture into prebaked pie shell, chilling about 3 hours

BANANA CREAM PIE

CRUST:
use nut crust recipe for "Fluffy Lime Pie" on page 256.

FILLING:
1 mashed banana   1 cup whipped cream
vanilla custard (see recipe on page
260)

1. Press banana into prebaked pie shell, pour custard on top, and chill till firm
2. Top with whipped cream or half whipped cream and half yogurt, with honey to taste and ½ tsp vanilla

LEMON MERINGUE PIE

CRUST:
¼ cup sesame flour   1 T honey
2 T butter   1¼ cup ground coconut

1. Mix all ingredients and prebake 12–15 min. at 350°

FILLING:
1¼ cups water   3 egg yolks, beaten
7 T arrowroot   ⅓ cup lemon juice
½ cup honey   2 tsp lemon rind (undyed)

1. Mix arrowroot with water. In a saucepan bring water, arrowroot, and honey to a boil; reduce heat and cook till mixture thickens; add lemon juice and rind
2. Add a dab of hot mixture to beaten egg yolks and then pour eggs into honey mixture; cook for an additional 2–3 min.
3. Remove from heat and pour mixture into prebaked pie shell

MERINGUE:
3 egg whites (room temp)   ½ tsp vanilla
2 tsp honey

1. Beat egg whites till frothy; add honey and vanilla slowly as you continue beating egg whites till stiff
2. Top filled pie with meringue and bake at 325° for 15–20 min. or until meringue is lightly browned. Cool before cutting; refrigerate

CRISPY APPLE PIE

CRUST:

1¾ cups soy flour
¼ cup arrowroot
pinch of sea salt

½ cup butter
2 cups finely grated cheese
4 T ice water

1. Mix soy flour, arrowroot, and sea salt; cut in butter
2. Mix cheese in well, then add water
3. Divide ball in half; roll out each half between two sheets of foil to form top and bottom crusts
4. Remove top foil sheet; turn pie pan upside down on top of crust; flip over; peel off foil

FILLING:

⅓ cup apple-juice concentrate
2 T arrowroot
½ tsp cinnamon

4½ cups sliced, unpeeled apples
½ cup chopped nuts
1 T butter

1. Mix apple-juice concentrate and arrowroot; add cinnamon. Stir in apples and chopped nuts
2. Pour apple mixture on top of dough-lined pie pan, dotting filling with butter
3. Put top of dough on top of filling, crimp edges, and cut decorative holes on top
4. Brush top with egg white and water mixture, then bake at 350° for about 1 hour

CHERRY COBBLER

FILLING:

3 cups cherries (frozen or fresh)
1 cup cherry juice (make by blending ½ cup cherries with water

2 T arrowroot
⅓ cup honey

1. Mix cherry juice with arrowroot, then heat this mixture in a saucepan along with honey till thickened
2. Stir in cherries
3. Pour into lightly oiled glass or Corningware baking dish

TOPPING:

1 T melted butter
½ cup milk or milk alternative
1 egg, beaten
¼ cup millet flour or alternative
1 cup seed flour

½ cup milk powder or protein powder
2 T arrowroot
2 tsp baking powder
½ tsp cinnamon

1. Mix first three ingredients
2. Combine dry ingredients and mix with egg mixture
3. Drop portions of batter on top of cherry mixture with a large spoon and gently spread evenly over mixture
4. Bake at 350° for ½ hour

PEACHY PECAN CRISP

FILLING:

5 sliced ripe peaches (or any fruit)
½ cup chopped pecans

½ tsp cinnamon
2 tsp lemon juice

1. Place sliced peaches in a low baking dish; sprinkle on nuts, cinnamon, and lemon juice

TOPPING:

½ cup rolled oats
⅓ cup oat flour
½ cup wheat germ or sesame flour
½ cup pecan flour

1 T arrowroot
¼ cup cold-pressed oil
¼ cup honey
½ tsp cinnamon

1. Combine all dry ingredients; blend in oil and honey
2. Sprinkle this mixture on top of apple mixture and bake at 350° for ½ hour

CUSTARD, GELATIN, PUDDING

For custard, gelatin, and pudding desserts, you can convert the many sugar-loaded recipes you probably already have to healthy versions. The following are the basic recipes, which can be flavor-adjusted to your family's tastes. Try new flavors they can't resist, like Banana Mint, Maple Pecan, or Cherry Almond (for custards or pudding), or Strawberry Coconut, Papaya Pineapple, or Lemon Lime (for gelatin).

What to call natural gelatin desserts brings up an interesting controversy. My son calls them "Jell-O," even though he understands that we do not use commercial gelatins, which may contain 85 percent sugar plus artificial colors and flavors. Some take a different stand, however, on precise terminology. When a friend of mine served her three-year-old son a natural gelatin dessert and her husband asked if he might have a bite of Jell-O, the child firmly replied, "I'm eating gel-a-tin, not Jell-O. Want some?"

BASIC CUSTARD *(yield: 4 servings)*

1 T unflavored gelatin   4 eggs
2½ cups milk   1 tsp vanilla
¼ cup sweetening

1. Soften gelatin in ½ cup of milk; then dissolve gelatin in milk in a saucepan over med/low heat
2. Add remaining ingredients and stir until slightly thickened
3. Remove from heat and stir in any desired flavorings such as ½ cup pureed cooked pumpkin, carrot, or dried or fresh fruit. Ground or chopped seeds and nuts may also be added

BASIC PUDDING WITH MILK AND EGGS
(yield: 4 servings)

1½ cups milk   optional flavoring: 1–2 cups of
½ cup milk powder   fruit or vegetables; small quantity
3 T arrowroot   of nuts, carob, seeds, extracts
¼ cup sweetening (optional)   1–2 eggs, beaten

1. In the blender combine milk and arrowroot, then add sweetening. Stir in flavoring and cook over med/low heat till thickened (about 6–7 min)
2. Pour a bit of hot mixture into beaten eggs, stir, combine eggs with mixture and pour into pan. Continue cooking and stirring for about 2 min. longer
3. Cool in refrigerator till firm

BASIC PUDDING WITHOUT MILK AND EGGS
(yield: 6 servings)

3 cups any fruit or vegetable—   ¼ cup sweetening (optional)
  pureed   ½ cup chopped fruit, nuts, seeds,
3 T arrowroot   or any desired flavoring

1. Blend pureed fruit or vegetable and arrowroot; stir in any additions
2. Cook over low heat till thickened
3. Refrigerate till firm

BASIC GELATIN *(yield: 4 servings)*

1 T gelatin   2 cups of liquid (juice)

1. Soak gelatin in 1 cup of liquid
2. Bring remaining cup of liquid to a rolling boil and combine with gelatin mixture

BASIC FINGER GELATIN

4 T gelatin   ¼ cup sweetening (optional)
2¾ cups liquid

1. Soften gelatin in ¾ cup liquid
2. Bring 1 cup of liquid to a rolling boil and stir into gelatin mixture till gelatin is dissolved
3. Stir in remaining cup of liquid
4. Pour into square 9-inch oiled pan and chill till firm. Extra layers of different-colored gelatin may be added (repeat above procedure). Any juice works well for Finger Gelatin
5. When firm, slice into small squares

ICES AND ICE CREAM

A birthday party just isn't complete without an ice or ice cream. Snacks, for that matter, are frequently a matter of ice cream or Popsicles, so obtaining or preparing natural ices and ice cream is a must.

Naturally sweetnened ice cream, ices on a stick, and novelties may be found in many health-food stores and natural–ice cream parlors across the country, and those allergic to milk can buy soy and rice ice cream variations. But often the purchased product seems a little too sweet or not the flavor we wish to have. Thus making your own ice cream permits you to adjust the sweetness and flavoring to just the way you like it most. Many different ice cream makers are now on the market. Some are quick and easy to use; many children, however, find the traditional crank model fun at parties, giving everyone a chance to help turn out the ice cream!

Ices, like ice cream, are made in a machine, but without milk products. Ice cream novelties are things you can do with ices and ice cream to make them even more fun for kids to eat.

BASIC VANILLA ICE CREAM

½ cup milk   ⅓ cup honey or other sweetener
½ cup milk powder   2 cups cream
2 tsp gelatin plus ¼ cup water   2 tsp vanilla

1. Blend milk and milk powder in the blender
2. Soften gelatin in water and pour into a saucepan with milk mixture; add honey and stir over medium heat until gelatin is dissolved, cool
3. Combine cooled honey-milk mixture with cream and stir in vanilla
4. Chill mixture and freeze in an ice cream machine

I GOTTA HAVE ICE CREAM NOW!

1 cup half-and-half or soy milk
2 T honey or other sweetener
1 T milk powder or protein powder

flavoring: vanilla, carob, mint, fruit, etc.
crushed ice

1. Put all ingredients (except ice) in blender and blend until smooth
2. Add crushed ice slowly as blender is going
3. Continue to blend and add ice till a thick, creamy consistency is formed
4. Eat on the spot

BUTTER PECAN ICE CREAM

1 recipe basic vanilla ice cream (use maple syrup for sweetening)

½ cup chopped pecans sautéed in butter

CAROB ALMOND ICE CREAM

1 recipe basic vanilla ice cream
4–6 T carob powder

1 cup chopped, sautéed almonds

EGGNOG ICE CREAM

1 recipe basic vanilla ice cream
4 egg yolks

1 tsp nutmeg
1 tsp rum extract

MISTY MINT CHIP ICE CREAM

1 recipe basic vanilla ice cream
½ cup unsweetened carob chips

½ tsp peppermint extract

SPUMONI ICE CREAM

1 recipe basic vanilla ice cream
½ cup chopped Bing cherries
½ cup drained crushed pineapple

¼ cup chopped nuts
¼ cup shredded coconut

FRUIT-FLAVORED ICE CREAM

1 recipe basic vanilla ice cream
2–3 cups blended fruit

1 cup chopped fruit

ANY FLAVOR ICE

1 T gelatin plus ¼ cup water
2 cups juice or fruit puree

1 cup crushed or chopped fruit

1. Soften gelatin in water
2. Combine gelatin, water, and juice or puree in a saucepan and heat until gelatin is dissolved; stir in fruit; chill
3. Freeze mixture in an ice cream machine

CHERRY ICE

2 cups cherry/apple juice
1 cup chopped Bing cherries

1 T gelatin plus ¼ cup water

MELON ICE

2 cups watermelon, cantaloupe, or other melon, pureed

1 T gelatin plus ¼ cup water

LEMON ICE

1 cup water
1 T gelatin plus ½ cup water

½ cup honey
¼ cup lemon juice

ROLLING ICE CREAM BALLS

Scoop out rounds of ice cream with a melon scoop (small) or ice cream scoop (large). Coat heavily with chopped nuts, coconut, and/or whatever you wish.

HONEY PIES

Spread honey ice cream or frozen yogurt between two natural cookies. May be dipped in carob syrup, or sides may be coated with carob chips. Freeze to harden.

BAKED ALASKA À LA NECTARINE

6 nectarines	4 egg whites
6 balls (ice cream—scoop size) of honey ice cream—freeze overnight so they will be firm	½ tsp vanilla 2 tsp honey

1. Prepare nectarines by cutting off tops (¼ of fruit) and scooping out the seeds
2. Place balls of ice cream in prepared fruit and put into freezer
3. Make a meringue with egg whites by beating and adding honey and vanilla very slowly as you beat egg whites till stiff
4. Seal tops of nectarines containing ice cream with meringue
5. Bake at 500° till lightly browned, about 2 min.

ANY FLAVOR FROZEN YOGURT

½ cup milk	½ cup honey or other sweetener
½ cup milk powder	2½ cups plain yogurt
1 T gelatin plus ¼ cup water	¾–1 cup blended fruit

1. Blend milk and milk powder in the blender
2. Soften gelatin in water
3. Combine blended milk, gelatin, water, and honey in a saucepan over low heat till gelatin is dissolved; cool
4. Mix in yogurt and fruit with milk/honey mixture
5. Chill mixture; freeze in an ice cream machine

"POPSICLES"

Freeze any fresh fruit or vegetable juice, with or without chopped fruit or vegetables added, in Popsicle molds.

NUTRA-SICLES

Freeze any milkshake, smoothie, or other beverages in the beverage section of this book.

BANANA GONE NUTS

Dip banana in melted, unsweetened carob chips (just add a little milk to the chips and heat gently till melted), then roll in finely chopped nuts.

CINNAMON NUT SURPRISE

Whip 1 cup of cream and beat in 2 tsp honey and 1 tsp vanilla. Next grind 1 cup of walnuts, mix in 1 tsp cinnamon, and add a bit of honey to keep mixture together. Using a muffin tin lined with cupcake papers, fill bottom of papers with walnut mixture. Add a spoonful of crushed fruit or natural jam and then a dollop of whipped cream. Top with a Bing cherry or strawberry; then freeze.

MAIN DISHES

Protein foods such as meat, fish, fowl, milk, cheese, and eggs are usually the center around which meals are made. Where breakfast and lunch can be pretty well individualized, dinner poses a special problem since it must appeal to the entire family. The following dinner and lunch ideas may appeal to some but not all family members and can be adjusted according to your family's needs and tastes.

When purchasing food, try to vary the proteins. Remember, protein is not necessarily beef; instead of ground beef you can use ground turkey, ground lamb, ground veal, or shredded chicken. If you are concerned about pickiness over the different taste of burgers, meat loaf, and the like, use half turkey/half veal. Many favorite recipes can be modified to fit your child's new food diet and still be enjoyed by the rest of the family. Fish is essential in an optimal diet and should be used four to five times per week. But children usually have to develop a taste for fish, so make this introduction a gradual one.

Children can be little imps about what they will and will not eat, so the appearance of as well as the combination of foods that you serve is important. Sometimes "their own" of something tends to interest them much more than a portion of a large dish. The recipe for Chicken Pot Pie that appears in this section is an excellent example: My son was not impressed with chicken pot pie when I made it in one large casserole, but when I made it in six small tins he was delighted and ate every bite! The name of a recipe can make a difference in a child's interest in the food, as can the table setting or the interesting way food is arranged on a plate. There is more to food than the way it tastes!

TORTILLA TEMPTER *(serves 4)*

1 bag of natural tortilla chips
10 green chilis, sliced open
2 cups blended fresh tomatoes
12 oz natural cheese

1 ripe avocado, chopped
1 small can pitted black olives
1 cup yogurt

1. In a low baking dish layer tortilla chips, chilis, tomato puree, cheese, avocado, and olives. Finish off with a layer of cheese and top with a few crushed tortilla chips
2. Bake for about 45 min at 350°
3. Serve with a dollop of yogurt

TINY TUNA SOUFFLÉS *(serves 4–6)*

2 T arrowroot
1 cup milk
3 T butter or cold-pressed oil
3 egg yolks
5 egg whites, beaten stiff
1 cup natural cheese, shredded
(optional)

3 cheese biscuits or soy buns,
split
2 cans water-packed dark tuna
plus mayonnaise to moisten
and ¼ cup sesame seeds

1. Mix arrowroot with milk, pour mixture into a saucepan, add butter, and stir over medium heat till thickened. Stir in egg yolks and heat for a few minutes, stirring constantly; set aside
2. Gently fold egg whites into arrowroot mixture, then fold in shredded cheese
3. Place split buns or biscuits in a shallow baking dish and place a generous portion of tuna mixed with mayonnaise and sesame on each bun. Then top buns completely with soufflé mixture
4. Bake at 425° for 15–20 min; top will be nicely browned

SALAD CRUNCH-OUT *(serves 4)*

1 lb. ground cooked turkey, veal,
or chicken
8 oz. natural chips (corn, potato,
or whichever)
2 whole ripe avocado, chipped
¼ cup cooked kidney beans
¼ cup black olive halves
1 head lettuce, chopped

1 handful spinach, chopped
1 handful alfalfa sprouts
1 tomato, chopped
12 oz. shredded natural cheese
dressing: ½ cup yogurt, ½ cup
mayonnaise, 1 T natural
ketchup, 1 chopped, cooked
egg

1. Combine all salad ingredients
2. Mix dressing ingredients and stir into salad, serve

PIZZA EXTRAVAGANZA *(serves 6)*

2 cups brown rice flour
    or 2½ cups oat flour
½ cup seed flour
3 T arrowroot powder
2 tsp baking powder

¼ cup cold-pressed oil
¾ cup water
1 egg
1 tsp sea salt

1. Combine dry ingredients
2. Mix liquid ingredients and combine the two mixtures
3. Knead dough slightly, adding more flour if needed
4. Separate into 6 equal portions, then roll and stretch into small rounds for small-sized pizzas (or just make one large pizza)
5. Place rounds on a baking sheet and bake for 15 min. at 350
6. For the topping use a natural sauce and any other desired toppings, such as olives, natural turkey sausage, ground veal, mushrooms, onion, green pepper, shredded vegetables, natural cheeses
7. Bake at 350° for 15–20 min. or until cheese melts. (Extra pizza may be frozen before baking for another meal)

SEAFOOD QUICHE *(serves 4)*

CRUST:
2 cups nut flour
2 T butter

1–2 T ice water
pinch of sea salt

FILLING:
8 eggs
⅓ cup cream or half-and-half
2 cups grated cheese

½ cup avocado, chopped
¼ cup steamed spinach
1–2 cups shrimp and crab
season to taste

1. Prepare crust (cut butter into flour, add water until a cohesive ball is formed) and press into a pie pan. Crimp edges and pop into the oven for about 15 min.
2. Mix eggs and cream, then add remaining ingredients; pour into crust and bake for 1 hour

LITTLE SHEPHERD PIES *(serves 6)*

1½ lbs. ground turkey, veal, or
    chicken
¼ cup grated parsnip
¼ cup grated yellow squash

1½ cups blended ripe tomato
1 cauliflower, steamed till soft
2 large potatoes, cut and cooked
preferred seasoning

1. Brown ground meat and sauté parsnip and squash
2. Blend fresh tomatoes for tomato puree and add to meat/vegetable mixture. Season and simmer for about ½ hour
3. Cook cauliflower and potatoes till tender, then mash with a little milk and butter to make fluffy mashed potatoes. Cauliflower may be used alone if potato is a problem
4. Pour meat mixture into 6 small tins or a low casserole dish. Pipe potato/cauliflower mixture through a pastry bag around the edges of the meat mixture. Bake at 375° for about 20 min. or until potato is browned

TACOS EL SUPREMO! *(serves 4)*

8 crisp natural taco shells
1½ lbs. ground meat or shredded chicken
chopped avocado

chopped tomato
sprouts and shredded lettuce
shredded cheese

1. Brown meat—may add Hain natural taco seasoning mix if tolerated, or use one or two tolerated seasonings
2. Prepare tacos by filling shells with meat or chicken, avocado, tomato, sprouts, cheese

LEMONY BAKED SALMON

Wrap salmon filet pieces in tinfoil; top with a sauce of 2 T lemon juice, 2 tsp Robbie's natural Worcestershire sauce, cube of butter, and a sprinkle of garlic.

CHICKEN-BROCCOLI CREPES *(serves 3–4)*

6 oat or rice crepes (see recipe)
2 T arrowroot
2 cups milk or milk alternative
2 T butter
1 cup shredded cheese (optional)

2 cups cooked chicken, cubed
½ cup steamed, chopped broccoli
¼ cup sautéed bok choy
¼ cup slivered, sautéed almonds
season to taste

1. Prepare cheese sauce by mixing arrowroot in milk, then pouring into saucepan; cook till thickened and add butter and cheese, stirring well (may leave out cheese if sensitive to it)
2. Combine chicken, broccoli, bok choy, and almonds in cheese sauce
3. Fill crepes with chicken mixture and place in a low baking dish
4. Bake at 350° for 20 min.
5. Serve with a dollop of yogurt and a sprinkle of slivered almonds

CHOPSTICKS TONIGHT! *(serves 4)*

2 tsp arrowroot plus 2 T water
2 T wheat-free tamari soy sauce
1 lb. shrimp or chicken cut into
  thin strips
¼ cup sliced water chestnuts
chopped Chinese cabbage

¼ cup broccoli (or any preferred
  vegetable)
⅓ cup cashews
1 cup cubed pineapple
handful of dried seaweed (optional)

1. Mix arrowroot with water, add soy sauce, add chicken or shrimp, and let stand about 15 min.
2. Heat 2 T of olive oil in your wok over high heat and stir-fry all ingredients
3. Serve with brown rice and chopsticks!

SHISH KEBABS

chunks of chicken
pineapple chunks
zucchini

mushrooms
small red potatoes

1. Arrange on skewers and brush with soy sauce and pineapple juice; broil or roast over grill

PIGGIES *(for a crowd of kids)*

6 rice or oat crepes (see recipe)
natural mustard and mayo
thin strips of Jack cheese (optional)

2 pkg. natural chicken, turkey, or
  beef hot dogs

1. Cut each crepe into 4 or 5 long strips, spread each with mayo and mustard, then place one cheese slice on each strip
2. Cut hot dogs in half so that you have 2 short ones, then roll each mini hot dog up in a crepe with cheese
3. Bake at 425° for about 15 min.

CHICKEN POT PIE *(serves 6)*

CRUST:
3 T butter
2¼ cups almond (or other nut)
  flour

pinch of sea salt
2 T ice water

FILLING:

1½ cups chicken stock
2 cups cooked, cubed chicken
1½ cups minced sautéed vegetables
(may use any available—
carrot, bok choy, yellow

squash, broccoli, asparagus,
and so on)
2 T butter
3 T arrowroot plus ¼ cup water
1½ cups shredded cheese (optional)
preferred seasoning

1. Prepare crust (mix sea salt into almond flour, cut in butter, add water till mixture forms a cohesive ball) and roll out dough between two sheets of foil. Form 1 large crust or 6 small crusts for little tins; crust is delicate, so don't worry if it cracks a little—just press pieces together

2. Cook chicken, cool, and cut into small pieces; preserve liquid chicken was cooked in

3. Mince and sauté vegetables

4. Mix water and arrowroot, then add chicken stock. Stir and cook till thickened

5. Add butter to chicken stock mixture, then stir in chicken, vegetables, and shredded cheese (optional); cook till cheese melts

6. Pour cooked mixture into one low casserole dish or into 6 small tins. Fit on crust, prick with a fork in a few places, then bake at 350° for about 45 min.

VEGETABLES AND FRUITS

Vegetables have earned a reputation for causing many eating problems. Children through the ages have refused to open their mouths when a plateful of spinach is set before them. Fruit, on the other hand, is willingly accepted by most children and requires less preparation. The vegetable problem can be dealt with, though! Here are a few ways that might help you avoid such horrors as force feeding. To get vegetables into mouths, you may try:

1) *Picking vegetables from a garden.* Vegetables grown in a garden taste far better (besides being much more nutritious) than the produce in the grocery store. In the excitement of seeing vegetables grow and picking them, your child may forget any aversions, may even get hooked on the taste of fresh veggies (but don't count on it; have other ideas ready if this one bottoms out).

2) *Serving vegetables raw with dip.* Some children can't stand cooked vegetables and prefer them raw. (I seem to recall feeling exactly this way as a child.) Vegetables are much better for you raw than cooked anyway, so serve veggies and dip before dinner, for lunch, or as snacks. Cut vegetables in interesting shapes for eye appeal.

3) *Mixing grated vegetables into main dishes.* Finely grated vegetables can be

easily and deliciously added to many main dishes such as omelettes, meat loaf, spaghetti, any casserole. My son devours any vegetable when it's in homemade vegetable soup, and even spinach in an omelette, but if I steam spinach—or any vegetable, for that matter—he pretends it is invisible and will not eat it. So combining vegetables with other foods can often help.

4) *Replacing bread or crackers with vegetables.* You can accomplish this by using lettuce leaves for bread or making hors d'oeuvre with slices of carrot, zucchini, cucumber, jicama, and so on topped with nut butter, cheese, tuna, salmon salad, or whatever. Some vegetables (such as celery and hollowed-out cucumber) invite fillings. Fruits can also be used creatively in much the same way.

5) *Preparing Salads.* Sometimes children prefer salads to other forms of vegetables. Salads may be a mixed green type with lots of chopped vegetables on top or a shredded type like carrot/pineapple/coconut or cole slaw, or a Waldorf. One of my family's favorite dinners is my Super Salad. I place a scoop of tuna or salmon, chicken, and egg salad in the center of each plate. Then I decorate the plate with lettuce, small scoops of shredded vegetables (squash, carrot beets, and the like), cooked kidney and garbanzo beans, strips of cheese, slices of avocado, alfalfa sprouts, jicama chunks, and so on. Arranged interestingly, this can be a special treat. A hot dog salad is also enjoyed by many children—chop and mix lettuce, sprouts, natural chicken hot dogs, avocado, cucumber, cheese cubes, sunflower seeds, olives, and so on with natural mayonnaise or salad dressing.

6) *Letting them grow their own.* If you have the time and space for a garden, plant one! But if not, sprouting beans, grains, and seeds in your home is fun too. Sprouts are extremely nutritious and are easy to grow whether you use a Mason jar or a Biosnacky (a three-tiered sprouter than makes sprouting more fun for children).

7) *Juicing vegetables.* Vegetables can be juiced and combined with fruit juices or you may blend vegetables into drinks in your blender. Freshly squeezed juices offer optimal nutrients.

You can bake, sauté, stir-fry, or steam vegetables, but boiling (unless you're making soup) can mean a loss of valuable nutrients when the water used is thrown away.

YELLOW AND GREEN FRITTATA SUPREME

1. Blend 1 T butter, 1 clove of garlic (put through a garlic press), and 2 T parsley. Set aside

2. Sauté 3 small yellow squash and 3 small zucchini (sliced thinly) in a few tablespoons of olive oil or butter. Season squash with 1 tsp oregano, pinch of sea salt, basil, marjoram, and rosemary. Blend butter-garlic mixture with squash into a casserole dish with high sides and grate 1½–2 cups of cheese on top of squash

3. Beat 5 eggs until frothy and pour over squash mixture

4. Bake at 350° for about 25 min.

EGGPLANT CRISPS

1. Cut an eggplant into thin slices; the larger slices may be cut in half
2. Dip in beaten egg
3. Coat both sides of each slice with seed flour or potato flour (or any alternative)
4. Sauté in olive oil till lightly brown

VEGETABLE MELODY

1. Slice a variety of vegetables on hand, such as broccoli, asparagus, celery, bok choy, water chestnuts, corn, squash, cabbage, turnips, carrots, cauliflower
2. Steam vegetables and place in a baking dish, mixing in chopped avocado, 1 cup mung bean sprouts (optional), and shredded cheese.
3. Bake at 350° till cheese is melted

BROCCOLI-SESAME CASSEROLE

1. Chop 1 large bunch of broccoli and steam 5 mins.
2. Grate 1 cup cheese
3. Grind ½ cup of sesame seeds
4. Layer a casserole dish with broccoli, shredded cheese, and ground sesame seeds, making a few layers; add a splash of milk, season to taste
5. Bake at 350° for 20 min.

LOOK-ALIKE POTATOES

1. For the child sensitive to potatoes, steam 1 head of cauliflower till tender
2. Mash and season as you would mashed potatoes

ASPARAGUS ALMONDINE

1. Sauté slivered almonds and steam asparagus
2. Mix and serve

MIXED-UP GREEN BEANS

1. Sauté sliced green beans, bamboo shoots, and mushrooms
2. Season to taste; serve

CINNAMON ACORN SQUASH

1. Slice an acorn squash in half
2. Prick pulp with a fork, then butter generously
3. Drizzle on 1 T honey or maple syrup
4. Bake at 350° for about 45 min.
5. Sprinkle with cinnamon before serving

Fruit is not limited to apples, oranges, and bananas. Offer as much variety as possible so that fruit doesn't become boring. Has your child tasted a kiwi? pomegranate? starfruit? mango? papaya?

Stick to fresh fruit whenever possible, but in winter, when fruit choices are limited, you can use frozen unsweetened fruit.

Fruits, like vegetables, are much more appealing when cut into interesting shapes. My son, at six, liked to make his own moon-launching sundae by cutting out the core of a slice of fresh pineapple, peeling a banana and placing it in the hole of the pineapple, then spooning yogurt (add vanilla, 1 tsp honey) around the pineapple slice and sprinkling sunflower seeds and coconut over the yogurt.

Some fruits may be too concentrated in carbohydrate for your child to handle—dried fruit often falls into this category.

BEVERAGES

Your beverage purchasing will change somewhat when sugar and chemicals are eliminated from your child's diet. As with all foods, drinks should reflect as much variety as possible. Juices should be freshly squeezed, although some bottled natural juices are okay. Health-food stores often carry some unusual varieties of juices—loganberry, passion fruit, mango, papaya, cranberry. Juices should always be diluted with 50 percent water. The best "juice" is fresh-squeezed juice or fresh fruit blended with water and ice in the blender.

Aside from juices, do some experimenting with blender drinks. Ground seeds, ground nuts, nutritional yeast, lecithin, protein powder, eggs, sprouts, cold-pressed oils, liver powder, acidophilus powder, vitamin and mineral powders, and the like can be added to milkshakes and smoothies for optimal nutritional value along with good taste. Try some of the following suggestions; but better yet, urge your family to create some of their own drinks:

SMOOTHIES

A smoothie is a blend of fruit and crushed ice that comes out slushy and icy in the blender. It consists of any possible combination of fruit with just enough juice to get the blender going and then the addition of crushed ice. My introduction to smoothies was in California, where vendors made up these fruity drinks in a variety of ways. The favorite seemed to be a mixture of orange juice, banana, strawberries, and ice. Smoothies are good, though, no matter what fruits or juices you add! Supplement additions to smoothies are a little more difficult than to shakes (they don't mask the taste of yeast, liver powder, and so on very well), but some high-nutrient additions such as protein powder, sprouts, and lecithin work if blended well.

MAPLE EGGNOG SHAKE

1 cup milk or milk alternative
1 T maple syrup
½ tsp vanilla
½ tsp rum flavoring
¼ tsp nutmeg

2 egg yolks
¼ cup protein powder
1 tsp lecithin
2–3 T ground seeds
bit of crushed ice

CAROB BANANA WALNUT SHAKE

1 cup milk or milk alternative
1 T carob powder
1 T honey or other sweetner
½ tsp vanilla
1–2 tsp nutritional yeast

½ tsp liver powder
½ ripe banana
small handful of walnuts
bit of crushed ice

ICE CREAM MILKSHAKES

Use homemade or honey ice cream only when making ice cream milkshakes. Protein powder, milk powder, ground seeds, carob, and ½–2 tsp of nutritional yeast, liver powder, or lecithin may be added, but taste before offering it to your child; the taste of supplements can be too strong.

PEACH VELVET SHAKE

1 cup yogurt
2 large ripe peaches
1 tsp vanilla
1 T protein powder

1 tsp lecithin
sweetner if needed
bit of crushed ice

JUICY DELIGHT SHAKE

½ cup carrot juice
½ cup coconut juice
¼ cup pineapple juice
¼ cup papaya juice

1 egg
1 tsp. nutritional yeast
1 tsp protein powder
crushed ice

PEANUT BUTTER SHAKE

1 cup milk or milk alternative
¼ cup peanut butter, almond
    butter, or cashew butter
1 egg

1–2 T honey or maple syrup
1–2 tsp nutritional yeast
1 T protein powder
bit of crushed ice

APPENDICES

A. The Vital Nutrients

Supplying the body with an optimal molecular environment in the form of essential nutrients ensures the achievement of healthy body and a healthy mind. Protein, carbohydrates, fats, vitamins, minerals, fiber, and water are the essential components of an optimal diet.

Protein

Protein is the primary building material of the body and is of the utmost importance in the growth and development of every part of the body, including the brain. The involvement of protein in the formation of enzymes, hormones, and antibodies is crucial.

Proteins are composed of many combinations of amino acids, which the body breaks down during normal digestion. There are 22 amino acids, nine of which are essential (which means they cannot be produced by the body) for children. Adults require eight, but for children histidine is additionally essential for growth and development. The content of essential amino acids determines whether a protein is complete or incomplete. Low-levels of missing essential amino acids in foods indicate incomplete proteins; those which contain rich amounts in the proper proportion are complete proteins. Meat (especially liver and kidney), eggs, fish, fowl, milk products, nutritional yeast, and soybeans are complete proteins. Grains, legumes, most nuts, seeds, fruit, and vegetables are among the incomplete proteins.

The quantity of protein required in the diet is directly dependent on the availability of amino acids. Obviously, an insufficient quantity of protein in the diet can lead to amino acid deficiencies. But even consuming huge amounts of protein may fail to supply the proper quantity and spectrum of amino acids if there are digestive disturbances or metabolic errors.

The availability of amino acids from protein foods is greatly impaired in allergic conditions. If an individual is allergic to chicken, for example, it then becomes an inappropriate protein source (unless therapeutic digestive aids are administered), since the protein is not broken down properly into separate amino acids. Instead, the protein remains in large polypeptide molecules (large molecules rather than the free amino acids which should be absorbed) and are absorbed into the bloodstream while in this form. These polypeptide molecules act as foreign matter by combining with antibodies and lodging in target areas of the body (the brain, the lungs, or any other vulnerable area). This may induce an allergic, or sensitivity, response.

Enzymes that digest protein are formed from amino acids, thus setting up a vicious circle in allergic conditions. To overcome this phenomenon, a physician may administer a specific formulation of free-form amino acids in a powder which is believed to be absorbed directly into the bloodstream through blood vessels under the tongue, thus helping to bypass the inadequate digestive system. Proper digestive support in the form of therapeutic supplementation (of pancreatic enzymes, HCL, and the like) may also be administered to those with digestive difficulties (whether they have allergies or not). Protein-rich (and potentially allergenic) foods need to be monitored more closely, with emphasis on fish rather than meat and fowl for the sensitive individual.

Carbohydrates

Carbohydrates provide the primary source of energy for all body functions and aid in the digestion and assimilation of food. Carbohydrates exist as starches and sugars (simple and double), which are broken down into glucose during digestion. Glucose must always be available to the brain, nervous system, and muscles; glucose that is not immediately needed is stored as fat. Refined carbohydrates act as severe stress factors to the human body by draining nutrient reserves and overtaxing the pancreas; therefore refined carbohydrates should be strictly avoided. Natural carbohydrates are necessary components of the diet, but like all nutrients, they must be balanced.

Water

Water, the most abundant nutrient in the body, serves as a transporter of all other nutrients. It helps keep the body temperature normal, assists in the removal of waste products, and plays a part in nearly all bodily processes.

A source of pure water is an absolute necessity for optimal health. Tap water, often the vehicle for chemicals, heavy metals, and other contaminents which play havoc with the body's well-being, is best avoided. However, finding a source of pure water can be a problem. Many people use bottled spring water or distilled water for their drinking needs. Bottled water should always be contained in glass rather than plastic to ensure purity.

Fats

Fats exist in nature in two basic forms—unsaturated and saturated. During digestion, fat is broken down into glycerin and fatty acids. A healthy body can produce most of the needed fatty acids on its own, but those it cannot manufacture are termed essential fatty acids (linoleic acid, arachidonic acid, and alpha-linolenic acid) and must be supplied by the diet. Fat plays an integral part in optimal nutrition, but the types of fat consumed are of vital importance, as is true of the consumption of protein and carbohydrates.

Essential fatty acids are supplied to the body through unsaturated fats such as pure, unprocessed oils (evening primrose, safflower, soy, linseed, walnut, wheat germ, sunflower, sesame, marine/fish oils), fish, whole grains, legumes, seeds, and nuts.

Saturated fats are easily available in the American diet through the ingestion of butter, meat, poultry, cream, milk, coconut (however, a small percentage of unsaturated fat is contained in these foods).

A third kind of "fat" has appeared in the American diet that is seriously threatening our well-being. Manufactured, altered fats are labeled hydrogenated fats and are widely distributed throughout processed foods to help extend shelf life. Fats are also altered when heated to high temperatures. This is especially so in deep-fried foods, which are possible carcinogens. Oils or unsaturated fats are unstable and may become peroxidized or rancid if not handled carefully (refrigeration). Thus manufacturers add hydrogen to keep their products more stable—but unfortunately, the nourishment in the oil is lost. These hydrogenated fats found in margarine and processed foods are termed "trans fats." These are foreign to the body and can produce considerable harm by blocking essential-fatty-acid metabolism and therefore prostaglandin (or local hormonallike messengers on a cellular level) production. Essential fatty acids in the diet (CIS-form unsaturated fats) are crucial for the production of prostaglandins and the proper structure of all cellular membranes. Special essential fatty acids such as long-chain fatty alcohols (octocosanol having shown dramatic clinical significance) supplied in unrefined oils (especially wheat-germ oil) are "capable of stimulating the repair of damaged neurons even in the brain, where such repair is classically described as unachievable."[1] The clinical results of using octocosanol (wheat-germ-oil derivative) in the case of brain injury have been astonishingly positive.

To supply the body with a wide spectrum of essential fatty acids and accompanying fatty-acid factors, the diet should contain natural, unprocessed oils such as soy, wheat-germ, linseed, safflower, lecithin, sunflower, evening primrose, sesame, fish (marine), walnut, and olive oils, and generous portions of seeds (raw), nuts, fish, legumes, and whole grains.

To protect unsaturated fats from peroxidation (combining with oxygen and becoming rancid, therefore harmful to the body by inducing free radical formation), antioxidant nutrients such as zinc, beta carotene, pantothenic acid, thiamine, selenium, pyridoxine, glutathione, and Vitamins E and C should be supplied liberally throughout the diet.

Food fried at high temperatures (french-fries, for example), hydrogenated oils, margarine, lard, and canned shortenings should be strictly avoided to maintain an optimal health level.

Vitamins

Vitamins are organic food substances contained in minute quantities in animals and plants. They are free of caloric value, but have a profound influence on the body. About 20 vitamins have been isolated, but it is believed there are more yet to be discovered. Whereas proteins, fats, and carbohydrates are broken down into other substances during digestion, vitamins remain largely unchanged by the body. Working as constituents of enzymes—as coenzymes—vitamins help to regulate nearly all bodily processes.

Vitamins exist in two forms—oil-soluble and water-soluble. The water-soluble vitamins (B complex and C) cannot be stored in the body and therefore must be replenished frequently. As with all nutrients, individual requirements for vitamins vary considerably, and they are best obtained from food so that all of them—known and unknown—are supplied to the body.

Vitamin A, a fat-soluble vitamin, exists in two forms: Provitamin A (carotene, such as that supplied by carrots) and Preformed A (retinol, such as that supplied by fish-liver oil). The body must convert carotene into Vitamin A, whereas retinol is Vitamin A that has been preconverted by an animal which has ingested carotene. To be properly absorbed, Vitamin A requires the presence of fat. However, a new form of Vitamin A is now on the market called micellated A (as is also true of Vitamin E) which is soluble in water and believed to have a much higher absorption rate across the intestinal wall. A micelle is a very small cluster of water-soluble fat molecules normally produced in the small intestine when ingested fat mixes with bile and enzymes that spit fat. Thus the micellated Vitamin A is especially helpful for those with digestive and absorption difficulties. Provitamin A, or beta carotene, appears to be a more effective antioxidant than performed Vitamin A and less apt to be toxic in therapeutic doses.

Vitamin A offers a powerful protection against infections by maintaining the strength of the cellular walls and the health of the mucous membranes in the mouth, nose, throat, and lungs. It is also essential for protein synthesis, formation of teeth—bones—blood, sensory function, growth and repair of body tissues, proper digestion, healthy skin—hair—nails, the formation of the protective sheathing around nerve fibers, the production of antibodies, and a potent blocking agent in the liberation of arachidonate from the phospholipid pool in mast cells.

Vitamin A has been found useful in handling stress, which can cause the need for Vitamin A (as well as other nutrients) to skyrocket, especially during illness or prolonged exposure to fluorescent lighting. Dr. Eli Seifter of the Albert Einstein Medical College in New York has observed that the administering of large doses of Vitamin A can reduce the amount of shrinkage of the thymus gland under stress. He also found Vitamin A useful in restoring the thymus to its original size after shrinkage had occurred. Beta carotene, along with Vitamin E, may help to block the liberation of the arachidonic cascade and therefore inflammatory substances.

Since Vitamin A is stored in the body, toxicity to it may occur when exceptionally large amounts are consumed over many months. This toxic amount is likely to be obtained not from food but rather from an overdose of supplements over a prolonged period of time. Beta carotene is the safest from of Vitamin A to be used in therapeutic doses.

Deficiency symptoms: One of the first signs of Vitamin A deficiency is a bumpiness on the elbows, back, buttocks, back of the upper arms, and knees. A more serious deficiency may include night blindness, retarded growth, dull dry hair, dandruff, skin disorders (blemishes, roughness, dryness, acne), frequent infections (especially those involving the respiratory tract), fatigue, loss of sense of smell and appetite, itching and burning of the eyes, weak tooth enamel, diarrhea, softening of the bones.

Sources: Deeply colored fruits and vegetables (spinach, kale, carrots, broccoli, apricots, melons, yams, and the like) liver, kidney, whole milk, eggs, fish-liver oils

B₁ (thiamine), like the entire B complex, is vital for proper functioning of the nervous system, the metabolism of fats, carbohydrates, and protein, and the production of enzymes and digestive juices. Thiamine is essential for growth, mental alertness, carbohydrate digestion (changing carbohydrates into glucose), muscle tone and maintenance, stamina, function of the nerves and brain, formation of acetylcholine (a neurotransmitter), conversion of glucose into energy or fat, and the manufacture of hydrochloric acid.

Thiamine is also closely involved in the oxidation process (burning of glucose) that goes on in every body cell to supply energy. Like all B vitamins, thiamine is water-soluble and cannot be stored within the body; it must be replenished frequently.

Deficiency symptoms: Loss of appetite, muscular weakness, low pulse, constipation, fatigue, numbness, digestive disturbances, insomnia, headaches, aching or burning sensation in hands or feet, diarrhea, sensitivity to noise, nausea due to motion (air or sea sickness). Mental symptoms include apathy, confusion, loss of memory, irritability, inability to concentrate, depression, mental instability, aggression, hostility, fear of impending doom, hallucinations

Sources: Nutritional yeast, wheat germ, rice polish, seeds, nuts, soybeans, milk products, beets, potatoes, leafy green vegetables, mushrooms, blackstrap molasses.

B₂ (riboflavin), another member of the B complex, is essential for normal growth; healthy eyes-skin-nails-hair, and the metabolism of fatty acids, amino acids, and glucose, is involved in the utilization of oxygen by the cells (cellular respiration); and assists in the formation of antibodies and red blood cells.

Deficiency symptoms: Digestive disorders, insomnia, dizziness, trembling, sore tongue, eczema, cracks at the corners of the mouth, oily skin, mental sluggishness, blurred vision, bloodshot eyes, sensitivity to light, eye fatigue, burning and dryness of the eyes, sense of grittiness under the eyelids, scaling around the mouth—nose—forehead—ears, burning feet, impairment of liver function.

Sources: Nutritional yeast, wheat germ, milk products, almonds, kidney, heart, avocado, liver, sunflower seeds, leafy green vegetables, eggs

B_3 (**niacin**) is helpful in stabilizing blood-sugar levels, relieving special sense dysperceptions (such as the delusion of moving letters), improving concentration and brain metabolism, and maintenance of the skin, nervous, and digestive systems. Niacin increases the oxygen in red blood cells, thereby helping to supply optimal amounts of oxygen to these cells for every part of the body and brain. It is also one of the principal constituents of megavitamin therapy used in the treatment of mental disorders (autism, some learning disorders and schizophrenias, and others).

Deficiency symptoms: Coated tongue, abdominal pain, fatigue, digestive disturbances, diarrhea, skin lesions, recurring headaches, nausea, vomiting, insomnia, canker sores, muscular weakness, tension, depression, irritability, nervousness, disorientation, impaired memory, apprehension, confusion, moodiness, and hyperactivity; in acute deficiency, visual and auditory hallucinations may occur as well as hostility, suspiciousness, hyperacute sense of smell, dulled sense of taste, mental dullness, and extreme sensitivity to light.

Sources: Liver, heart, kidney, beef, turkey, chicken, tuna, wheat germ, halibut, swordfish, sunflower seeds, nutritional yeast.

B_6 (**pyridoxine**) seems to be involved in more bodily functions than any other nutrient. It works closely with its counterparts, magnesium and zinc, in many functions. Thus supplementation of pyridoxine should always include magnesium and zinc. Pyridoxine activates many enzymes and enzyme systems, aids in the synthesis of nucleic acids, is vital for the normal function of the brain and nervous system, is essential for the absorption, synthesis, and metabolism of protein, regulates body fluids, and is necessary for the production of red and white blood cells, antibodies, and hormones (adrenaline, insulin). Pyridoxine has an antihistamine effect (along with Vitamin C, pantothenic acid, and Vitamin E), thus is helpful to the immune system. It has proved useful in blocking or diminishing allergic reactions when used with Vitamin C and has been found to stimulate B and T lymphocyte function. Reactions to monosodium glutamate (MSG is found in processed food and Chinese food) have become known as the "Chinese-restaurant syndrome" (dizziness, headaches, mental changes, uncoordination) and may actually be due to a deficiency of pyridoxine, as well as being indicative of a disturbed amino acid metabolism.

Pyridoxine has been found to prevent tooth decay, greatly relieve

asthma attacks, and in some cases, alleviate walking and speech disturbances. In a study of autistic children, Dr. Bernard Rimland found dramatic
results in using supplements (high doses) of pyridoxine, pantothenic acid,
and niacinamide. Pyridoxine is essential for the metabolism of fats and
carbohydrates, needed by the liver and muscles in the conversion of glycogen (stored glucose) into energy, and is essential for the production of the
neurotransmitter serotonin (and other neurotransmitters as well) from the
amino acid tryptophan. Some individuals have a diminished ability to convert pyridoxine into the coenzyme form, pyridoxal-5-phosphate; thus supplements must be in the latter form. Therapeutic doses should be closely
monitored by a physician and balanced with other supplementation (especially magnesium and zinc).

Deficiency symptoms: Headaches, halitosis, dizziness, nausea, insomnia, nervousness, lethargy, inability to concentrate, low glucose tolerance (low blood-sugar
level), numbness, cramps, tooth decay, eczema, depression, visual and auditory
disturbances, edema, convulsions, motion sickness, absence of dreams, bed-wetting.

Sources: Meat, whole grains, liver, nutritional yeast, sunflower seeds, beans,
tuna, bananas, walnuts, peanuts, salmon, pecans

B_{12} (**cyanocobalamin**) is a chemically complex vitamin containing cobalt. Its assimilation by the body is difficult, since B_{12} (the extrinsic factor)
requires the presence of a secretion called the intrinsic factor within the
body. The intrinsic factor ensures that B_{12} is absorbed through the small
intestine. This factor is undersupplied or lacking in many people, which is
why injections of B_{12} are frequently given. Calcium contributes to the absorption of B_{12}, as does hydrochloric acid.

B_{12} is necessary in the production of RNA and DNA, helps maintain the
myelin sheath around nerve cells, offers resistance to infections, is necessary
for the production and regeneration of red blood cells (prevents anemia),
promotes growth, and is involved in many metabolic and enzymatic processes. As a root of some mental illnesses, a B_{12} deficiency is involved in
disturbances of memory, perception, thinking, behavior, and emotions even
when anemia is not present. B_{12} has been shown to be especially helpful in
asthmatic conditions by stimulating the immune system.

Deficiency symptoms: Pernicious anemia, poor appetite, retarded growth, inability to learn and concentrate, insomnia, fatigue, lack of balance, depression, sore
mouth and tongue, unpleasant body odor, rapid heartbeat, shortness of breath,
diarrhea, numbness/tingling, confusion with paranoid delusions, auditory hallucinations, hypersensitivity to noise and light, severe agitation, diminished reflex response, speech and walking difficulties, disturbed carbohydrate metabolism

Sources: Liver, kidney, heart, muscle meat, milk products, egg yolk, sardines,
oysters, crab, salmon, trout, mackerel.

Pantothenic acid, a B vitamin, is termed the stress vitamin because it is
vital to the health of the stress glands in the body, the adrenals. Pantothenic
acid is involved in every vital function of the body, and is most highly
concentrated in the brain. It is necessary for the synthesis of lipids (fats),

helps maintain the function of the digestive tract (stimulates intestinal mobility), helps build antibodies, is essential to the growth and development of the nervous system, prevents fatigue, helps protect the body from radiation, plays an important role in cellular metabolism, and is crucial in helping the body withstand stress.

Pantothenic acid assists in the production of the neurotransmitter acetylcholine (important in memory and concentration) and helps protect against allergic reactions (a lack of pantothenic acid may aggravate or bring about an allergic response). The blood-sugar level stays abnormally low with a deficiency of pantothenic acid because adrenal hormones are not adequately produced. Thus the conversion of glucose and fat into energy is markedly crippled, since the adrenal hormones stimulated by pantothenic acid are considerably reduced.

Deficiency symptoms: Loss of appetite, insomnia, irritability, sullenness, depression, tension, dizziness, numbness, vomiting, restlessness, abdominal pains, burning feet, fatigue, constipation, gastrointestinal disturbances, muscular weakness and cramping, retarded growth, decreased formation of antibodies, prolonged respiratory infections; decreased adrenal production may lead to or aggravate low blood-sugar level and allergies or adrenal exhaustion.

Sources: Nutritional yeast, liver, egg yolk, molasses, wheat germ, peas, beans, peanuts, brain, kidney, herring, buckwheat, soy, sesame seeds, sunflower seeds; pantothenic acid may be synthesized in the body by the intestinal flora but still needs to be supported with pantothenic acid–rich foods in the diet.

Folic acid, a part of the B complex, is necessary for the formation of red blood cells, the production of RNA and DNA, production of antibodies, the proper function of the liver, growth and healing, the health of the skin and hair, the proper functioning of the immune system, and the utilization of glucose and amino acids. Folic acid also increases the appetite, is vital for proper brain functioning, is essential for the growth and division of all body cells, functions as a part of numerous enzymes, and is crucial for emotional and mental well-being. Low folic acid levels have been found in a large percentage of psychiatric patients.

Deficiency symptoms: Fatigue, dizziness, shortness of breath, irritability, paleness, mouth sores and sore tongue, forgetfulness, mental sluggishness, depression, nervousness, anemia, intestinal disorders, low white-blood-cell count, skin disorders.

Sources: Liver, nutritional yeast, wheat germ, egg yolk, green leafy vegetables, asparagus, mushrooms, nuts, lentils, lima beans, peanuts.

Inositol, another B vitamin, assists the liver in the production of lecithin, a fatlike substance involved in fat metabolism (emulsifying fats in the bloodstream; digestion, absorption, and carrying of blood lipids and Vitamins A-D-E-K; transporting fats from the liver to the cells), and is a primary constituent of the protective covering, the myelin sheath, of nerve cells. The spinal cord, nerves, and brain contain high concentrations (four times that of blood) of inositol. Early research shows that inositol has a calming effect on the brain, but further work is needed on its involvement with brain-cell nutrition. Inositol is concentrated in the lens of the eye, thus is necessary for the health of eye membranes. It also is needed for the growth of cells in bone marrow and the intestines.

Deficiency symptoms: Constipation, eczema, abnormalities of the eyes, insomnia, anxiety.

Sources: Lecithin, nutritional yeast, liver, wheat germ, molasses, oatmeal, corn, brains, heart, bulgur wheat, nuts.

Choline, a B vitamin which, like inositol, is a part of lecithin and has many functions in unison with inositol. Choline is essential to the health of the liver and kidneys and the myelin sheath covering the nerve cells; is a principal component of the nerotransmitter acetylcholine (important in memory and concentration; may be helpful for hyperactive children), thus essential for the transmission of nerve impulses; and is necessary for the synthesis of nucleic acid and the production of RNA and DNA. Along with folic acid, B_{12}, and methionine (an amino acid), choline has been found effective in the development of the immune system. Choline may be obtained in its phosphatidyl form for optimal utilization.

Deficiency symptoms: Dysfunctions of the immune and nervous systems are suspected, but exact symptoms in children are unexplored at this time.

Sources: Lecithin, liver, nutritional yeast, egg yolk, wheat germ, brains, kidneys, green leafy vegetables

Biotin is a member of the B complex that is synthesized within the intestine by friendly bacteria, which may produce sufficient quantities for good health. Sulfa drugs, antibiotics, and *Candida albicans* infection disrupt this friendly bacterial action, however, and it must be reinstated with the use of acidophilus. Raw egg whites eaten in large quantities can interfere with the absorption of biotin by binding it with avidin (a protein found in raw egg whites).

Biotin promotes growth, assists in the metabolism of fatty acids and glucose, and is necessary for the health of skin-hair-nerves-bone marrow-glands.

Deficiency symptoms: Fatigue, depression, muscle pains, hypersensitive sensory responses, poor appetite, disturbed nervous system, skin disorders (dermatitis, eczema, dandruff, dry skin), lassitude, nausea, pallor

Sources: liver, egg yolk, nutritional yeast, brown rice

D,d-dimethylglycine, the speech nutrient (not really a vitamin, even though it may be referred to as B_{15}), appears important for cellular respiration, including respiration of brain tissue. Its major contribution seems to be to increase the oxygen intake of all tissues. D,d-dimethylglycine is believed to stimulate glandular, immune, and nervous functions, regulate fatty acid–amino acid–glucose metabolism, increase the quantity of oxygen in the bloodstream, and stimulate the oxidation (burning) of glucose. It has been used to help regulate blood-sugar levels, stimulate speech in autistic children, help relieve respiratory difficulties, and activate IgA response to bacterial antigens.

Deficiency symptoms: Much of the research involving d,d-dimethylglycine has been conducted in Russia, where it has been used in the treatment of asthma, heart difficulties, hypoxia (inadequate oxygen supply to the tissues), and disturbed children. Deficiency symptoms involving immune and nervous disorders need to be researched more fully in relation to d,d-dimethylglycine

Sources: Rice bran and polish, whole grains, nutritional yeast, pumpkin and sesame seeds

Vitamin C, a water-soluble vitamin, effective in the treatment of infectious and noninfectious disorders, necessary for the health of bones—teeth —gums, promotes healing of burns—wounds—fractures, helps protect against poisoning from heavy metals (such as mercury, lead, cadmium, copper), activates T-lymphocytes, stimulates interferon production, acts as a detoxicant, has antihistamine properties, is essential to the adrenals in the production of hormones, is necessary for the formation of red blood cells, maintains normal vision, aids in the absorption of iron and has an antianxiety effect on the brain.

Vitamin C is used up at a tremendous rate during stress. It seems to increase alertness and sociability in disturbed children and is helpful in the treatment of both allergic and mental disturbances. Vitamin C is essential for the formation and maintenance of collagen (intercellular "cement") which connects and holds together all the cells in the body. Weakening of this protective living cement due to a deficiency often results in bleeding gums and excessive bruising. The permeability of cellular walls is decreased when Vitamin C is inadequately supplied. When permeability of the cellular wall occurs (this can also be caused by a lack of any number of other nutrients), essential nutrients seep out and toxic matter enters, severely disrupting the health of cells.

Deficiency symptoms: Tooth decay, soft and bleeding gums, nose bleeds, bruising, listlessness, confusion, allergies, slow healing, lowered resistance to infection, abnormal bone development, glandular insufficiencies, digestive disturbances, depression, mental disorders

Sources: Most fresh fruits and vegetables, especially rose hips, citrus, black currants, acerola cherries, persimmons, strawberries, broccoli, cabbage potatoes, green bell pepper, apples

Bioflavinoids—Vitamin P—are close counterparts of Vitamin C which greatly enhance its effectiveness. The bioflavinoids consist of citrin, hesperidin, rutin, flavones, flavonals. They strengthen the capillary walls, intensify the antihistamine effect of Vitamin C, and help relieve respiratory infections.

Deficiency symptoms: Bleeding gums, eczema, asthma, bruising

Sources: Buckwheat, green bell pepper, the pulp of citrus, strawberries, apricots, plums, rose hips, cherries

Vitamin D, the sunshine vitamin, is fat-soluble and stored within the liver. It aids in the absorption of calcium and phosphorus, is essential for normal growth, requires fat for proper absorption, prevents tooth decay, and is essential for the normal function of the parathyroid glands, which regulate the transport of calcium.

Deficiency symptoms: Poor bone growth (the extreme would be rickets), tooth decay, muscular weakness; may contribute to myopia, tooth malformation

Sources: Fish-liver oils, liver, egg yolk, sunflower seeds, sunlight

Vitamin E is an oil-soluble vitamin consisting of a group of tocopherols —alpha, beta, gamma, delta, epsilon, zeta, eta. However, the known active form of Vitamin E is alpha. Vitamin E is needed in the formation of the nucleus of all body cells (in addition to RNA and DNA); is essential to the cells' utilization of oxygen; protects cell membranes (so that unsaturated fatty acids contained in the membrane are not damaged by oxygen); promotes stamina and endurance by improving cellular respiration in muscles and nerves (used to relieve muscular cramps); has antihistamine properties; helps to block the liberation of the arachadonic cascade, thus inflammatory substances; assists in the absorption of unsaturated fatty acids; is necessary for the proper focusing of the eyes, is vital to glandular activity (especially concentrated in the pituitary gland); works closely with selenium in some of its functions; and prevents fat-soluble vitamins, fatty acids, and hormones from being destroyed by oxygen.

Vitamin E has been found helpful in reducing the transmission of anxiety impulses to the brain cortex in mental disturbances, the treatment of asthma, increasing alertness and learning ability, and promoting healing when applied topically.

Deficiency symptoms: Anemia, diarrhea, muscle weakness, nervous disorders, headaches, skin disorders, glandular dysfunction, weak eye muscles

Sources: Wheat-germ oil, wheat germ, safflower oil, peanuts, rice, oats, outer portion of cabbage, spinach, broccoli, asparagus, nuts, seeds, soybeans

Vitamin K is necessary for the normal clotting of blood and normal liver function. It is synthesized by intestinal flora when the diet is relatively free of refined carbohydrates and adequately supplied with unsaturated fatty acids. As with production of B vitamins, Vitamin K is destroyed with the use of sulfa drugs and antibiotics. Acidophilus culture helps to reinstate favorable intestinal flora so that Vitamin K can be produced once again.

Deficiency symptoms: Hemorrhaging in any part of the body

Sources: Egg yolk, fish-liver oil, molasses; synthesized by the body

Minerals

Minerals may be obtained from both organic and inorganic sources and constitute 4 to 5 percent of the body's weight. They are essential to overall mental and physical health and participate in nearly all bodily processes.

Minerals required in large amounts by the body are termed macrominerals (calcium, phosphorus, magnesium, potassium, sodium, chloride, and sulfur). Those needed in much smaller amounts but of no less importance are called trace minerals (zinc, manganese, iron, chromium, selenium, silicon, iodine, lithium, fluorine, molybdenum, copper, cobalt, and many others with functions yet unknown).

Like all nutrients, minerals must be balanced. Supplementation of one or two correspondingly increases the need for others. Proper balancing is best achieved through use of nutrient-rich foods and the avoidance of processed ones.

Calcium is the most plentiful mineral in the body. Working with phosphorus, it builds and maintains bones and teeth. Ninety-nine percent of the body's calcium is found in bones and teeth and 1 percent in soft tissues and body fluids. This 1 percent is vitally important for blood-clotting mechanisms, excitability of nerves and muscles (contraction), and the activity of the parathyroid hormone. Calcium is also one of several nutrients necessary for the movement of nutrients in and out of cells, activation of several enzymes, regulation of heartbeat, erect posture, healing, maintaining acid/alkaline balance, and cell division. Vitamins A, C, and D, phosphorus, and hydrochloric acid are helpful for calcium's absorption. The calcium/phosphorus ratio is often disturbed in children because of a high intake of processed foods and soft drinks resulting in too much phosphorus and too little calcium in their diets.

Deficiency symptoms: Cramping of muscles in any part of the body, but especially legs, and feet; heart palpitations; tooth decay; insomnia; elevated pain sense; retarded growth; irritability; depression; nervousness; poor posture

Sources: Milk products, sesame seeds, broccoli, bone meal (from animals in a pure environment), balanced nutritional yeast

Phosphorus, second only to calcium in abundance in the body, is found in every cell, with about 86 percent being located in bones and teeth. It is essential for maintenance and division of cells, and necessary for proper growth, energy production, kidney function, carbohydrate metabolism, maintaining acid/alkaline balance along with calcium and other minerals, muscle contraction, utilization of carboyhydrates—protein—fat, and proper brain and nerve function. Phosphorus esixts in a fine balance with calcium (and Vitamin D) which must be respected by the avoidance of processed foods.

Deficiency symptoms: Retarded growth, muscle weakness, fatigue, dysfunctions of brain and nervous system, increased susceptibility to infection, lack of appetite

Sources: Nutritional yeast, lecithin, wheat germ, seeds, meat, poultry, fish, nuts, milk, eggs, whole grains, legumes

Potassium is concentrated mostly in soft tissues, rather than in bones as are phosphorus and calcium. It is found primarily inside cells, while sodium occurs primarily in extracellular fluid, outside the cellular walls. Potassium is essential for growth, protein assimilation, health of the digestive tract, cellular metabolism, normal secretions of hormones, muscle contraction, healthy skin, regulating the heartbeat and body fluids (along with sodium), and acid/alkaline balance. Potassium increases cell uptake of oxygen, activates enzymes, helps rid the body of toxins, has been effectively used in allergic conditions, and is needed by red blood cells to expel carbon dioxide through the lungs. It is especially important in the conversion of glucose into glycogen (stored sugar), thus in energy production.

Deficiency symptoms: Listlessness, slow irregular heartbeat, poor reflexes, confusion, insomnia, hypersensitivity to cold, edema, constipation, extreme fatigue, apathy, muscle weakness, low blood sugar, and allergic manifestations (deficiency may aggravate or contribute to bringing about)

Sources: All fresh fruits and vegetables, melons, oranges, bananas, sunflower seeds, nuts, potato peelings, nutritional yeast, lentils, soybeans

Magnesium is essential as an enzyme catalyst for hundreds of enzymes and enzyme systems—more so, in fact, than any other mineral. It is particularly involved in the conversion of glucose into energy and works closely with pyridoxine in many functions within the body. Magnesium is essential for the synthesis of ATP (energy production in the body). Seventy percent of magnesium is concentrated in bones and teeth, 30 percent in soft tissues and body fluids. Magnesium is essential for muscle contraction, protein synthesis, nerve excitability, carbohydrate and amino and fatty acid metabolism, regulation of body temperature, formation of hard tooth enamel, lecithin production, absorption of other minerals (calcium, potassium, sodium, phosphorus), and the health of every cell, as every transfer of nutrients into or out of the cell requires a magnesium ion. Magnesium is vital for normal function of the endocrine system (the pituitary in particular) and the brain, spinal cord, and nerves. It is vital for the immune system, as it appears to activate T-lymphocyte function.

Magnesium, like potassium, remains largely within cells. When a deficiency of magnesium occurs, potassium levels also are diminished and do not return to normal until magnesium is reinstated. A deficiency of magnesium also causes severe losses of calcium. Fluorine (added to drinking water) and synthetic Vitamin D (added to pasteurized milk) tend to bind with magnesium, rendering it useless to the body; thus it is best to avoid these exposures. A deficiency of magnesium is hard to diagnose unless intracellular tests are performed, since the serum may show normal levels of this mineral even during a severe deficiency.

Deficiency symptoms: Tantrums, apathy, rashes, irritability, hypersensitivity to noise, apprehension, twitching, tremors, muscular tics, irregular pulse, insomnia, muscle weakness, restlessness, nervousness, jerkiness, cramps, confusion, disorientation, depression, tooth decay, poor bone development

Sources: Nutritional yeast, fresh green vegetables, wheat germ, soybeans, seeds, nuts, figs, corn, apples, seafood

Zinc is a vital constituent of insulin. It is essential for the action of numerous enzymes, formation of the nucleus of every cell (RNA and DNA), fatty-acid metabolism, protein synthesis, health of eye membranes (zinc is concentrated in the eye), energy metabolism, growth, tissue respiration, bone formation, carbohydrate metabolism, and health of the thymus gland (thus the immune system). Like magnesium, zinc works closely with pyridoxine in many of its functions. The Brain Bio Center in Princeton, New Jersey, has found zinc deficient in many hyperactive and autistic children. Zinc absorption is best obtained with a picolinic acid source.

Deficiency symptoms: Distortions of taste and smell, lethargy, apathy, slow healing, low resistance to infection (including ear infections), retarded growth, white spots on the nails, dandruff, loss of interest in learning, stretch marks, fatigue, poor hair and nail growth, and atrophy of the thymus gland

Sources: Oysters, nutritional yeast, herring, seafood, onions, eggs, pumpkin seeds, sunflower seeds, nuts, wheat germ, green leafy vegetables

Iron in the body is always present in combination with protein. Iron combines with protein and copper to form hemoglobin, which transports oxygen in the blood from the lungs to the tissues. Iron also is involved in protein metabolism. Iron deficiency has recently been implicated in impairing behavior and cognitive function in young children. The absorption of iron is difficult, but the use of Vitamin C taken with iron supplementation aids in iron uptake.

Deficiency symptoms: Anemia, pallor, constipation, apathy, brittle nails, lowered resistance to stress and disease, shortness of breath, extreme fatigue, muscle weakness, impairment of memory and cognitive functioning, functional hyperactivity

Sources: Liver and other organ meats, dried fruit, shellfish, blackstrap molasses, eggs, oysters, green leafy vegetables

Manganese is a trace element essential for insulin production, the synthesis of fatty acids and cholesterol, formation of the hormone thyroxin in the thyroid gland, normal growth, and protein—carbohydrate—fatty-acid metabolism and is involved in maintaining normal nerve and immune functions. Manganese also activates many enzymes and helps in the regulation of several brain neurotransmitters.

Deficiency symptoms: Retarded growth, tooth decay, hyperactivity, uncoordinated movements, poor equilibrium, low glucose tolerance, digestive disturbances, asthma, aching in joints and muscles, ataxia, dizziness

Sources: Nuts, seeds, egg yolk, green leafy vegetables, wheat germ, bran, oranges, blueberries, brussels sprouts, spinach, beets

Chromium works closely with insulin, helping it function properly, and is vital for energy metabolism. Chromium is exceptionally concentrated in the brain, activates several enzymes and hormones, plays a role in the synthesis of fatty acids and cholesterol, is necessary for utilization of carbohydrates, and forms many complexes with protein. Very little inorganic chromium can be absorbed; thus it is necessary to obtain chromium in its organic form—usually labeled Glucose Tolerance Factor, or GTF, chromium—which is found in foods like nutritional yeast and liver.

Deficiency symptoms: Depressed growth rate and blood-sugar difficulties

Sources: Nutritional yeast, liver, whole grains, mushrooms, beets

Selenium from organic sources (such as kelp or other seaweed) is preferred when it is used as a supplement in the diet. Selenium is an antioxidant that works closely with Vitamin E in many of its metabolic activities. It helps maintain tissue elasticity, prevents destruction of fatty acids by oxygen, helps to protect the body against mercury toxicity, and is vital to the immune system in its involvement as an antioxidant in the enzyme glutathione peroxidase. Selenium is often quite helpful in allergic conditions.

Deficiency symptoms: May be expressed as allergic responses and physical degeneration; more research is needed

Sources: Seafood, nutritional yeast, wheat germ, bran, organ meats, seaweed, garlic

Sulfur is contained in every body cell, but is especially concentrated in the cells of hair, skin, nails. Sulfur is a component of insulin, is necessary for the health of the nerves and tissue respiration, is involved in the secretion of bile, and may help in elimination of heavy metals (copper, mercury, lead) from the body.

Deficiency symptoms: Skin disorders, brittle hair and nails

Sources: Meat, fish, eggs, garlic, nuts, brussels sprouts, soybeans, watercress, celery, onions, radishes, turnips

Sodium works closely with chloride and potassium in many body functions and is found predominantly in extracellular fluids. It is necessary for proper glandular function, regulation of body fluids (regulates the distribution of fluids on either side of the cellular walls), helps keep other minerals in the blood soluble, is beneficial to muscular and nervous-system activity, and is necessary for normal digestion (production of hydrochloric acid) and the health of the lymph glands. Deficiencies are rare—a result of the overconsumption of salt in the American diet.

Deficiency symptoms: Nausea, vomiting, muscualr weakness, apathy, heat exhaustion, respiratory dysfunction, intestinal gas

Sources: Celery, seaweed, watermelon, lettuce, asparagus, cheese, sea salt

Iodine, converted to iodide in the body, it vital to the health of the thryroid gland and formation of the thyroid hormone thyroxin. Iodine participates in regulation of energy production and body metabolism.

Deficiency symptoms: Fatigue, anemia, lethargy, nervousness, restlessness, irritability, mental dullness, dryness of hair and skin

Source: Seaweed, garlic, seafood, citrus, artichoke, pineapple, watercress, turnip greens

Cobalt is an integral constituent of Vitamin B_{12} and aids in formation of hemoglobin.

Deficiency symptoms: Pernicious anemia

Sources: Liver, clams, oysters, green leafy vegetables

Chloride, existing in the body in combination with sodium or potassium, helps in the removal of toxic wastes by the liver, regulates acid/alkaline balance, is involved in fluid and electrolytic balance, stimulates production of hydrochloric acid, and participates in assimilation of minerals and in the digestion of protein.

Deficiency symptoms: Digestive disturbances, poor muscular contraction

Sources: Seaweed, watercress, avocado, chard, olives, pineapple, oats, seafood, asparagus, celery, turnips, rye

Copper is involved along with iron and protein in the formation of hemoglobin in red blood cells. Copper is necessary for production of RNA, the synthesis of phospholipids, activation of many enzyme systems, bone formation and maintenance, and protein metabolism. Too much copper is a problem for many people because of water supplies' being routed through copper pipes. Too much copper depresses zinc levels. Copper has a stimulant effect on the brain, and too much copper in the diet may be a factor in hyperactivity, aggression, and other mental changes in children.

Deficiency symptoms: anemia, impaired respiration, digestive disturbances, weakness

Sources: liver, kidney, brains, almonds, beans, peas, green leafy vegetables, prunes, whole grains

Molybdenum, a trace element, works closely with copper. It is a necessary constituent of enzymes that are involved in the oxidation of fats and the mobilization of iron from liver reserves (thus helps to prevent anemia).

Deficiency symptoms: Possibly some involvement with anemia

Sources: Nutritional yeast, millet, wheat germ, brown rice, sunflower seeds, liver, lima beans, lentils, soybeans

Lithium appears to be involved in the function of the nervous system and brain.

Deficiency symptoms: May be involved in some mental disorders
Sources: Seaweed

Silicon is a trace element that has not received much attention from researchers. It is involved in the formation and health of the teeth, hair, and nails.

Deficiency symptoms: Possibly retarded bone development
Sources: Seaweed, alfalfa, strawberries, oats, apples, sunflower seeds, beets, almonds

Fluorine exists in nature as calcium fluoride and has been indicated to be useful in strengthening of bones and helping to prevent tooth decay. The fluoride added to water supplies is sodium fluoride, and evidence indicates that this form is much more toxic and likely to cause problems. Ingestion of fluorides does *not* free children to consume copious amounts of refined sugar without fear of tooth decay.

Calcium fluoride appears beneficial to the body when supplied through food, but an unnatural form of fluorine, especially in excess, may result in mottling of teeth as well as toxicity. Fluoride may act as an inhibitor (interferes with the activity) of numerous enzymes, especially of some enzymes in the brain.

Deficiency symptoms: May contribute to tooth decay; under investigation
Sources: Seafood, seaweed, gelatin, sunflower seeds, almonds, garlic, green vegetables

Supplementary Foods

Tablets, powders, or capsules can be quite supportive to an optimal diet, but owing to the unknown functions, interactions, and requirements of many nutrients, a pill or potion cannot be depended on to completely nourish children. Therefore, high-quality, concentrated food that offers a wide spectrum of nutrients needs careful consideration.

The following is a list of high-quality supplementary foods that can enhance any diet. Some foods may be inappropriate because of sensitivity and should be avoided. Those tolerated may be consumed alone or added to other foods:

Unrefined cold-pressed oils—
    safflower, sesame, soy,
    sunflower, linseed, walnut,
    olive, marine, evening primrose,
    and wheat-germ oil
Eggs
Bran—from oat, rice, wheat

Rice polish
Nutritional yeast
Alfalfa and comfrey powder
High-quality protein powder
Organ meats—fresh or dried,
    chemical-free
Garlic

Sprouts—from seeds, grains, beans
Lecithin granules
Milk powder, yogurt, kefir, and
  acidophilus cultures
Seeds and nuts
Wheat germ, corn germ

Raw fruits and vegetables and their
  fresh-squeezed juices
Aloe vera
Seaweed
Beans

Food Supplements

The supportive use of individual nutrients has been found to be beneficial when the body's demand cannot be met by food. This may result from a diminishing (from any form of stress) of the body's reservoir of nutrients or from an inordinate predisposed (hereditary) need. Regardless of cause, the need must be fulfilled or the body will fall short of performing optimally. Just how body and brain respond to nutrient inadequacies is influenced by many factors. So determining which nutrients are lacking should always be approached with an awareness of the interaction of all nutrients. An orthomolecular physican can help with this balancing of nutrients and may administer any of the following in treating nutritional insufficiencies:

Vitamins and minerals may be administered in megadoses or small doses, singularly or in combination, by injection or by mouth, for extended periods of time or only once. The child's history, symptoms, and test results direct the physician to what dosage and particular nutrients will need to be applied. Under no circumstances should megadoses be given to your child unless directed by a physician.

Digestive support is crucial because even when the best possible diet is consumed, if it is improperly digested and assimilated it cannot properly nourish. Some digestive difficulties require the support of pancreatic enzymes, bile salts, hydrochloric acid, bicarbonate. With the aid of a test called the Heidelberg gastrogram an assessment of digestive problems can be made, and the physician may use any number of digestive aids such as acidophilus, aloe vera, bicarbonate, bromelain, papain, bile salts, hydrochloric acid, and pancreas compound. William Philpott, M.D., has established[2] that pancreatic insufficiency is of vital consideration in allergic manifestations. The pancreas (which normally releases bicarbonate and enzymes into the small intestine) may fail to neutralize the acidity from the stomach, in which case proper digestion cannot take place. Therefore, proteins (as well as carbohydrates and fats) cannot be broken down into amino acids, and these partly digested protein molecules are absorbed into the bloodstream and are regarded by the body as invaders—allergenic material.[3]

Many of the B vitamins are synthesized by the intestinal flora. In cases where the child is given antibiotics, sulfa drugs, or large amounts of sugar, all of which disrupt this production, acidophilus culture will be needed to reestablish friendly bacteria in the intestine. Some physicians and clinical ecologists advise use of pancreatic enzymes and bicaronate compound (a mixture of sodium, potassium, and calcium bicarbonates called trisalts) to be taken one-half hour after meals to ward off allergic attacks. This helps to ensure the correct pH in the intestine so that proper digestion can take place. Long-term encouragement of enzyme production may be accomplished by the use of free-form amino acids.

The aminos have recently come to the nutritional forefront. Abram Hoffer, Ph.D., writes in the *Journal of Orthomolecular Psychiatry*[4] that vitamins and minerals are not exclusive additions in the orthomolecular approach. Certain amino acids also have been found deficient in some individuals. Dr. Hoffer calls the use of amino acids the Mega Amino Acid Treatment. It involves administration of essential as well as nonessential amino acids.[5] The body can, under normal circumstances, produce the nonessential from the essential aminos, but some individuals lack this ability. Thus, those amino acids considered to be nonessential may actually be essential for some people because of this error in metabolism. Essential aminos may also be required in larger-than-average quantities.

Some amino acids are converted into neurotransmitters necessary for proper brain function. Proper conversion, however, may be interrupted by errors in amino acid metabolism, nutrient deficiencies (like pyridoxine and manganese), or the production of "false neurotransmitters" in a *Candida albicans* infection.

Individual amino acids should not be added to the diet unless a special test called an amino acid assay is performed, because amino acid needs are as unique as other nutrient needs. Once again we view the close interactions and balance of nutrients that must be respected if answers to children's problems are to be found. A broad-spectrum free-form amino acid supplement that dissolves under the tongue may be prescribed by your child's physician. This approach has proved to be of tremendous benefit in stabilizing blood sugar, controlling allergic conditions, and stimulating enzyme production.

Raw-glandular therapy has been used to support the endocrine system with some success when particular glands are under severe stress, such as the thymus gland in a severe allergic condition. Used with vitamins and minerals, glandular therapy may speed healing. However, it should be used with caution, as a specific level and balance of raw-glandular supplementation must be implemented for each individual under a physician's care.

Essential-fatty-acid supplementation in the diet is vital in reaching an optimal health level. The membrane, or structure, of every cell in the human body is made up of essential fatty acids. These essential-fatty-acid building blocks are available in whole grains, seeds, beans, fish, and oils such as cold-pressed safflower, soy, sesame, linseed, sunflower, evening primrose, wheat-germ, chestnut, walnut, and marine (fish) oils from both warm and cold climates.

Even with proper availability of nutrients in the diet, some individuals have errors in their fatty-acid metabolism whereby (to various degrees) they are unable to effectively convert one essential fatty acid into another. A prime example is the impaired ability to convert linoleic acid (Omega 6) into gamma-linolenic acid. This may be mediated for many reasons: a nutrient deficiency (niacin, phyridoxine, C, zinc), a defective delta-6-desaturase enzyme (needed to make the conversion from linolenic to gamma-linolenic acid), trans (hydrogenated) fats in the diet like margarine, high beef intake (arachidonic acid), or errors in metabolism. When gamma linolenic acid is not adequately available, impairment of immune function may occur[6] with subsequent symptoms such as eczema, acne, hyperactivity, abnormal brain development and function, inflammatory disorders, endocrine imbalances, and so on. Therefore, direct supplementation of gamma-linolenic acid in the form of evening primrose oil (the only other source being mother's milk) may be necessary to supply the missing link.

Other essential-fatty-acid studies led by Donald Rudin, M.D., former director of molecular biology at the Eastern Pennsylvania Psychiatric Institute and author of the forthcoming book *The Omega Factor* (Rodale Press, 1986) have indicated that omega-3 fatty acids (cold-weather linseed, walnut, soy, and fish oils, beans) are grossly deficient in the American diet. According to Dr. Rudin, "The dominant illnesses in modernized societies, which range from bowel and heart disease to cancer and psychoses, may be gene-controlled alternative expressions of a lipid-deficiency disease resulting from dietary depletion of newly recognized trace nordic omega-3 essential fatty acids (as in fish oil—particularly salmon oil) augmented by synergistic fiber and vitamin deficiencies."[7] The deficiency of omega-3 fats in the American diet, Rudin states, may cause impairment of nerve and brain, endocrine, immune, cardiovascular, and weather-adaption functions.

First, we must make available to our cells these essential-fatty-acid building blocks by ingesting a diet that liberally offers them (cold-pressed oils, raw nuts and seeds, whole grains, fish, beans) instead of draining our store of essential fatty acids by ingesting diets high in beef and manmade, burned, and rancid fats (margarine, fried foods, hydrogenated vegetable oils). Once essential fatty acids are ingrained in the membrane of the cell, however, they still require protection from combining with oxygen and the threat to cellular integrity. Antioxidant nutrients (zinc, selenium, glutathione, pantothenic acid, pyridoxine, beta carotene, Vitamins C and E) are those nutrients which guard against "free radical attack of amino acids, proteins, and lipid membranes necessary for functional and structural integrity of cells and tissues."[8]

In addition to forming the structures of cell membranes, activated essential fatty acids (both omega-3 and omega-6 forms, which relate to the number of carbon atoms from the methyl terminal and to the first double bond in the essential fatty acid) form prostaglandins, which act as local chemical messengers regulating vital metabolic processes thoughout the entire body. There are three series of prostaglandins, grouped according to the number of their chemical bonds. The prostaglandins in the 2 series are far too prevalent—a result of a diet high in meat and trans (hydrogenated) fats—repressing prostaglandins in the 1 and 3 series, from primrose oil and fish oils respectively. Prostaglandins must be constantly replenished, as they act locally on the same tissue or organ that produces them.

It is crucial that specific medical testing (membrane-lipid profile, essential-fatty-acid profile) be performed to ascertain unique essential-fatty-acid needs in seriously ill individuals so that proper availability and balance of omega-6 (from safflower and evening primrose oil) and omega-3 (from linseed and fish oils) essential fatty acids can be achieved in the diet.

Other fatty-acid research has led to therapeutic applications of octocosanol, a long-chain, waxy alcohol derived from wheat-germ oil which has

ESSENTIAL FATTY ACID PATHWAYS TO PROSTAGLANDINS

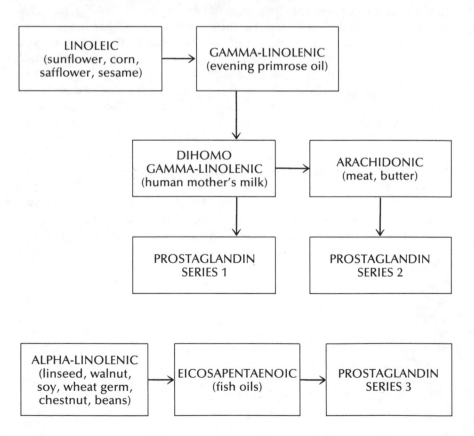

been successful in the treatment of brain-injured children. Dr. Carlton Fredericks has worked with many physicians in treating nerve/muscle disorders and has had some astonishing results. Octocosanol is a nutrient, not a drug, and used in conjunction with evening primrose oil, an optimal diet, and mega-nutrient therapy may prove to be the most important contribution of our time in treating brain injury.

The Protective Plus

To offer special protection against deficiencies, many parents give their children vitamin and mineral supplements in the form of liquids, powders, and tablets. But food supplements for children with sensitivities should be chosen carefully. Whether a product is of natural or synthetic origin, its fillers, binders, colorings, and flavorings can cause problems. It may be difficult to find supplements that taste good, are made from natural ingredients, are free of natural substances like corn, wheat, soy, and milk that may cause sensitivities, and are balanced properly. (See listing in "The Finish Line" of companies that offer supplements for allergic people.) Pure powders and capsules are available for acutely sensitive individuals.

Like love, a healthy body and a healthy mind are a basic need for all children. And children are much too precious to waste.

B. A Nutritional Directory

Rotation Diet Services

Diet Design
Sally Rockwell
Seattle, Washington 98115
(206)527–0877

Rotation diet ideas
Books, newsletter
Rotation game

Environmental Allergy Consulting
Joy Underwood
1202–1175 Broadview Avenue
Toronto, Ontario CANADA M4K2S9
(416)425–7072

Series of books on all aspects of allergy,
including rotation

Jessica Denning
4160 Friendly Lane
Lincoln, California 94648

Food Family Wheels
Rotation diet planners for 4,5,6,7,8 day
rotation diets

Product Source List

Czimer Food Inc.
Route 7, P.O. Box 285
Lockport, Illinois 60441
(312)460–2210

Exotic meats, organic foods
Free brochure

Kennedy Natural Foods
1050 West Broad Street
Falls Church, Virginia 22046
(703)533–8484

Organic foods, game meats
Extensive catalog ($2.00)

Walnut Acres
Penns Creek, Pennsylvania 17862
(717)837–0601

Organic foods
Free catalog

Special Foods
Karen Slimack
9207 Shotgun Court
Springfield, Virginia 22153
(703)644–0991

Many unusual foods—pasta, fruit roll-
ups, cookies, flours, cereals, breads,
crackers, etc. made from rare foods

Shiloh Farms White Oak Road Martindale, Pennsylvania 17549 (717)354–4936	Meats, seafood, nuts, grains, juices
Sunburst Farms Natural Foods 20 South Kellog Goleta, California 93017 (805)964–8681	Organic produce and natural foods
Timbercrest Farms 4791 Dry Creek Road Healdsburg, California 95448 (707)433–8251	Sonoma dried fruits
Vita Green Farms 217 Escondida Avenue Vista, California 92083 (619)724–2163	Organic produce

Allergy Supplement Companies

To order:
Nutracology/Allergy Research
400 Preda/P.O. Box 489
San Leandro, California 94577
(800)545–9960

Klaire Labs/Vital Life
P.O. Box 618
Carlsbad, California 92008
(619)744–9680

The Dews Company
Crystal Springs
Bald Mountain
Biochem
P.O. Box 147
Mineral Wells, Texas 76067–0147
(817)325–0771

Bronson Pharmaceuticals
4526 Rinetti Lane
La Canada, California 91011
(213)790–2646

Cardiovascular Research, Ltd.
1060-B Shary Circle
Concord, California 94518
(800)351–9429
(415)827–2636

Tru-Vita Corporation
4324 Sunbelt Avenue
Dallas, Texas 75248

Metagenics
23180 Del Lago
Laguna Hills, California 92653
(800)692–9400 or (714)844–1718

Available in health food stores:
Natren, Inc./Ethical Nutrients

Twinlab

Nature's Plus

Viobin

Efamol (bottled under various
companies but look for the word
Efamol on the label to make sure you
are purchasing a supplement with
GLA)

Books:
Biosocial Publications
P.O. Box 1174
Tacoma, Washington 98401
(206)627–7237 or (800)523–1234

Organizations

American Institute for Biosocial
  Research, Inc.
505 Broadway, P.O. Box 1174
Tacoma, Washington 98401

Linus Pauling Institute of Science and
  Medicine
440 Page Mill Road
Palo Alto, California 94025

Northwest Academy of Preventive
  Medicine
15 Bellevue-Redmond Road, Suite E
Bellevue, Washington 98008

The Orthomolecular Medical Society
6151 West Century Blvd., Suite 1114
Los Angeles, California 90045

Academy of Orthomolecular Psychiatry
P.O Box 372
Manhasset, New York 11030

Huxley Institute for Biosocial Research
219 East 31st Street
New York, New York 10016

Institute for Bio-Ecologic Medicine
6106 Central Avenue
St. Petersburg, Florida 33710

Society for Clinical Ecology
2005 Franklin Street, Suite 490
Denver, Colorado 80205

Institute for the Achievement of
  Human Potential (Brain Injury)
8801 Stenton Avenue
Philadelphia, Pennsylvania 19118

New York Institute for Child
  Development
215 Lexington Avenue
New York, New York 10016

Human Ecology Action League (HEAL)
P.O. Box 1369
Evanston, Illinois 60204

Gesell Institute of Human Development
310 Prospect Street
New Haven, Connecticut 06511

New England Foundation for Allergic
  and Environmental Diseases
3 Brush Street
Norwalk, Connecticut 06850

Institute for Child Behavior Research
  (Autism)
4756 Edgeware Road
San Diego, California 92116

Human Ecology Research Foundation
720 North Michigan Avenue
Chicago, Illinois 60611

Critical Illness Research Foundation
  (Candida albicans)
2614 Highland Avenue
Birmingham, Alabama 35205

Center for Science in the Public Interest
1755 South Street, NW
Washington, D.C. 20009

La Leche League International, Inc.
9616 Minneapolis Avenue
Franklin Park, Illinois 60131

Price-Pottenger Nutrition Foundation
P.O. Box 2614
La Mesa, California 92041

International Academy of Preventive
  Medicine
Suite 469, 34 Corporate Woods
10950 Grandview
Overland Park, Kansas 66210

References

CHAPTER TWO

1. Iverson, L. "Neurotransmitters and Central Nervous System Disease." *Lancet,* pp. 914–18, October 23, 1982.
2. Wurtman, R. "Behavioral Effects of Nutrients." *Lancet,* pp. 1145–47, May 21, 1983.
3. Dhopeshwarkar, G. *Nutrition and Brain Development.* New York: Plenum Press, 1983.
4. Myron Brin in Iverson, L. "Chemistry of the Brain." *Scientific American,* June, 1980, pp. 139–49.
5. Hemmings, W. A. "Dietary Proteins Reach the Brain." *Journal of Orthomolecular Psychiatry* 6:304, 1977; and "The Entry into the Brain of Large Molecules Derived from Dietary Protein." *Proceedings of the Royal Society* (England) 200, pp. 175–92, 1978.
6. Lonsdale, D., and Shamberger, R. "Red Cell Transketolase as an Indicator of Nutritional Deficiency." *American Journal of Clinical Nutrition* 33(2): 205–11, 1980.
7. Hambridge, M. K., and Baum, J. D. "Low Levels of Zinc in Hair of Children with Poor Growth and Appetites." *Pediatric Research* 6,868, 1972.

CHAPTER THREE

1. Olson, C., and Richey, N. "Study on Sugar Consumption." *Journal of the American Dietetic Association* 84:1506, 1984.
2. Morgan, K. J., and Zabik, M. E. "Amount and Food Sources of Total Sugar Intake by Children 5–12 Years." *American Journal of Clinical Nutrition* 34, 404, 1981.
3. U.S. Dept. of Agriculture/U.S. Dept. of Health, Education and Welfare, *Nutrition and Your Helath,* February, 1980.
4. Brewster, L., and Jacobson, M. F. *The Changing American Diet.* Center for Science in the Public Interest, Washington, D.C., p. 78, 1982.
5. Pao, E. M., and Mickle, S. J. "Problem Nutrients in the United States." *Food Technology* 35(9):58, 1981.
6. Fishbein, D. "Refined Carbohydrate Consumption and Maladaptive Behaviors: An Experiment." *International Journal of Biosocial Research,* Vol. 2, pp. 21–24, 1981.

7. Schoenthaler, S. J. "Diet and Delinquency: A Multi-State Replication." *International Journal of Biosocial Research,* Vol. 5 (2), pp. 70–78, 1983.
8. Smith, Lendon. *Improving Your Child's Behavior Chemistry,* Englewood Cliffs, N.J.: Prentice-Hall, 1976.
9. Philpott, W. H.; Philpott, K. M.; Bridges, E.; and Stream, M. A. "Ecologic-Metabolic Profile of Schizophrenia." *Journal of Orthomolecular Psychiatry,* Vol. 8, No. 2, 1979.
10. *Ibid.*
11. *Ibid.*
12. Selye, Hans. *Stress Without Distress.* New York: J. B. Lippincott, 1974
13. Fredericks, Carlton. *New Low Blood Sugar and You.* New York: Putnam, 1985
14. Yaryura-Tobias, J., and Neziroglu, B. A. "Violent Behavior, Brain Dysrhythmia and Glucose Disfunction." *Journal of Orthomolecular Psychiatry,* Vol. 4, No. 3, pp. 182–88, 1975.
15. Hemmings, W. A. "The Entry into the Brain of Large Molecules Derived from Dietary Protein." *Proceedings of the Royal Society,* (England) 200, pp. 175–92, 1978.
16. Roy-Feiler, B., and Starzinski, T. "Phosphates as a Factor in Hyperaggression and Juvenile Delinquency." West German Society for Criminology, Heidelberg, 1979 (in German); and Wakler, M. "Phosphates and Hyperactivity: Is There a Connection?" *Academic Therapy,* 17:4, 1982.
17. Hafer, Hertha. *The Heavenly Drug: The Effects of Phosphates.* Heidelberg: West German Society for Criminology, 1984 (in German).

CHAPTER FOUR

1. Rie, H. and Rie, E. "Effects of Ritalin on Underachieving Children: A Replication." *American Journal of Orthopsychiatry,* Vol. 46, No. 2, 1976.
2. Rapp, D. *Allergies and the Hyperactive Child.* New York: Cornerstone Books, 1979.
3. *Ibid.;* and leaflets in Ritalin and Dexadrine boxes.
4. Feingold, B. *Why Your Child Is Hyperactive.* New York: Random House, 1974.
5. Printz, R., *et al.* "Double Blind Study Implicates Sugar, Questions Feingold." *Journal of Behavioral Ecology,* Vol. 2, No. 1, 1981.
6. Printz, R., *et al.* "Dietary Correlates of Hyperactive Behavior in Children." *Journal of Consulting and Clinical Psychology,* Vol. 48, No. 6, 760–69, 1980.
7. Franklin, A. J. "Diet and Behavior." *Archives of Disturbed Children* 59:799, 1984.
8. Fredericks, C. *New Low Blood Sugar and You.* New York: Putnam, 1985.
9. O'Shea, J., and Porter, S. "Double Blind Study of Children with Hyperkinetic Syndrome Treated with Multi-Antigen Extract Sublingually." *Journal of Learning Disabilities,* 14:189–91, 1981.
10. Rapp, D. "Does Diet Affect Hyperactivity?"*Journal of Learning Disabilities,* 11:383, 1978.
11. Rapp, D. "Food Allergy Treatment for Hyperkinesis." *Journal of Learning Disabilities,* 12(9):45-50, Nov., 1979.

12. Langseth, L., and Dowd, J. "Glucose Tolerance and Hyperkinesis." *Food and Cosmetic Toxicology* 16, pp. 129–33, August, 1977.

13. Egger, J.; Carter, C. M.; Graham, P. J.; Gumley, D.; and Soothill, J. F. "Controlled Trial of Oligoantigenic Treatment in the Hyperactive Syndrome." *Lancet,* pp. 540–45, March 9, 1985.

14. Ott, J. "Influence of Fluorescent Lights on Hyperactivity and Learning Disabilities." *Journal of Learning Disabilities,* Vol. 9, No. 7, pp. 417–22, August-September, 1976; and "School Lighting and Hyperactivity." *Journal for Biosocial Research,* Vol. 8, pp. 6–7, Summer, 1980.

15. Ott, J. *Light, Radiation and You.* Old Greenwich, Conn.: Devin-Adair, 1982.

16. Colquhoun, I., and Bunday, S. "A Lack of Essential Fatty Acids as a Possible Cause of Hyperactivity in Children." *Medical Hypotheses* 7:673, 1981.

17. Wright, S., and Burton, J. L. "Oral Evening Primrose Oil Improves Atopic Eczema." *Lancet* 2:1120, 1982.

18. See Appendix A for more information on essential fatty acids.

19. Horrobin, D. F. *Clinical Uses of Essential Fatty Acids.* Montreal: Eden Press, 1982.

20. This raises the question of the effect of feeding infants formula: infants also lack the ability to convert linoleic acid to dihomo-gamma-linolenic acid, and therefore immune suppression may result when formula instead of breast milk is used.

21. Efamol evening primrose oil has been used in therapeutic trials.

22. Thatcher, R. W., *et al.* "Effects of Low Levels of Cadmium and Lead on Cognitive Functioning in Children." *Archives of Environmental Health* 37 (3): 159–66, 1982.

23. David, O.; Clart, J.; and Voeller, K. "Lead and Hyperactivity." *Lancet,* 2:900–903, 1972.

24. ———"The Relationship of Hyperactivity to Moderately Elevated Lead Levels." *Archives of Environmental Health* 38(6): 341–46, 1983.

25. Pfeiffer, C. *Zinc and Other Micro-Nutrients.* New Canaan, Conn.: Keats, 1978.

26. *Ibid.*

27. Millar, J. A., *et al.* "Lead and d-Aminolevulinic Acid Dehydratase Levels in Mentally Retarded Children and in Lead Poisoned Suckling Rats." *Lancet* 2:695–98, 1970.

28. *Ibid.*

29. *Ibid.*

30. Pfeiffer, *op. cit.*

31. Lester, M. L.; Thatcher, R. W.; and Monroe-Lord, L. "Refined Carbohydrate Intake, Hair Cadmium Levels, and Cognitive Functioning in Children." *Nutrition and Behavior* 1:3–13, 1982.

32. Pfeiffer, *op. cit.*

CHAPTER FIVE

1. Frazier, C. *Parents' Guide to Allergy.* New York: Grosset & Dunlap, 1978.

2. Wright, S., and Burton, J. L. "Oral Evening Primrose Oil Improves Atopic Eczema." *Lancet* 2:1120, 1982.

3. Frazier *op. cit.*

4. Abrahamson, E., and Pezet, A. *Body, Mind and Sugar.* New York: Holt, Rinehart & Winston, 1951
5. USDA Federal Proceedings 43:470, 1984.
6. Egger, J.; Carter C. M.; Wilson J.; Turner, M. W.; and Soothill, J. F. "Is Migraine Food Allergy?" *Lancet* 2:865–69, 1983.
7. Rapp, D. *Allergies and the Hyperactive Child.* New York: Cornerstone Books, 1979.

CHAPTER SIX

1. Schauss, A. G., and Simonsen, C. E. "A Critical Analysis of the Diets of Chronic Juvenile Offenders, Part I." *Journal of Orthomolecular Psychiatry,* 8(3): 149–57, 1979; Schauss, A. G.; Bland, J.; and Simonsen, C. E. "A Critical Analysis of the Diets of Chronic Juvenile Offenders, Part II." *Journal of Orthomolecular Psychiatry,* 8(4): 222–26, 1979; Schauss, A. G. "Differential Outcomes Among Probationers Comparing Orthomolecular Approaches to Conventional Casework/Counseling." *Journal of Orthomolecular Psychiatry,* 8(3): 158–68, 179; ———. "Food, Environment and the Criminal Mind." *Panhandle* 2:19–22, 1983; ———. "Nutrition and Antisocial Behavior" (special article). *International Clinical Nutrition Reviews,* 4(4): 172–77, 1984; ———. "Nutrition and Behavior: Complex Interdisciplinary Research." AB Academic Publishers, London, 3:9–37, 1984; ———. "Research Links Nutrition to Behavior Disorders." *School Safety* (publication of the U.S. Department of Education and the U.S. Department of Justice) 3:20–28, 1985.
2. Yaryura-Tobias, J. A., and Neziroglu, F. "Violent Behavior, Brain Dysrhythmia and Glucose Dysfunction: A New Syndrome," *Journal of Orthomolecular Psychiatry,* Vol. 4, No. 3, pp. 182–88, 1975.
3. Schoenthaler, S. J. "The Effects of Sugar on the Treatment and Control of Antisocial Behavior: A Double-Blind Study of an Incarcerated Juvenile Population." *International Journal of Biosocial Research* 3(1), 1982; ———. "Diet and Crime: An Empirical Examination of the Value of Nutrition in the Control and Treatment of Incarcerated Offenders." *International Journal of Biosocial Research* 4(1):25–39, 1983; ———. "The Alabama Diet-Behavior Program: An Empirical Evaluation at the Coosa Valley Regional Detention Center," *International Journal of Biosocial Research* 5(2): 79–87, 1983; ———. "The Los Angeles Probation Department Diet-Behavior Program: An Empirical Evaluation of Six Institutional Settings." *International Journal of Biosocial Research* 5(2):88–98, 1983; ———. "Diet and Delinquency: A Multi-State Replication." *International Journal of Biosocial Research,* 5(2): 70–78, 1983; ———. "The Northern California Diet-Behavior Program: An Empirical Evaluation of 3,000 Incarcerated Juveniles in Stanislaus County Juvenile Hall." *International Journal of Biosocial Research* 5(2): 99–106, 1983; ———. "The Effects of Citrus on the Treatment and Control of Antisocial Behavior: A Double-Blind Study of an Incarcerated Juvenile Population." *International Journal of Biosocial Research* 5(2):107–117, 1983; and ——— and Doraz, W. E. "Types of Offenses Which Can Be Reduced in an Institutional Setting Using Nutritional Intervention: A Prelim-

inary Empirical Evaluation." *International Journal of Biosocial Research* 4(2):74–78, 1983.
4. Schmidt, K.; Brajkovich, W.; and Asch, M. "Clinical Ecology Treatment Approach for Juvenile Offenders." *International Journal of Biosocial Research* 2:15–20, 1981.
5. Bryce-Smith, D. "Anorexia, Depression, and Zinc Deficiency." *Lancet,* November 17, 1984.
6. "Case of Anorexia Nervosa Responding to Zinc Sulfate." *Lancet,* August 1, 1984.
7. Bakan, A. "Anorexia and Zinc." *Lancet,* October 13, 1984.

CHAPTER EIGHT

1. Pauling, Linus. *Orthomolecular Psychiatry,* 160, 265–71, April 19, 1968.
2. Pfeiffer, C. *Mental and Elemental Nutrients.* New Canaan, Conn.: Keats, 1975.
3. *Ibid.*
4. Mandell, M., and Scanlon, L. *Dr. Mandell's 5-Day Allergy Relief System.* New York: Thomas Y. Crowell, 1979.
5. Pfeiffer, C. "Psychiatric Hospital vs. Brain Bio Center in Diagnosis of Biochemical Imbalances." *Journal of Orthomolecular Psychiatry,* Vol. 5, No. 1, pp. 28–34, 1976.
6. ———. "Testing the Spoor of the Gray Behemoths—The Schizophrenias." *Journal of Orthomolecular Psychiatry,* Vol. 6, No. 2, pp. 165–70, 1977.
7. *Ibid.*
8. ———. *Mental and Elemental Nutrients, op. cit.*
9. ———. "The Schizophrenias '76." *Biological Psychiatry,* Vol. 11, No. 6, pp. 773–75, 1976.
10. ———. *Mental and Elemental Nutrients, op. cit.*
11. *Ibid.*
12. *Ibid.*
13. Philpott, W., and Kalita, D. *Brain Allergies.* New Canaan, Conn.: Keats, 1980; and ———. *Victory over Diabetes,* Keats, 1983.
14. Horrobin, D. F. "Prostaglandins and Schizophrenia." *Lancet* 1:706–7, 1980.
15. Rudin, D. "The Three Pellagras." *Journal of Orthomolecular Psychiatry,* Vol. 12, No. 2, 1982.
16. Horrobin, *op. cit.*
17. Rudin, *op. cit.*
18. Coleman, M., *et al.* The Autistic Syndromes. New York: North Holland Publishing, 1976.
19. Information on fenfluramine was presented at the National Autistic Conference (Omaha, Nebraska) in 1982 by Edward Ritvo of the UCLA Medical Center. Research on the effects of fenfluramine in autistic children was continued through the Autism Research Project at Stanford.
20. American Academy of Environmental Medicine Conference, October, 1984.
21. Rimland, B. "High Dosage Level of Certain Vitamins in the Treatment of Children with Severe Mental Disorders." *Orthomolecular Psychiatry,* 1971.
22. Pfeiffer, C. *Zinc and Other Micro-Nutrients.* New Canaan, Conn.: Keats, 1983.
23. O'Banion, D.; Armstrong, B.; Cummings, R. A.; and Stange, J. "Disruptive

Behavior: A Dietary Approach." *Journal of Autism and Schizophrenia,* Vol. 8, No. 3, 1978.

24. The Kaplan Foundation, 7150 Santa Juanita, Orangevale, Calif. 95662.

25. Philpott and Kalita, *Brain Allergies, op. cit.*

26. Rapp, D. *Allergies and the Hyperactive Child.* New York: Cornerstone Books, 1979.

27. Philpott, W. "Chemical Defects, Allergic and Toxic States as Causes and/or Facilitating Factors of Emotional Reactions, Dyslexia, Hyperkinesis, and Learning Problems." *Journal of the International Academy of Metabology* 2:58, 1973.

28. Warden, N.; Duncan, M.; and Sommars, E. "Nutrional Changes Heighten Children's Achievement." *International Journal of Biosocial Research* 3:72, 1982.

29. Wunderlich, R. "Nutrition and Learning." *Academic Therapy* 16:3, pp. 303–7, January, 1981.

30. Kershner, J., and Hawke, W. "Megavitamins and Learning Disorders: A Controlled Double Blind Experiment." *Journal of Nutrition* 109, pp. 819–26, 1979.

31. Mandell, M., and Scanlon, L. *op cit.*

32. The Doman-Delacato method of patterning was developed to accelerate the activation of brain cells. Based on a reenactment of normal development to stimulate neurological growth, patterning is a procedure by which the arms and legs and head of the brain-injured child are moved in a precise, rhythmical pattern to simulate motion of mobility (truncal patter), crawling (homolateral pattern), creeping (cross pattern), and walking (cross pattern). Patterning is not an exercise but an attempt to "organize the hurt brain so that it might perform its own functions" as described by Glenn Doman in the book *What to Do About Your Brain Injured Child.* New York: Doubleday, 1974.

33. Powers, H. "Dietary Measurements to Improve Behavior and Achievement." *Academics and Therapeutics* IX 3, pp. 203–14, Winter, 1973–74.

34. Johnson, D. L., and McGowen, R. J. *"Anemia and Infant Behavior."* Nutrition *and Behavior,* Vol. 1, No. 2, 1983.

35. Pollitt, E.; Leibel, R. L.; and Greenfield, D. B. "Iron Deficiency and Cognitive Test Performance in Preschool Children." *Nutrition and Behavior,* Vol. 1, No. 2, 1983.

36. Tucker, D. M., *et al.* "Iron Status and Brain Function." *American Journal of Clinical Nutrition* 39:105–13, 1984.

37. Pollitt, E., *et al.* "Cognitive Effects of Iron Deficency Anemia." *Lancet* 1:158, 1985.

CHAPTER NINE

1. Langseth, L., and Dowd, J. "Glucose Tolerance and Hyperkinesis." *Food and Cosmetic Toxicology* 16, pp. 124–33, August, 1977.

2. Spiller, G. *Nutritional Pharmacology.* New York: Alan Liss, 1982.

3. Williams, Roger, J. *Nutrition Against Disease.* New York: Pitman, 1971.

4. *Ibid.*

5. Harte, R. A., and Chow, B. "Dietary Interrelationships," in Whol, M., and

Goodhart, R. *Modern Nutrition in Health and Disease.* Philadelphia: Lea and Febiger, pp. 534–44, 1964.

CHAPTER TEN

1. Horrobin, D. *Clinical Uses of Essential Fatty Acids.* Montreal: Eden Press, 1982; and *Prostaglandins: Physiology, Pharmacology and Clinical Significance.* Eden Press, 1978.
2. Loose, L. D., *et al.* "Environmental Chemical Induced Macrophage Dysfunction." *Environmental Health Perspectives,* 39:79–91, 1981; and "Assessment of Environmental Contaminant–Induced Lymphocyte Dysfunction." *Ibid.,* 105–28, 1981.
3. Beisal, W. R., *et al.* "Single Nutrients and Immunity." *American Journal of Clinical Nutrition,* Vol. 35, No. 2, 1982 (entire volume on this subject); and "Single Nutrient Effects on Immunologic Function." *JAMA,* 245:53, 1981.
4. Anderson, R., and Van Rensberg, A. J. "The Effects of Increasing Weekly Doses of Ascorbate on Cellular and Immune Function in Normal Volunteers." *American Journal of Clinical Nutrition,* 33:71, 1980.
5. Rudin, D. "The Dominant Diseases of Modernized Societies as Omega-3 Essential Fatty Acid Deficiency Syndrome." *Medical Hypothesis* 8:17–47, 1982.
6. Nelson, N. A.; Kelly, R. C.; and Johnson, R. A. "Prostaglandins and the Arachidonic Cascade." *Chemical and Engineering News* 80, August 16, 1982.
7. Horrobin, D., *et al.* "The Nutritional Regulation of T Lymphocyte Function." *Medical Hypothesis* 5:969–85, 1979.
8. Goodwin J. S., and Webb, D. R. "Regulation of the Immune Response by Prostaglandins." *Clincial Immunologic Immunopthology* 15:106–22, 1980.
9. Kunkel, S. L; Ogawa, H.; Ward, P. A.; and Zurrier, R. B. "Suppression of Chronic Inflammation by Evening Primrose Oil." *Progressive Lipid Research* 20:885–9, 1982.
10. Truss, O. "The Role of Candida Albicans in Human Illness." *Journal of Orthomolecular Psychiatry,* Vol. 10, No. 4, 1981.
11. Published by author. Order by Mail to: *The Missing Diagnosis,* P.O. Box 26508, Birmingham, Ala. 35226.
12. Truss, O. "Restoration of Immunologic Competence to Candida Albicans." *Journal of Orthomolecular Psychiatry,* Vol. 9, No. 4, 1978.
13. Truss. *The Missing Diagnosis, op. cit.*
14. Article appearing in the *San Francisco Examiner* October, 1983, on Duffy Mayo.
15. Philpott, W. H.; Philpott, K. M.; Bridges, E.; and Stream, M. A. "Ecologic-Metabolic Profile of Schizophrenia." *Journal of Orthomolecular Psychiatry,* Vol. 8, No. 2, 1979.
16. Philpott, W. H.; Khaleeluddin, K.; and Philpott, K. "The Role of Addiction in the Mental Disease Process on the Chemistry of Addiction." *Journal of Applied Nutrition* 32:30–36, 1980.
17. Buisseret, P. D. "Allergy." *Scientific American,* June, 1982.
18. Philpott, W., and Kalita, D. *Brain Allergies.* New Canaan, Conn: Keats, 1981.
19. King, D. S. "Can Allergic Exposure Provoke Psychological Symptoms? A Double Blind Test." *Biological Psychiatry* 16:3–19, 1981.

20. Potkin, S. G.; Weinberger, D.; Kleinman, J.; *et al.* "Wheat Gluten Challenge in Schizophrenic Patients." *American Journal of Psychiatry* 138:1208–11, 1981.
21. Singh, M., and Kay, S. R. "Wheat Gluten as a Pathogenic Factor in Schizophrenia." *Science* 191:400–401, 1976.
22. Dohan, F. C., and Grasberger, J. C. "Relapsed Schizophrenia: Earlier Discharge from the Hospital After Cereal-Free Milk-Free Diet." *American Journal of Psychiatry* 130:85–88, 1973.
23. Philpott. *Brain Allergies, op. cit.*
24. Rea, W., *et al.* "Elimination of Oral Food Challenge Reaction by Injection of Food Extracts: A Double Blind Evaluation" *Archives of Otolaryngology* 110:248–52, 1984.
25. Rapp, D. "Sublingual Provocative Food Testing (letter)." *Annals of Allergy* 46:176, 1981.
26. Watson, G. *Nutrion and Your Mind.* New York: Harper and Row, 1972.

CHAPTER THIRTEEN

1. Write to NUTRA, Sara Sloan, P.O. Box 13825, Atlanta, Ga. 30324.
2. Books that can be ordered include *Is Nutrition Served at Your School? Yuk to Yum Snacks, From Classroom to Cafeteria,* and *A Guide for Nutra Lunches and Natural Foods,* all by Sara Sloan. A film has been made of Ms. Sloan's work and is available to any school interested in the Nutra Lunch program. Order from NUTRA, *ibid.*

CHAPTER FOURTEEN

1. Oils, for instance, may be stated as "oil" on a label, but no mention may be made that the oil contains BHT and BHA as additives.
2. Do not be misled into thinking that fructose is derived from fruit—its origin is refined corn or beet sugar. Sucrose—white "table" sugar—contains glucose and the fructose that is usually employed.
3. Food families were developed by Dr. Warren Vaughan in 1930 and modified by other researchers (Randolph and Ellis in particular).

CHAPTER FIFTEEN

1. Saifer, P., and Saifer, M. *Human Ecologist,* Volumes 13 and 14, 1981.
2. Carson, R. *Silent Spring.* Greenwich: Fawcett Books, 1962.
3. *Ibid.*
4. Faith, R. E.; Luster, M. I.; and Vos, J. G. "Effects on Immune Competence by Chemicals of Environmental Concern." *Review of Biochemical Toxicology* 2:173–211, 1980.
5. This estimate by the EPA was prepared for Senator Edward Kennedy, D.-Mass.
6. Cohn, Victor. "EPA Study Shows Millions in Peril From Toxic Waste Dumps." *The Washington Post,* June, 1980, quoting Senator Kennedy.
7. Mandell, M., and Scanlon, L. *Dr. Mandell's 5-Day Allergy Relief System.* New York: Thomas Y. Crowell, 1979.
8. Saifer and Saifer, *op. cit.*

9. The odors of foods to which a child is sensitive may initiate an allergic response.
10. Cellophane rolls are available from various paper distributors such as the Crown Zellerbach Corporation. Cellophane bags may be obtained from the Nuvita Food Company, 7524 S.W. Macadam Avenue, Portland, Ore. 97219, in a variety of sizes.
11. Soyka, F., and Edmonds, A. *The Ion Effect.* New York: E. P. Dutton & Company, 1977.
12. Neutralization techniques can be applied by a clinical ecologist in severe cases of sensitivity to natural substances such as pollen.
13. Levine, S., and Reinhardt, J. "Biochemical Pathology Initiated by Free Radicals, Oxidant Chemicals, and Therapeutic Drugs in the Etiology of Chemical Hypersensitivity Disease." *Journal of Orthomolecular Psychiatry,* Vol. 12, No. 3, 1983.

The Vital Nutrients (Appendix A)

1. Fredericks, C. *Eat Well, Get Well, Stay Well.* New York: Grosset & Dunlap, 1981.
2. Philpott, W., and Kalita, D. *Brain Allergies.* New Canaan, Conn.: Keats, 1980.
3. Jackson, P. G.; Lessof, M. H.; Baker, R. W. R.; *et al.* "Intestinal Permeability in Patients with Eczema and Food Allergy." *Lancet* 1:1285–86, 1981. A more recent article on intestinal permeability appeared in *Lancet* on February 2, 1985, as well as the work of Hemmings discussed previously.
4. First Quarter, Vol. 9, No. 1, 1980.
5. Bessman, S. P. "The Justification Theory: The Essential Nature of the Non-Essential Amino Acids." *Nutritional Review* 37:209, 1979.
6. Horrobin, D. *Clinical Uses of Essential Fatty Acids.* Montreal: Eden Press, 1982.
7. Rudin, D. "The Dominant Diseases of Modernized Societies as Omega-3, Essential Fatty Acid Deficiency Syndrome." *Medical Hypothesis* 8:17-47, 1982.
8. Levine, S., and Reinhardt, J. "Biochemical Pathology Initiated by Free Radicals, Oxidant Chemicals, and Theraputic Drugs in the Etiology of Chemical Hypersensitivity Disease." *Journal of Orthomolecular Psychiatry,* Vol. 12, No. 3, 1983.

Suggested Reading

General Nutrition Information

Bland, J. *Nutraerobics*. New York: Harper and Row, 1985.

Pfeiffer, C. *Mental and Elemental Nutrients*. New Canaan, CT: Keats, 1976.

Pfeiffer, C. *Zinc and Other Micro-Nutrients*. New Canaan, CT: Keats, 1978.

Williams, R. *Nutrition Against Disease*. New York: Pitman Publishing, 1977.

Smith, L. *Feed Your Kids Right*. New York: McGraw Hill, 1979.

Bland, J. *Your Health Under Siege*. Brattleboro, VT: Stephen Greene Press, 1981.

Fredericks, C. *Nutrition Guide for the Prevention and Cure of Common Ailments and Diseases*. New York: Fireside Books, 1982.

Sloan, S. *A Guide for Nutra Lunches and Natural Foods*, c/o Sara Sloan, P.O. Box 13852, Atlanta, GA 30324.

Davis, A. *Let's Eat Right to Keep Fit*. New York: Harcourt, Brace, Jovanovich, 1970.

McEntire, P. *Mommy, I'm Hungry*. Sacramento, CA: Cougar Books, 1982.

Hoffer, A. and Walker, M. *Orthomolecular Nutrition*. New Canaan, CT: Keats, 1978.

Hunter, B. *The Sugar Trap and How to Avoid it*. Boston: Houghton Mifflin Co., 1982.

Bershad, C. and Bernick, D. *Bodyworks: The Kid's Guide to Food and Physical Fitness*. New York: Random House, 1979.

Goodwin, M. and Pollen, G. *Creative Food Experiences for Children*. Washington D.C.: Center Science in the Public Interest, 1980.

Fredericks, C. *New Low Blood Sugar and You*. New York: Putnam, 1985.

Rudin, D. *The Omega Factor*. Emmaus, PA: Rodale Press, 1986.

Wunderlich, R. and Kalita, D. *Nourishing Your Child*. New Canaan, CT: Keats, 1984.

Nutrition/Behavior

Walsh, R. *Treating Your Hyperactive and Learning Disabled Child*. New York: Anchor Press/Doubleday, 1979.

Smith, L. *Improving Your Child's Behavior Chemistry*. Englewood Cliffs, NJ: Prentice-Hall, 1976.

Fredericks, C. *Psycho-Nutrition*. New York: Grosset and Dunlap, 1976.

Doman, G. *What to do About Your Brain-Injured Child*. New York: Doubleday, 1974.

Cott, A. *The Orthomolecular Approach to Learning Disabilities.* San Rafael, CA: Academic Therapy, 1977.

Ilg, Ames, Baker. *Child Behavior.* New York: Harper & Row, 1981.

Hoffer, A. and Osmond, H. *How to Live with Schizophrenia.* Secaucus, NJ: Citadel Press, 1974.

Schauss, A. *Diet, Crime, and Delinquency.* Berkeley, CA: Parker House, 1980.

Philpott, W. and Kalita, D. *Victory Over Diabetes.* New Canaan, CT: Keats, 1983.

Cheraskin, E. *Psychodietetics.* New York: Bantam Books, 1976.

Stevens, L. and Stoner, R. *How to Improve Your Child's Behavior Through Diet.* New York: Signet Books, 1979.

Sheinkin, Schachter, Hutton. *Food, Mind, and Mood.* New York: Warner Books, 1979.

Schauss, A. *Nutrition and Behavior.* New Canaan, CT: Keats, 1985.

Watson, G. *Nutrition and Your Mind: The Psychochemical Response.* New York: Harper & Row, 1972.

ALLERGY INFORMATION

Philpott, W. and Kalita, D. *Brain Allergies.* New Canaan, CT: Keats, 1980.

Crook, W. *Tracking Down Hidden Food Allergy.* Jackson, TN: Professional Books, 1978.

Crook, W. *The Yeast Connection.* Jackson, TN: Professional Books, 1983.

Mandell, M. *Dr. Mandell's 5-Day Allergy Relief System.* New York: Thomas Y. Crowell Publishers, 1979.

Golos, Golbitz, Golos. *Coping With Your Allergies.* New York: Simon and Schuster, 1979.

Rapp, D. *Allergies and the Hyperactive Child.* New York: Simon and Schuster, 1979.

Randolph, T. *An Alternative Approach to Allergies.* New York: Lippincott and Crowell Publishers, 1980.

Bell, I. *Clinical Ecology: A New Approach to Environmental Illness.* Bolinas, CA: Common Knowledge Press, 1982.

Yoder, E. *A Guide for an Allergen-Free Elimination Diet.* New York: Healthful Living Company, 1982.

Dadd, D. and McGovern, J. *Nutritional Analysis System.* San Francisco, CA: Nutritional Research Publishing Company, 1980.

Golos, N. and Golbitz, F. *If It's Tuesday It Must Be Chicken.* New Canaan, CT: Keats, 1983.

Levin, A. and Zellerbach, M. *Type One, Type Two Allergy Relief System.* Los Angeles, CA: Jeremy P. Tarcher, 1983.

Dadd, D. *Nontoxic and Natural.* Los Angeles, CA: Jeremy P. Tarcher, 1984.

Eagle, R. *Eating and Allergy.* New York: Doubleday, 1980.

Frazier, C. *Coping with Food Allergy.* New York: Quadrangle, 1974.

ENVIRONMENTAL INFORMATION

Ott, J. *Light, Radiation, and You*. Old Greenwich, CT: Devin-Adair, 1982.

Zamm, A. *Why Your House May Endanger Your Health*. New York: Simon and Schuster, 1980.

Carson, R. *Silent Spring*. Boston: Houghton Mifflin, 1962.

INDEX

sandwiches, 180
sausage, 178, 179–80
Schauss, Alexander, 68, 69
schizophrenia, 78, 79–82, 112–14,
 135
Schmidt, K., 68
Schoenthaler, S. J., 32, 68
school:
 diets in, 140–43
 potential allergens in, 165–66
seafood quiche, 267
seasonings, 96, 229
seed(s), 96, 155
 -cinnamon cereal, 243
 crackers, coconut, 241
 flour, 228
 milk, 226
Seifter, Eli, 39, 279–80
selenium, 290
serotonin, 83
sesame:
 -broccoli casserole, 272
 crunch bread, 231
 flour crust, 257
 seeds, 155
Shambaugh, George, 58–59
Shamberger, R., 27
shellfish, food families of, 149
shish kebabs, 269
silicon, 292
skin allergies, 59, 60, 109, 162
sleeping patterns, 45, 46, 72–
 77
Sloan, Sara, 141–42, 143
Smith, Lendon, 74
smoking, 53–54, 164, 165
smoothies, 274–75
smothered response, 23
snacks, 181
sodium, 290–91
soft drinks, 42, 43, 177
soufflés, tiny tuna, 266
soy:
 bread, super, 231
 flour, 228
 flour crust, 258
 milk, 226
 pretzels, 241–42
soya carob dessert crepes, 239
sprouts, 96
spumoni ice cream, 263
squares, 248–50
 carob cherry nut, 248–49
 fudgy nut brownies, 249

lemon coconut, 248
raspberry-jam, 249–50
squash:
 cinnamon acorn, 273
 yellow and greet frittata supreme,
  271
stomach problems, 17, 59
stress, 65
 vitamins for, 64, 279–80, 282, 283,
  285
sugar:
 addiction to, 27–28
 allergy to, 109, 116–17, 124–26
 average consumption of, 29–30
 hyperactivity and, 49–51
 substitutes for, 177, 225–26
 see also blood-sugar levels
sulfur, 290
supplements, nutritional, 96, 120–32,
  137, 139, 155, 292–97
suppressor T cells, 101, 102, 103, 104

Tacos el Supremo!, 268
T cells, 100, 101, 102, 103, 104
tea, 42–43
tearful response, 20
teenagers, 65–71
 alcohol use of, 66–67
 diet of, 67–71
 drug use of, 66
telephone handset, 164
television, hyperactivity and, 52
tension-fatigue syndrome, 63–64
thiamine, 27
thirst, as symptom of hyperactivity, 52–
 53
throat problems, 19, 109
thumbprints, 246
thymus, 38, 40, 101, 102, 103, 280
thyroid, 38, 40, 108
toast, 31
tofu, 226
tortilla tempter, 266
Tracking Down Hidden Food Allergy
 (Crook), 115
trip response, 19
Truss, Orian, 106
tuna soufflés, tiny, 266

urea formaldehyde, 162, 164
urinalysis, 92
utilization factor, 97